Treatment of Non-infectious Uveitis

Phoebe Lin • Eric Suhler
Editors

Treatment of Non-infectious Uveitis

Springer

Editors
Phoebe Lin, MD, PhD
Oregon Health and Science University
Casey Eye Institute
Portland, OR
USA

Eric Suhler, MD, MPH
Oregon Health and Science University
OHSU-PSU School of Public Health
Portland Veterans Administration
Medical Center
Portland, OR
USA

ISBN 978-3-030-22825-5 ISBN 978-3-030-22827-9 (eBook)
https://doi.org/10.1007/978-3-030-22827-9

This Springer imprint is published by the registered company Springer Nature Switzerland AG
The registered company address is: Gewerbestrasse 11, 6330 Cham, Switzerland

Foreword

The history of the therapeutic approach to inflammation, in general, and to uveitis, in particular, contains many curios. Aspirin was synthesized in 1897, and for decades, it was virtually the only known pill that reliably treated inflammation. In the 1930s, the theory that uveitis resulted from an occult infection inspired some to recommend hysterectomy or prostatectomy as treatment for uveitis [1]. Another popular approach during this era was fever therapy as could be induced by typhoid vaccine [2]. Philip Hench from the Mayo Clinic began to use adrenal derivatives to treat rheumatoid arthritis in 1948 and received the Nobel Prize for this discovery only 2 years later. Hench died of suicide, and many believe that much of his depression resulted from the realization that cortisone therapy was fraught with toxicities that he had never appreciated on the basis of the short-term studies for which he was appropriately honored. Methotrexate is now a popular immunosuppressive whose mechanism of action is partially due to poisoning leukocytes. It was developed to treat leukemia. The suggestion that methotrexate should be used to treat inflammation was greeted by many with skepticism.

In the 1950s, growing up in Portland, Oregon, I would make hospital rounds with my father. He had been trained by Hench and then came west to become arguably the first rheumatologist in the state. But his bag of therapeutic magic for rheumatoid arthritis was nearly empty. A mainstay was the injection of gold, based in part on the concept that heavy metals could be toxic to bacteria like tuberculosis. As I write today, the contribution of tuberculosis to certain inflammations within the eye still often provokes heated debate. My father's most effective therapies might have been bedrest and his ever optimistic personality which continually encouraged improvement. Our current rheumatology fellows have never met a patient who received gold therapy even though that was standard of care when I did my rheumatology fellowship in the late 1970s.

Editors, Phoebe Lin and Eric Suhler, have assembled a collection of manuscripts which thoroughly describe the state of the art for noninfectious uveitis therapy in 2018. Each contribution is written by an expert or experts. It is impossible for me to hold the volume without thinking how much has changed since I founded a uveitis clinic in a tertiary medical center in 1985. Even more pleasant to imagine is how much more will change thanks to the careers of the editors, authors, and readers of this collection.

Portland, OR, USA James T. Rosenbaum, M.D.

March, 2018

References

1. Rosenow EC, Nickel AC. Elective localization in determining the etiology of chronic uveitis. Am J Ophthalmol. 1932;15:1–18.
2. Solomon HC, Kopp I. Fever therapy. N Engl J Med. 1937;217:805–14.

Preface

The field of uveitis is considered by many ophthalmologists to be among the most challenging to deal with among the broad panoply of ophthalmic diseases. While uveitic differential diagnoses are broad and require consideration of systemic diseases infrequently considered or encountered by ophthalmologists, we would submit that perhaps the most intimidating aspect of uveitis care to those not well-steeped in it would be the treatment aspect of uveitis, especially when systemic therapy is required. Many patients, and some providers, are very fearful of the use of systemic "poisons," and the monitoring of these patients for potential toxicity gives pause to providers not well versed in their use.

This book was carefully designed to fill a previously unmet need: to provide one single reference for all of the reader's questions on the treatment of noninfectious uveitis. From topical treatment to locally administered therapy, including drug-releasing implants, to systemic immunosuppressive treatments both tried and new, as well as surgical management, this reference expertly covers all of it. Each chapter highlights important practice pearls as well as provides an easy-reference dosing table, side effects, and lab monitoring pertinent to the agents discussed. *Treatment of Non-infectious Uveitis* provides salient information for the resident or fellow as well as practice tips and higher-level information that comprehensive ophthalmologists and subspecialists in uveitis and retina will also appreciate.

We had the very distinct pleasure in the production of this text to work with respected leaders in the field of uveitis and clinical ocular immunology, many of whom were former fellows at our institution, Oregon Health and Science University, or who have been longtime friends and collaborators, and we thank and honor them for their scholarly contributions.

While no volume can be completely comprehensive in this rapidly changing field, we hope this text will find a home on the shelves of uveitis-interested medical providers and that its well-referenced chapters will serve as a primer for those wishing to learn more about the topical, local, and systemic treatment of uveitis.

Portland, OR, USA

Phoebe Lin, MD, PhD
Eric Suhler, MD, MPH

Contents

Contributors

Alfredo Adán, MD, PhD Institut Clinic d'Oftalmologia, Hospital Clinic de Barcelona, Universitat de Barcelona, Barcelona, Spain

Himanshu K. Banda, MD Department of Ophthalmology, Uveitis and Vasculitis Service, Emory Eye Center, Emory University School of Medicine, Atlanta, GA, USA

Andrea D. Birnbaum, MD, PhD Department of Ophthalmology and Visual Sciences, University of Illinois at Chicago, Chicago, IL, USA

Department of Ophthalmology, Northwestern Feinberg School of Medicine, Chicago, IL, USA

Durga S. Borkar, MD Harvard Medical School, Massachusetts Eye and Ear Infirmary, Department of Ophthalmology, Boston, MA, USA

Nicholas J. Butler, MD Department of Ophthalmology, Harvard Medical School, Massachusetts Eye and Ear, Boston, USA

Veterans Affairs Boston Healthcare System, Boston, MA, USA

Andrew W. Francis, MD Department of Ophthalmology and Visual Sciences, University of Illinois at Chicago, Chicago, IL, USA

Debra A. Goldstein, MD Department of Ophthalmology, Northwestern University Feinberg School of Medicine, Chicago, IL, USA

John A. Gonzales, MD University of California, San Francisco, Francis I. Proctor Foundation, San Francisco, CA, USA

Laura J. Kopplin, MD, PhD Department of Ophthalmology and Visual Sciences, University of Wisconsin – Madison, Madison, WI, USA

Kara C. LaMattina, MD Department of Ophthalmology, Boston University School of Medicine, Boston, MA, USA

Lyndell Lim, MBBS, DMedSci Royal Victorian Eye and Ear Hospital, Centre for Eye Research Australia, University of Mellbourne, East Melbourne, VIC, Australia

Phoebe Lin, MD, PhD Oregon Health and Science University, Casey Eye Institute, Portland, OR, USA

Victor Llorenç, MD, MSc, PhD Institut Clinic d'Oftalmologia, Hospital Clinic de Barcelona, Universitat de Barcelona, Barcelona, Spain

Marina Mesquida, MD, PhD Institut Clinic d'Oftalmologia, Hospital Clinic de Barcelona, Universitat de Barcelona, Barcelona, Spain

Ophthalmology Clinical Research Unit, Fundació Clínic per a la Recerca Biomèdica, IDIBAPS, Barcelona, Spain

Abhiniti Mittal, MD New York Medical College - MS3, Valhalla, NY, USA

George R. Mount, MD Casey Eye Institute, Oregon Health and Science University, Portland, OR, USA

Madigan Army Medical Center, Tacoma, WA, USA

Sarju S. Patel, MD, MPH, MSc Uveitis and Ocular Immunology, Retinal Consultants Inc., Sacramento, CA, USA

Russell W. Read, MD PhD Uveitis and Ocular Inflammatory Diseases Service, Department of Ophthalmology and Visual Sciences, University of Alabama at Birmingham, Birmingham, AL, USA

Akbar Shakoor, MD Ophthalmology and Visual Sciences, Uveitis and Vitreoretinal Divisions, John A. Moran Eye Center, University of Utah Hospital, Salt Lake City, UT, USA

Amde Selassie Shifera, MD, PhD Division of Ocular Immunology, Wilmer Eye Institute, Johns Hopkins University School of Medicine, Baltimore, MD, USA

Justine R. Smith, FRANZCO, FRACS, PhD Flinders University College of Medicine and Public Health, Adelaide, SA, Australia

Eric Suhler, MD, MPH Oregon Health and Science University and OHSU-PSU School of Public Health, Portland, OR, USA

Portland Veterans Administration Medical Center, Portland, OR, USA

Albert T. Vitale, MD Ophthalmology and Visual Sciences, Uveitis and Vitreoretinal Divisions, John A. Moran Eye Center, University of Utah Hospital, Salt Lake City, UT, USA

Xia Ni Wu, MBBS (Hons), B. Med Sci (Hons) Lions Eye Institute, Nedlands, WA, Australia

Steven Yeh, MD Department of Ophthalmology, Uveitis and Vasculitis Service, Emory Eye Center, Emory University School of Medicine, Atlanta, GA, USA

Introduction

1

Phoebe Lin and Eric Suhler

The heterogeneity of uveitis is a much talked-about conundrum that ophthalmologists face when diagnosing and managing uveitis patients. The etiology of most clinical uveitic entities has yet to be fully elucidated, and each of these disease classifications likely has diverging triggers and possibly different intraocular cytokine profiles (as a single potential example of their heterogeneity). That said, one necessary and practical trend has been to identify the overlapping characteristics of uveitis that can allow us to study treatment in clinical trials and, also, identify successful treatment for the uveitis patient that presents to us in the clinic. Over the past decade, significant advances in how we study treatment for uveitis have been made, with the advent of uveitis clinical trials utilizing multifaceted combined imaging and clinical endpoints to include several anatomic subtypes of uveitis and to more powerfully investigate treatment efficacy. What these well-designed studies have taught us is that while we still have yet to understand the basic mechanisms of many types of non-infectious uveitis, we can successfully plunge forward with disease-modifying, sight-sparing treatment. At the same time, impactful developments in both systemic immunosuppressive therapy, particularly in the biologic realm, as well as advancements in surgical technology, have occurred. These developments have added greatly to our treatment armamentarium and have given us needed alternatives to the chronic use of corticosteroids, which if not tapered successfully may reduce the quality and sometimes the quantity of our patients' lives. Collaborative studies such as the Systemic Immunosuppressive Therapy for Eye Diseases (SITE) cohort and the Multicenter Uveitis Steroid Treatment (MUST) trial have provided us with valuable information to guide us on how to treat and counsel our patients. What remains a challenge is how we generalize this evidence to the patient sitting in front of us, every day.

We encourage the reader to use this book as a one-stop reference for treatments for uveitis ranging from anterior uveitis to intermediate, posterior, and panuveitis. We hope that it will provide an up-to-date knowledge base from which to make the complex decisions for you and your patient. Included is information regarding drug mechanism, drug dosing for children and adults, as well as evidence for efficacy based on studies that utilize visual acuity, inflammatory control, as well as complications

P. Lin (✉)
Oregon Health and Science University, Casey Eye Institute, Portland, OR, USA
e-mail: linp@ohsu.edu

E. Suhler
Oregon Health and Science University and OHSU-PSU School of Public Health, Portland, OR, USA

Portland Veterans Administration Medical Center, Portland, OR, USA
e-mail: suhlere@ohsu.edu

P. Lin, E. Suhler (eds.), *Treatment of Non-infectious Uveitis*,
https://doi.org/10.1007/978-3-030-22827-9_1

such as cystoid macular edema and retinal neovascularization, as outcomes. Practice pearls are highlighted in each chapter, and convenient drug tables are provided for quick reference. Treatment for infectious uveitis is not covered in this book, and any use of the medications covered in this manuscript presupposes that the treating clinician has ruled out infectious causes before treating uveitis patients with depot local steroids or systemic immunosuppression in order to prevent causing sight-threatening exacerbations of infectious disease. In addition, we have included a chapter on novel and emerging therapies on the horizon for uveitis, an area which, by its very definition, is constantly changing and expanding.

While this reference includes detailed information on individual therapies and evidence for each therapy, special scenarios should be highlighted. We have all encountered the refractory patient who cannot taper down to a safe dosage of systemic steroids without recurrent sight-threatening inflammation. Adjunctive therapies can be tried in the latter scenario including combination systemic therapy such as adding cyclosporine to an anti-metabolite or co-treatment with an anti-metabolite and a biologic such as a TNF-alpha inhibitor. The latter combination is often used to decrease the rate of anti-adalimumab or anti-infliximab antibody formation, but can also be dosed for treatment effect. While simultaneous treatment with multiple biologics is not recommended outside the context of a clinical trial, switching from one biologic to another is commonly necessary after failure of one biologic. If multiple biologics from a single class have already been tried without treatment response, or if class-specific toxicity is encountered, then one can switch to another class of biologic. In our practices, as long as there are no contraindications for their use, TNF blockers are the first biologics that are initiated after anti-metabolites fail or are only partially effective. If TNF blockers fail, then tocilizumab, rituximab, or other agents can be tried. Other treatments such as interferon therapy can be effective, alternatively. Another strategy would be to pair local corticosteroid adjunctive treatment with systemic immunosuppressive therapy, which can be effective as well.

Other special scenarios pertain to treatment of pediatric uveitis (which is highlighted in a separate chapter), as well as considerations of treatment in pregnant and lactating women. In children, the clinician should pay special attention to dosing and special concerns for side effects that might impact growth and/or future fertility. While there is no separate chapter in this reference for pregnant and lactating women, we would like to summarize and highlight several pearls: systemic corticosteroids are used in pregnancy and lactation despite its category C status; cyclosporine is also category C but is used in low doses during pregnancy, taking care to pay attention to blood pressure and renal function; the anti-metabolites are category D or X drugs. Among this latter class, azathioprine has not definitely shown evidence of increased rates of miscarriage or congenital malformation; however, methotrexate and mycophenolate are known teratogens. The TNF inhibitors are category B drugs and can be considered in pregnancy although to be safe, one might consider holding until the start of the third trimester [1].

Quality of life in uveitis is another topic that is pertinent to treatment of uveitis patients, and is not covered as a separate topic in this book. We would like to highlight several recent studies showing the impact of treatment in quality of life in uveitis patients. The MUST study has shown similar significant improvements in vision-related quality of life measures in patients treated with either a surgical steroid implant or systemic immunosuppressive therapy [2], although the steroid implant group experienced immediate improvements compared to the gradual improvement in the systemic therapy group. It should be noted, however, that a separate study showed that while both methotrexate and mycophenolate equally improved the vision-related quality of life in patients (similar to the MUST study), the overall health-related quality of life measures including the mental health component declined over the treatment course

[3], suggesting the burden of treatment side effects (such as due to headache, nausea, diarrhea, fatigue, and vomiting, all side effects that are not necessarily identified as serious adverse events in larger trials such as the MUST trial). The importance of treatment and the dogma of sustained control of inflammation to achieve the best visual acuity results must thus always be tempered by assessing the patient's overall quality of life.

We and the international group of experts who have authored these chapters hope that you will find the detailed information about each type of uveitis treatment illuminating and as a helpful guide in treating your non-infectious uveitis patients, of course not to be supplanted by the irreplaceable value of consultation with your colleagues and continuing educational efforts.

References

1. Grotting LA, Papaliodis GN. A review of the course and treatment of non-infectious uveitis during pregnancy. Semin Ophthalmol. 2017;32:75–81.
2. Sugar EA, Venugopal V, Thorne JE, et al. Longitudinal vision-related quality of life for patients with non-infectious uveitis treated with fluocinolone acetonide implant or systemic corticosteroid therapy. Ophthalmology. 2017;124:1662–9.
3. Niemeyer KM, Gonzales JA, Rathinam SR, et al. Quality-of-life outcomes from a randomized clinical trial comparing antimetabolites for intermediate, posterior, and panuveitis. Am J Ophthalmol. 2017;179:10–7.

2 Topical Therapy in Uveitis

Andrew W. Francis and Andrea D. Birnbaum

Pearls

- Topical prednisolone acetate 1% and difluprednate are the most effective topical treatments for anterior uveitis in the United States in the absence of infectious keratitis.
- Intraocular pressure should be monitored at 1–2 weeks after initiating topical steroids.
- Twice daily or less of prednisolone acetate 1% contributes minimally to complications such as cataract.
- NSAIDs are not usually effective in treating anterior uveitis.
- Cycloplegics are important adjunctive topical therapy in moderate to severe anterior uveitis.

Introduction

Treatment of ocular inflammation is often initiated during the diagnostic stage, before potential infectious etiologies have been identified or a diagnosis is assigned. Therapy at this stage is intended to control symptoms, decrease inflammation, and reduce the risk of structural damage and permanent vision loss. Initial management of the most common uveitic disorders typically includes topical therapy, which may be the only treatment required in cases of anterior uveitis. For more severe disease involving the posterior segment, topical therapy is used in conjunction with periocular or systemic treatment. Corticosteroids, nonsteroidal anti-inflammatory drugs (NSAIDS), and cycloplegic agents are the most commonly prescribed topical medications.

Corticosteroids

Corticosteroids have been the mainstay of therapy for ocular inflammatory disease since the early 1950s [1]. They are effective in controlling inflammation and reducing symptoms of pain, photophobia, and redness associated with inflammation of the anterior segment. Reducing anterior segment inflammation decreases the risk of synechiae formation and permanent structural damage. Some topical corticosteroids penetrate the anterior chamber, providing targeted therapy

A. W. Francis
Department of Ophthalmology and Visual Sciences, University of Illinois at Chicago, Chicago, IL, USA

A. D. Birnbaum (✉)
Department of Ophthalmology and Visual Sciences, University of Illinois at Chicago, Chicago, IL, USA

Department of Ophthalmology, Northwestern University, Chicago, IL, USA

P. Lin, E. Suhler (eds.), *Treatment of Non-infectious Uveitis*,
https://doi.org/10.1007/978-3-030-22827-9_2

and reducing the risks associated with systemic corticosteroids. Although short-term application of topical corticosteroids is relatively safe, potentially serious side effects may occur with long-term use, including cataract formation and elevation in intraocular pressure [2, 3]. There are several different corticosteroid preparations available for topical administration with varying potencies and ocular penetration. The most common topical ophthalmic corticosteroids utilized clinically are listed in Table 2.1 [4, 5]. It should be noted that prednisolone acetate and difluprednate are the only topical steroids available in the United States that appear to penetrate the anterior chamber effectively enough to treat anterior uveitis.

Indications

Specific indications for topical corticosteroid therapy are numerous, although general considerations include anterior segment inflammation, posterior synechiae in an inflamed eye, and cystoid macular edema. To rapidly reduce intraocular inflammation, many clinicians begin treatment with frequent dosing of topical corticosteroids. The medication can then either be tapered, with the goal of utilizing the lowest possible dose required to control inflammation, or completely discontinued, depending on whether the disease process is acute or chronic in duration. During the course of treatment, patients should undergo frequent examinations to check

Table 2.1 Topical corticosteroid agents

Generic name	Trade name	Strength	Treatment frequency[a]
Dexamethasone sodium phosphate	Maxidex	Suspension, 0.1%	4–6 times daily
	Ocu-Dex	Ointment 0.05%	
	Generic	Solution 0.1%	
Difluprednate	Durezol	Emulsion, 0.05%	4–6 times daily (used at approximately half the frequency of prednisolone)
Fluorometholone	FML S.O.P	Ointment, 0.1%	4–6 times daily in first 24–48 h; 1–3 times daily after
	FML Liquifilm	Suspension, 0.25%	4–6 times daily
	Fluor-Op	Suspension 0.1%	
	Gemeroc	Suspension 0.1%	
Fluorometholone acetate	Flarex	Suspension, 0.1%	4–6 times daily
Medrysone	HMS	Suspension, 1%	4–6 times daily
Prednisolone acetate	Econopred Plus Omnipred Pred Forte Generic	Suspension, 1%	3–4+ cell: every 1 h to every 2 h 2+ cell: at least 4–6 times daily
Prednisolone sodium phosphate	Inflamase Forte Prednisol Generic	Solution, 1%	4–6 times daily
Rimexolone	Vexol	Suspension, 1%	Hourly while awake for 1 week; every 2 h while awake in second week; taper

[a]Drops are often tapered rather than abruptly stopped

intraocular pressure and level of inflammation. As a general rule, treatment courses greater than 2 or 3 weeks should include a taper of the medication rather than an abrupt discontinuation to prevent rebound inflammation.

Mechanism

Corticosteroids are potent anti-inflammatory agents whose mechanism of action is inhibition of the enzyme phospholipase A2, preventing production of the two main mediators of inflammation, prostaglandins and leukotrienes [6]. Corticosteroids also block the cyclooxygenase/prostaglandin E2 isomerase (COX-1 and COX-2) enzymes, which are also inhibited by non-steroidal anti-inflammatory drugs (NSAIDs). In addition to reducing anterior chamber cell, corticosteroids are thought to reduce vascular permeability of the iris and ciliary body [7]. The multitude of actions of corticosteroids appear to be via the activation of anti-inflammatory gene expression downstream of binding to the glucocorticoid receptor [8].

Penetration

Topically applied corticosteroids penetrate the eye via the cornea [4, 9]. The rate-limiting step for penetration of hydrophilic molecules into the anterior chamber is the corneal epithelium, whereas the rate-limiting step for penetration of hydrophobic molecules is the corneal stroma [9–11]. Therefore, for a topical corticosteroid to effectively penetrate the cornea, it must be both lipophilic and hydrophilic with the relative potency of a glucocorticoid agent and its associated risk for side effects dependent on its bioavailability in vivo. Certain steroids, especially fluorinated agents, are less potent in vivo because their penetration is significantly reduced across the corneal epithelium. Additionally, acetate-based agents such as prednisolone acetate achieve much higher concentrations in the aqueous fluid than either alcohol-based agents such as dexamethasone or phosphate-based agents such as prednisolone phosphate. This is one reason that prednisolone acetate at a 1% concentration is much more effective in treating anterior uveitis than dexamethasone alcohol at a 0.1% concentration despite the fact that it is less potent on a molar basis [12].

Side Effects

A list of ophthalmic and systemic adverse effects from long-term corticosteroid therapy is listed in Table 2.2. Common side effects include local irritation and blurred vision. Clinically significant increases in intraocular pressure can be reported as early as 2 weeks after the initiation of treatment in susceptible patients [13, 14] with most topical preparations. This response can be seen even earlier with difluprednate [15]. The pediatric uveitis population is particularly susceptible to difluprednate, with 50% of patients in one report experiencing significant intraocular pressure elevation. Prolonged use of topical corticosteroid agents may result in cataract formation [15]. Patients using topical corticosteroids are at increased risk for corneal ulcers, particularly if they wear contact lenses; therefore, they should

Table 2.2 Corticosteroid adverse effects

Ophthalmic	Systemic
Glaucoma	Suppression of the pituitary-adrenal axis
Posterior subcapsular cataracts	Osteoporosis and muscle wasting
Worsening viral (especially herpetic) or fungal infections	Obesity/weight gain
Ptosis	Insomnia
Mydriasis	Aseptic necrosis of hip
Scleral melt	Peptic ulcers
Eyelid skin atrophy	Diabetes mellitus
Central serous retinopathy	CNS effects, including psychosis

be advised to avoid contact lenses while using the medication. All methods of corticosteroid administration have been linked to central serous retinopathy. Finally, an increased risk of reactivation of herpes simplex keratitis [16], worsening fungal keratitis [17], and the development of infectious crystalline keratitis have been reported with long-term topical corticosteroid use [18].

Evidence and Guidelines for Use

Despite the widespread use of topical corticosteroids in treating anterior uveitis, there are few randomized controlled trials in the published literature. Dunne et al [19] conducted a double-blind randomized controlled trial comparing the efficacy of betamethasone phosphate 0.1% (BP 0.1%), clobetasone butyrate 0.1% (CB 0.1%), and placebo in the treatment of acute unilateral nongranulomatous uveitis. They found that BP 0.1% was more effective than CB 0.1% in reducing clinical signs of uveitis. However, patients treated with BP 0.1% were also more likely to develop a significant increase in intraocular pressure than those treated with CB 0.1%.

More recent studies have compared the commonly used prednisolone acetate (PA) 1% to other corticosteroids, with a focus on reduction of inflammation and elevation of intraocular pressure. PA 1% and rimexolone 1% were studied in patients with acute, recurrent, or chronic anterior uveitis. Both drops were shown to be effective in decreasing ocular inflammation, but patients treated with PA 1% were more likely to develop an intraocular pressure response [20]. The Loteprednol Etabonate US Uveitis Study Group [21] compared topical PA 1% to loteprednol etabonate 0.5% (LE 0.5%). PA 1% reduced anterior chamber inflammation in patients with anterior uveitis more effectively than LE 0.5%. As in the previous study, patients treated with PA 1% were more likely to develop a clinically significant increase in intraocular pressure than those treated with LE 0.5%.

Difluprednate ophthalmic emulsion (DOE) 0.05% is a derivative of prednisolone acetate that has been modified for increased potency and penetration. Dosing of DOE 0.05% four times a day has been shown to be equivalent to dosing PA 1% eight times a day [22]. A phase III, multicenter, randomized, double-masked non-inferiority study of PA 1% dosed eight times a day versus DOE 0.05% dosed four times a day demonstrated that both medications were equally effective at decreasing inflammation in patients with anterior uveitis. However, DOE 0.05% was more likely to induce a steroid response than PA 1%.

These studies suggest that efficacy and intraocular steroid responses are related. In the future, the ophthalmology community would benefit from a topical preparation that provides excellent control of inflammation without the associated local side effects.

Standard Treatment Approach

Topical prednisolone acetate 1% and difluprednate are the most effective topical treatments for anterior uveitis in the United States in the absence of infectious keratitis. PA1% is typically employed for the initial treatment of anterior uveitis starting at 1 drop QID for anterior uveitis ≥1+ cell, with an increased frequency to Q1 h for ≥2+ cell (cell grading designated by the Standardization of Uveitis Nomenclature study group). The corresponding doses of difluprednate would thus be BID and Q2 h, respectively [23]. The tapering schedule of PA1% or difluprednate may differ depending on the chronicity and severity of presenting anterior uveitis, with the possibility of titrating doses from daily difluprednate down to daily PA1% upon improvement of anterior uveitis, prior to stopping [23]. Patients should be monitored for local side effects, specifically elevated intraocular pressure, in 2 weeks after initiating PA1% and 1 week for initiation of difluprednate, particularly in children. Chronic use of topical corticosteroids can also result in cataract formation, which can be consequential especially in the amblyogenic age range in children with anterior uveitis. The goal often is to maintain quiescence off of topical steroids. However, in one study by Thorne et al., ≤3 drops daily of topical steroids (largely PA1%, but a few received rimexolone 1%) was associated with an 87% lower risk of cataract formation in juvenile idiopathic arthritis-associated uveitis, with a 0/eye-year risk in eyes receiving ≤2 drops daily [24]. Therefore, long-term low-frequency PA1%, particularly BID or less, may be an effective means of maintaining quiescence, and in some cases, can obviate escalation to systemic immunosuppression. It is unknown whether or not these data generalize to elevations in intraocular pressure or to other effective topical steroids like difluprednate. In general, maintaining control of inflammation (either 0 cell or trace or less cells in some cases) should be the goal guiding treatment, with close attention to balance the side effects of these drugs [23].

Cycloplegics

Cycloplegic agents serve dual roles in the treatment of anterior uveitis. First, inducing cycloplegia reduces the symptoms of pain and photophobia often present in acute disease. Second, these agents help break existing posterior synechiae and prevent the formation of new synechiae in acutely inflamed eyes. However, in chronic disease, dilating drops are ineffective in cleaving synechiae; these adhesions must be removed surgically, which often occurs in conjunction with cataract surgery.

A list of common cycloplegic agents is displayed in Table 2.3. The different formulations have varying degrees of potency in reducing ciliary body spasm, paralyzing accommodation, and facilitating pupillary dilation. The most common cycloplegic agents utilized clinically include tropicamide 0.5% or 1% with a duration of action up to 6 h; cyclopentolate, available as 0.5%, 1%, and 2%, with a duration of action up to 24 h; homatropine, available as 2% and 5% solutions, with a duration of action up to 2 to 3 days; and atropine, available as 0.5% or 1%, with a duration of action up to 14 days. All cycloplegic agents are also mydriatic agents; however sympathetic agonists have more mydriatic action and are poor cycloplegics. Phenylephrine is a mydriatic that is available as 2.5% and 10% with duration of action from 3 to 6 h. Mydriatics are not often used in treatment of uveitis because they do not adequately control the pain and photophobia associated with acute uveitis.

Mechanism

The iris sphincter muscle is controlled by parasympathetic innervation, and the iris dilator muscle is controlled by sympathetic innervation. Anticholinergics, including atropine and homatropine, antagonize the muscarinic acetylcholine receptors in the eye resulting in sphinc-

Table 2.3 Mydriasis and cycloplegia of common topical mydriatic drops

	Time to maximum effect (min)		Duration of action (min)				
Agent[a]	Mydriasis	Cycloplegia	Mydriasis	Cycloplegia	Mechanism and effect	Treatment frequency	Side effects
Cyclopentolate 1%	15–30	15–30 min	12–24 h	12–24 h	Iris sphincter paralysis, moderate cycloplegic	2–4 times daily	Increased sensitivity to light, eye irritation, transient conjunctival hyperemia
Homatropine 5%	30–60	30–60 min	1–2 days	1–2 days	Iris sphincter paralysis, strong cycloplegic	2–3 times daily	
Atropine 1%	30–60	1 day	7–10 days	7–14 days	Iris sphincter paralysis, strongest cycloplegic	1–2 times daily	

[a]Phenylephrine and tropicamide were excluded given their weak cycloplegic properties

ter paralysis, pupillary dilation, and cycloplegia. Because the iris sphincter is a stronger muscle than the iris dilator, agents that paralyze the iris sphincter have a more prominent effect on pupillary dilation than sympathomimetics that activate the iris dilator muscle. The ciliary muscle controls accommodation and ciliary spasm resulting in pain during episodes of uveitis. Therefore, cycloplegic agents that exert a greater paralytic effect on the ciliary body result in reduced accommodation with relief of pain from uveitis.

Side Effects

Routine administration of topical cycloplegic agents, including tropicamide 1%, cyclopentolate 1%, scopolamine 0.25%, and atropine 1%, is not associated with significant ocular or systemic side effects in adults, such as alterations in heart rate or blood pressure [25, 26]. The most common side effect of topical cycloplegic agents is sensitivity to the increased amount of light passing into the eye. Other innocuous side effects include eye irritation and transient conjunctival hyperemia. Most topical cycloplegic agents are well tolerated in adults, but children younger than 6 years of age are at risk of central nervous system impairment following routine administration, possibly due to increased plasma concentrations and smaller body mass indices (BMI) [27, 28]. One study involving young children compared two drops of topical cyclopentolate 1% (C + C) versus one drop of cyclopentolate 1% and one drop of tropicamide 1% (C + T). Its findings showed moderate drowsiness was more frequent in the C + C group, suggesting that repeated doses of cyclopentolate may not be well tolerated in young children. This is particularly true in children with a low BMI [29]. Other side effects in children taking routine doses of common cycloplegic agents include moderate to severe excitation, hyperactivity, and behavioral problems [30].

Evidence and Guidelines for Use

At the present time, no randomized controlled trials have been conducted comparing the relative efficacies of different dilating agents used in the treatment of uveitis. Some uveitis specialists prefer stronger cycloplegic agents, such as atropine, which provide extended dilation and relief from pain and photophobia. Others prefer shorter acting agents, such as cyclopentolate or homatropine. These agents allow the pupil to alter size throughout the day and theoretically avoid the development of posterior synechiae of the fully dilated pupil. Typically, it is recommended to initiate cycloplegic use when there is ≥1+ anterior chamber cell, photophobia, or with progressive synechiae in the presence of anterior chamber flare even in the absence of anterior chamber cell. Many uveitis specialists will avoid atropine to prevent synechiae in the dilated position, and alternative agents are commonly preferred to allow for pupillary mobility during acute anterior inflammation.

Nonsteroidal Anti-inflammatory Drugs (NSAIDs)

Topical ophthalmic nonsteroidal anti-inflammatory drugs (NSAIDs) have a more limited role in the treatment of uveitis than topical corticosteroid agents. At present, a total of five agents are available for use in the United States. These agents include flurbiprofen, ketorolac, diclofenac, bromfenac, and nepafenac. Ophthalmic NSAIDs are currently FDA approved to reduce pain and inflammation following cataract surgery and corneal refractive surgery, to prevent intraoperative miosis, and to treat allergic conjunctivitis. They are also frequently used off-label in the treatment of postoperative cystoid macular edema. NSAIDs are not approved to treat inflammation associated with uveitis [31], although animal studies suggest that topical indomethacin (not commercially available in the United States) may prevent vascular

Table 2.4 Topical NSAIDs[a] currently approved for use in the United States

Drug	Trade name	Concentration	FDA indication	Treatment frequency	Side effects
Diclofenac sodium	Voltaren Ophthalmic	0.1%	Postoperative inflammation after cataract surgery and corneal refractive surgery	4 times daily	Surface irritation, hyperemia most common; keratitis and ulceration without loss of tissue, corneal and scleral melting, corneal and scleral perforations possible
Ketorolac tromethamine	Acular Acular LS Acular PF	0.4% Acular LS 0.5% Acular and PF	Seasonal allergic conjunctivitis, postoperative inflammation after cataract surgery (Acular);inflammation after corneal refractive surgery (LS and PF)	4 times daily	
Bromfenac	Xibrom	0.07%, 0.09%	Postoperative cystoid macular edema after cataract surgery	2 times daily	

[a]Flurbiprofen and nepafenac are additional topical NSAIDs that are only FDA approved for postoperative inflammation after cataract surgery

leakage [32]. A list of currently available topical NSAIDs is listed in Table 2.4.

Mechanism

NSAIDs inhibit cyclooxygenase (COX) enzymes 1 and 2, preventing the synthesis of prostaglandins and thromboxanes, both important mediators of inflammation.

Side Effects

NSAIDs for ophthalmic use are generally very well tolerated at standard doses with surface irritation and hyperemia being the two most common side effects reported in controlled trials [33, 34]. Keratitis and ulceration without loss of tissue, corneal and scleral melting, and corneal and scleral perforations have also been reported in patients using topical NSAIDs. High-risk patients for NSAID use include those with significant dry eye syndrome, epithelial surface irregularities, and recent keratorefractive surgery [35–37].

Evidence and Guidelines for Use

Several randomized controlled trials have evaluated topical NSAIDs in the treatment of uveitic disorders. Two studies found no difference between topical NSAIDs and topical corticosteroids for anterior uveitis. In the first study, Young et al [38] carried out a double-masked controlled clinical trial of unpreserved tolmetin 5% (T 5%) versus prednisolone 0.5% (P 0.5%) versus placebo in the treatment of acute endogenous nongranulomatous anterior uveitis. In the second study, Dunne et al [34] compared the anti-inflammatory efficacies of T 5%, prednisolone disodium phosphate 0.5% (PD 0.5%), and betamethasone disodium phosphate 0.1% (BS 0.1%) in a randomized controlled trial. In both studies, the topical corticosteroid decreased signs and symptoms of inflammation better than the NSAID, but no significant statistical difference was measured after 2 to 3 weeks of treatment.

Sand et al. [33] carried out a randomized controlled clinical trial comparing the effect of topical non-steroid versus potent steroid preparation in acute anterior nongranulomatous uveitis. Patients were randomized to either indomethacin 1% or dexamethasone 0.1% treatment six times a day. They reported a statistically significant improvement in the corticosteroid group versus the NSAID group during the first week. By the end of the second week, no statistically significant difference was noted. Most uveitis practices rely on topical corticosteroids rather than NSAIDs for treatment of anterior uveitis. Prednisolone acetate 1% is thought to be more effective at controlling intraocular inflammation than many of the preparations used in these studies. Topical NSAIDs are therefore not typically used to effectively treat anterior uveitis, but may have a role as an adjunctive to topical corticosteroids in the treatment of uveitic or post-cataract surgery cystoid macular edema.

References

1. Gordon DM, McLean JM, Koteen H, Bousquet FP, McCusker WD, Baras I, et al. The use of ACTH and cortisone in ophthalmology. Am J Ophthalmol. 1951;34(12):1675–86.
2. Becker B, Mills DW. Elevated intraocular pressure following corticosteroid eye drops. JAMA. 1963;185:884–6.
3. Urban RC, Cotlier E. Corticosteroid-induced cataracts. Surv Ophthalmol. 1986;31(2):102–10.
4. Awan MA, Agarwal PK, Watson DG, McGhee CN, Dutton GM. Penetration of topical and subconjunctival corticosteroids into human aqueous humour and its therapeutic significance. Br J Ophalmol. 2009;93(6):708–13.
5. McGhee CN. Pharmacokinetics of ophthalmic corticosteroids. Br J Ophthalmol. 1992;76(11):681–4.
6. Kragbelle K. Topical corticosteroids: mechanism of action. Acta Derm Venereol Suppl (Stockh). 1989;151:7–10.
7. Green K, Paterson CA, Cheeks L, Slagle T, Jay WM, Aziz MZ. Ocular blood flow and vascular permeability in endotoxin-induced inflammation. Ophthalmic Res. 1990;22:287–94.
8. Rhen T, Cidlowski JA. Antiinflammatory action of glucocorticoids—new mechanisms for old drugs. New Engl J Med. 2005;353(16):1711–23.
9. Rosenblum C, Dengler RE, Geoffory RF. Ocular absorption of dexamethasone phosphate disodium b the rabbit. Arch Ophthalmol. 1967;77(2):234–7.
10. Hosseini K, Matsushima D, Johnson J, Widera G, Nyam K, Kim L, et al. Pharmacokinetic study of dexamethasone disodium phosphate using intravitreal, subconjunctival, and intravenous delivery routes in rabbits. J Ocul Pharmacol Ther. 2008;24(3):301–8.
11. Watson D, Noble MJ, Dutton GN, Midgley JM, Healey TM. Penetration of topically applied dexamethasone alcohol into human aqueous humor. Arch Ophthalmol. 1988;106(5):686–7.
12. Awan MA, Agarwal PK, Watson DG, McGhee CN, Dutton GN. Penetration of topical and subconjunctival corticosteroids into human aqueous humour and its therapeutic significance. Br J Ophthalmol. 2009;93(6):708–13.
13. Sallam A, Sheth HG, Habot-Wilner Z, Lightman S. Outcome of raised intraocular pressure in uveitic eyes with and without a corticosteroid-induced hypertensive response. Am J Ophthalmol. 2009;148(2):207–13.e1.
14. Sallam A, Taylor SR, Lightman S. Review and update of intraocular therapy in noninfectious uveitis. Curr Opin Ophthalmol. 2011;22(6):517–22.
15. Slabaugh MA, Herlihy E, Ongchin S, van Gelder RN. Efficacy and potential complications of difluprednate use for pediatric uveitis. Am J Ophthalmol. 2012;153(5):932–8.
16. Kibrick S, Takahashi GH, Leibowitz HM, Laibson PR. Local corticosteroid therapy and reactivation of herpetic keratitis. Arch Ophthalmol. 1971;86(6):694–8.
17. Thomas PA, Kaliamurthy J. Mycotic keratitis: epidemiology, diagnosis and management. Clin Microbiol Infect. 2013;19(3):210–20.
18. Sharma N, Vajpayee RB, Pushker N, Vajpayee M. Infectious crystalline keratopathy. CLAO J. 2000;26(1):40–3.
19. Dunne JA, Travers JP. Topical steroids in anterior uveitis. Trans Ophthalmol Soc U K. 1979;99(4):481–4.
20. Foster CS, Alter G, DeBarge LR, Raizman MB, Crabb JL, Santos CI, et al. Efficacy and safety of rimexolone 1% ophthalmic suspension vs 1% prednisolone acetate in the treatment of uveitis. Am J Ophthalmol. 1996;122(2):171–82.
21. Loteprednol Etabonate US Uveitis Study Group. Controlled evaluation of loteprednol etabonate and prednisolone acetate in the treatment of acute anterior uveitis. Am J Ophthalmol. 1999;127(5):537–44.
22. Foster CS, Davanzo R, Flynn TE, McLeod K, Vogel R, Crockett RS. Durezol (difluprednate ophthalmic emulsion 0.05%) compared to Pred Forte 1% ophthalmic suspension in the treatment of endogenous anterior uveitis. J Ocul Pharmacol Ther. 2010;26(5):475–83.
23. Jabs DA, Nussenblatt RB, Rosenbaum JT, Standardization of Uveitis Nomenclature (SUN) Working Group. Standardization of uveitis nomenclature for reporting clinical data. Results of the First International Workshop. Am J Ophthalmol. 2005;140(3):509–16.
24. Thorne JE, Woreta FA, Dunn JP, Jabs DA. Risk of cataract development among children with juvenile idiopathic arthritis-related uveitis treated with topical corticosteroids. Ophthalmology. 2010;117(7):1436–41.
25. Lahdes K, Huupponen R, Kaila T, Salminen L, Iisalo E. Systemic absorption of ocular scopolamine in patients. J Ocul Pharmacol. 1990;6(1):61–6.
26. Lahdes K, Kaila T, Huupponen R, Salminen L, Iisalo E. Systemic absorption of topically applied ocular atropine. Clin Pharmacol Ther. 1988;44(3):310–4.
27. Lahdes K, Huupponen R, Kaila T, Monti D, Saettone MF, Salminen L. Plasma concentrations and ocular effects of cyclopentolate after ocular application of three formulations. Br J Clin Pharmacol. 1993;35(5):479–83.
28. Lahdes K, Huupponen R, Kaila T, Ali-Melkkilä T, Salminen L, Saari M. Systemic absorption of ocu-

lar cyclopentolate in children. Ger J Ophthalmol. 1992;1(1):16–8.
29. van Minderhout HM, Joosse MV, Grootendorst DC, Schalij-Delfos NE. Adverse reactions following routine anticholinergic eye drops in a paediatric population: an observational cohort study. BMJ Open. 2015;5(12):e008798.
30. Palmer EA. How safe are ocular drugs in pediatrics? Ophthalmology. 1986;93(8):1038–40.
31. Wilson DJ, Schutte SM, Abel SR. Comparing the efficacy of ophthalmic NSAIDs in common indications: a literature review to support cost-effective prescribing. Ann Pharmacother. 2015;49(6):727–34.
32. Bucolo C, Marrazzo G, Platania CB, Romano GL, Drago F, Salomone S. Effects of topical indomethacin, bromfenac and nepafenac on lipopolysaccharide-induced ocular inflammation. J Pharm Pharmacol. 2014;66(7):954–60.
33. Sand BB, Krogh E. Topical indometacin, a prostaglandin inhibitor, in acute anterior uveitis. A controlled clinical trial of non-steroid versus steroid anti-inflammatory treatment. Acta Ophthalmol. 1991;69(2):145–8.
34. Dunne JA, Jacobs N, Morrison A, Gilbert DJ. Efficacy in anterior uveitis of two known steroids and topical tolmetin. Br J Ophthalmol. 1985;69(2):120–5.
35. Lin JC, Rapuano CJ, Laibson PR, Eagle RC, Cohen EJ. Corneal melting associated with use of topical nonsteroidal anti-inflammatory drugs after ocular surgery. Arch Ophthalmol. 2000;118(8):1129–32.
36. Flach AJ. Corneal melts associated with topically applied nonsteroidal anti-inflammatory drugs. Trans Am Ophthalmol Soc. 2001;99:205–10; discussion 10-2.
37. Guidera AC, Luchs JI, Udell IJ. Keratitis, ulceration, and perforation associated with topical nonsteroidal anti-inflammatory drugs. Ophthalmology. 2001;108(5):936–44.
38. Young BJ, Cunningham WF, Akingbehin T. Double-masked controlled clinical trial of 5% tolmetin versus 0.5% prednisolone versus 0.9% saline in acute endogenous nongranulomatous anterior uveitis. Br J Ophthalmol. 1982;66(6):389–91.

3 Systemic Corticosteroids in the Treatment of Uveitis

Sarju S. Patel and Abhiniti Mittal

Pearls

- Prednisone is still a mainstay for the treatment of uveitis and four times more potent than cortisol with a biological half-life of 18–36 h.
- Long-term steroid use is associated with increased mortality rates, while short-term steroid use is associated with significant morbidity, including bone fractures and venous thromboembolism.
- The prescribing ophthalmologist must team with other care providers to screen and treat the various steroid-associated side effects and has the responsibility to use corticosteroids safely and limit long-term use.
- The most common immediate side effects after glucocorticoid initiation are fluid retention, blurred vision, mood changes, insomnia, and weight gain. The more serious gradual effects include those related to endocrine metabolism, especially hyperglycemia, osteopenia/osteoporosis, dyslipidemia, obesity, and adrenal suppression.
- Calcium intake (including dietary and oral supplementation) of 1200–1500 mg/day and vitamin D supplementation should be recommended if there is anticipated glucocorticoid use at any dose with duration of ≥3 months.

Introduction

Corticosteroids are a class of steroid hormones produced in the adrenal cortex and include both glucocorticoids, like cortisone, and mineralocorticoids, like aldosterone. These hormones regulate a wide range of physiologic processes. Synthetic corticoids have been created and exploited to treat various inflammatory processes, but given the wide-ranging physiologic effects, they typically come with both desired effects and undesired side effects.

Synthetic corticosteroids were first introduced in the 1940s with wide spread use in medicine by the 1950s. Given the impact of corticosteroids, the original scientific work was awarded the Nobel Prize in 1950. Within ophthalmology, corticosteroid use began in the 1950s and is largely credited to DM Gordon [1] and given its success has expanded into a variety of formulations and

S. S. Patel (✉)
Uveitis and Ocular Immunology, Retinal Consultants Inc., Sacramento, CA, USA

A. Mittal
New York Medical College - MS3, Valhalla, NY, USA
e-mail: Abhiniti_Mittal@nymc.edu

P. Lin, E. Suhler (eds.), *Treatment of Non-infectious Uveitis*,
https://doi.org/10.1007/978-3-030-22827-9_3

local modes of delivery. Due to the systemic nature of uveitis, systemic corticosteroids still remain the mainstay in the initial treatment of a variety of conditions and a very important part of the armamentarium in the treatment of complex conditions. Nevertheless, adverse side effects of long-term use can be limiting. As such, a thorough understanding of these drugs is necessary for judicious use in the treatment of uveitis.

Mode of Action

Both anti-inflammatory and immunosuppressive effects can be mediated by corticosteroids. This is primarily accomplished by interrupting pro-inflammatory cytokine-mediated signaling pathways and by the induction of apoptosis [2, 3], which broadly exerts its effect on T cells, macrophages, and neutrophils, among others.

At the cellular level, synthetic corticosteroids act as agonists and carry out most of their function by binding to glucocorticoid receptors (GR) in the cytoplasm. Upon binding and activation, the GR dissociates from the cell membrane and translocates to the nucleus where it stimulates or inhibits gene expression, affecting translation of protein mediators.

Once inside the nucleus, there are two possible mechanisms through which corticosteroids counter inflammation. Transcription activation primarily involves GR subunits interacting directly with GRE sequences within DNA, ultimately leading to the synthesis of anti-inflammatory molecules such as lipocortin-1 and IL-10. In contrast, transcriptional repression leads to the inhibition of pro-inflammatory mediators. This process mainly relies on direct protein-protein interaction between GR subunits and transcription factors like NF-kB and AP-1. Consequently, this prevents the synthesis of multiple pro-inflammatory cytokines such as TNF-alpha, IL-2, IL-3, IL-6, IL-8, and IL-11 [4]. The effects of corticosteroids employing GR receptor signaling pathway is evident in multiple cell types and tissues throughout the body. As such, immune cells such as T cells, B cells, and dendritic cells have altered expression and function as a result of corticosteroids [5].

Corticosteroids also inhibit two key steps in the production of prostaglandins, a pro-inflammatory molecule. First, the upregulation of lipocortin-1 prevents the enzyme phospholipase A2 from converting phospholipids into arachidonic acid, a precursor to prostaglandins. Lipocortin-1 binds directly with substrate phospholipids and prevents an enzyme-substrate complex. As such, the production of inflammatory molecules such as prostaglandins is greatly reduced under the influence of corticosteroids.

In addition, corticosteroids affect both transcriptional and post-transcriptional aspects of pro-inflammatory enzymes such as COX-2. Studies have shown a 25–40% decrease in COX-2 mRNA production, indicating the immense role corticosteroids play in blocking transcription. Transrepression also induces the MAP kinase phosphatase (MKP-1) pathway to further destabilize COX-2 mRNA [4]. In addition, post-transcriptional modification mechanisms like polyadenylation of COX-2 mRNA are inhibited, thereby destabilizing mRNA and rendering it useless [6].

Table 3.1 lists various sites and mechanism of action of corticosteroids in immunosuppression. Table 3.2 highlights the process through which corticosteroids enable anti-inflammatory activity.

Altogether, these effects lead to multiple effects on the functioning immune system. Lymphocyte distribution is altered, with less cells being recruited to sites of inflammation with a concomitant reduction in T-cell activation. Neutrophil migration and bactericidal activity are reduced, as is mononuclear phagocytic activity. There are additional effects, as well, that lead to robust anti-inflammatory and immunosuppressive activity that leads to their immense clinical utility.

Classification of Steroids

Steroids hormones are carbon ring structures derived from cholesterol and classified into four major categories, including *estrogens*, *androgens*, *progestogens*, and *corticoids*. The classification is based on the number of car-

Table 3.1 Various sites and mechanism of action of corticosteroids in immunosuppression

Corticosteroid sites of action (immunosuppression)	Cause	Effect
T cells	CD4+/CD8+ matured thymocytes within thymus	Highly sensitive to apoptosis
	Inhibit IL-2 production	Reduce # of circulating T cells
B cells	Inhibit NF-kB	Decrease B cell production and proliferation
	Decrease IL-2 and IL-2 receptor	Decrease expansion of B cell and antibody synthesis
Dendritic cells		Inhibit maturation and function
Corticosteroid sites of action (anti-inflammation)		
Prostaglandins	Activate lipocortin-1 synthesis to suppress phospholipase-A2 — >decrease prostaglandin production — >decrease leukocyte activity	
	Inhibit COX-1/COX-2 production	

Developed from Refs. [1–8]

Table 3.2 Process through which corticosteroids enable anti-inflammatory activity

Drug type	Potency (relative to cortisol)	Duration[a]	Equivalent doses	Common route for administration of drug
Cortisol	1	S	20 mg	Oral
Prednisone	4	I	5 mg	Oral
Methylprednisolone	5	I	4 mg	Oral Intravenous
Triamcinolone	5	L	4 mg	Periocular/intravitreal injection
Dexamethasone	25	L	0.75 mg	Topical, intravitreal implant

Developed from multiple sources

[a]S, short (8–12 h); I, intermediate (18–36 h); L, long (>36 h) [6]

bons in the backbone and variable side ring attachments within each molecule. These structural differences contribute to the different physiological functions of each class of steroid hormones.

Synthesis of steroid hormones is a complex process that is primarily controlled by the availability and transport of free cholesterol from the cytoplasm to the mitochondria. Within the mitochondria and smooth ER, cholesterol undergoes multiple enzymatic steps to ultimately produce steroid hormones and its intermediates (Fig. 3.1).

Steroid hormones are lipid soluble which allows them to pass freely through cell membranes. Steroid hormones bind to specific carrier proteins like corticosteroid-binding globulin to travel through bloodstream. Steroid hormones attach to their specific steroid hormone receptors on their target tissue to carry out their function.

Corticoids are a class of 21-carbon steroid hormones that includes mineralocorticoids, like aldosterone, and glucocorticoids (GCs), like cortisol. Synthesis of corticoids occurs primarily in the adrenal cortex via cytochrome P450 family of enzymes. Cortisol regulates metabolism and mediates anti-inflammatory processes like decreasing eosinophil production and preventing phospholipid release. Aldosterone maintains water and electrolyte balance by targeting kidney function. Synthetic corticoids like prednisone and dexamethasone are widely used to treat systemic and local inflammation. Drugs like prednisone have both mineralocorticoid- and glucocorticoid-like effects, while dexamethasone functions only as a glucocorticoid analog.

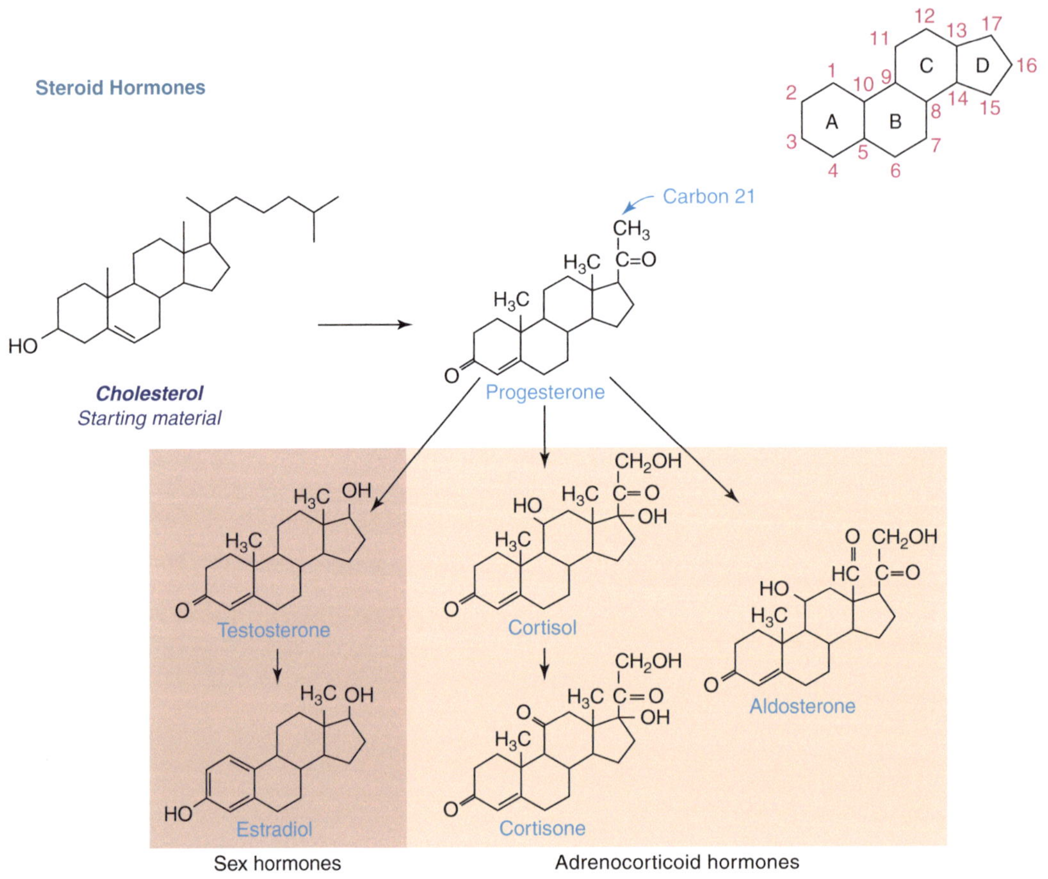

Fig. 3.1 Chemical structure and differentiation of steroid hormones

Various Preparations of Synthetic Corticosteroids Used to Treat Uveitis

Oral Formulations Prednisone is a widely used synthetic corticosteroid effective in the treatment of non-infectious uveitis among other systemic inflammatory conditions. Prednisone is four times more potent than cortisol and has a biological half-life of 18–36 hours. Oral administration of prednisone is a common practice in ophthalmology especially if the inflammation is resistant to local therapy. Oral prednisone is prepared in 1, 2.5, 5, 10, 20, and 50 mg tablets. Once ingested, it is converted to its active form, prednisolone, in the liver.

Oral prednisolone is also available and is also four times more potent than cortisol, but less commonly used, as is oral methylprednisolone, which is favored by some physicians as it may be better tolerated by certain patients. This is because methylprednisolone has less mineralocorticoid activity and, therefore, may be preferred when these effects, like water retention, are particularly undesirable [7].

Therapy with prednisone typically starts at 0.5–1 mg/kg and is slowly tapered as the inflammation is controlled; however in severe, vision-threatening disease, doses of 2 mg/kg may be required. High-dose steroids are used until a clinical response is seen and then a taper is initiated. With the administration of prednisone, or other systemic corticosteroids, it is important to monitor the patient's blood glucose, lipids, and blood pressure due to serious side effects, as will be discussed below [8]. Because of these side effects, it is preferable to start steroid-sparing immunotherapy for chronic disease with the goal of tapering off corticosteroids in 3–4 months. Ideally, corticosteroids would be completely stopped, but in some patients a low dose may still be required. While no particular dose is considered absolutely safe, it is currently preferable to get patients to doses less than or equal to 5 mg/day if longer-term use is necessary.

Intravenous Steroids Intravenous methylprednisolone (five times the potency of cortisol) is used in uveitis when vision is immediately threatened such as bilateral serous detachments or necrotizing scleritis, much like it is used in optic neuritis. Methylprednisolone sodium succinate is administered intravenously over the course of 3 consecutive days. The dose is typically 250–1000 mg/day given over 1–2 h and pulsed typically for 3–4 days and then continued on oral preparations with tapering over time.

Other Modes of Steroid Delivery Various topical and peri-/intravitreal steroid formulations are available and will be covered in depth in another chapter. Briefly, the most common topical formulations available include dexamethasone, fluorometholone, loteprednol, prednisolone acetate, and difluprednate. While dexamethasone is six times more potent than prednisolone, topical dexamethasone does not penetrate the cornea as effectively as prednisolone or difluprednate. The ocular side effects of long-term local steroid use include elevated intraocular pressure and cataract formation.

Complications in Short- and Long-Term Use of Systemic Corticosteroids

Numerous undesired physiologic effects typically occur with the use of corticosteroids. Most notably, an increased all-risk mortality has been observed with long-term corticosteroid use across multiple diseases and indications [9–11]. This risk was observed to correlate directly with dosage; although, there appeared to be no increased risk with long-term doses less than or equal to 5 mg of prednisone per day [9–11]. Additionally the concomitant use of steroid-sparing therapy may mitigate this risk in rheumatoid arthritis patients, as well [10]. Even short-term steroid use of less than 30 days is associated with increased morbidity with elevated rates of sepsis, venous thromboembolism, and fractures [12]. The glucocorticoid nature of the drugs commonly results in secondary Cushing's syndrome and metabolic side effects, while the mineralocorticoid nature of the medications can cause hypertension, electrolyte imbalance, and connective tissue changes, among other effects.

The most common *immediate* effects encountered are fluid retention, blurred vision, mood changes, insomnia, and weight gain. The more serious *gradual* effects include those related to endocrine metabolism, especially hyperglycemia, osteopenia/osteoporosis, dyslipidemia, obesity, and adrenal suppression.

A more complete list of the most common listed side effects include:

1. Metabolic: sodium and fluid retention, nephrolithiasis, metabolic syndrome, and central obesity/weight gain
2. Endocrine: glucose intolerance/diabetes mellitus, gonadal dysfunction, hirsutism, growth suppression in children, and Cushing's syndrome
3. Cardiovascular: arterial hypertension and hypercoagulability
4. Gastrointestinal: peptic ulcer disease/nausea and increased appetite
5. Musculoskeletal: osteoporosis, muscle weakness/steroid myopathy, tendon rupture, and aseptic necrosis of femoral/humeral heads
6. Immunological: susceptibility to infections
7. Neurological: psychiatric disorders, sleep disturbance, and mood lability
8. Ophthalmic: blurred vision, cataracts, glaucoma, and central serous chorioretinopathy
9. Dermatologic: skin thinning, poor wound healing, and bruising

Many of these effects are well known among practicing physicians, but the less common side effects are very important to be aware of as well, as they are just as important to consider and screen for when treating patients on corticosteroids.

Hypercoagulability Hypercoagulability is a lesser-known effect of systemic corticosteroids. The effects were explored when it was discovered that mortality rates in Cushing's syndrome were about two times higher than those in the general population and higher in those with cardiovascular disease [13]. It is thought that the activation of the hemostatic system contributes to the development of atherosclerosis and subsequent cardiovascular morbidity and mortality [14]. The mechanisms that are involved in the thromboembolic complications in hypercortisolism revolve around alterations in Virchow's triad: endothelial dysfunction, hypercoagulability, and stasis.

Most studies have demonstrated that the hypercoagulable state can be explained by increased levels of procoagulant factors, mainly factors VIII, IX, and von Willebrand factor, and also by an impaired fibrinolytic capacity, which mainly results from an elevation in plasminogen activator inhibitor-1 [14]. Consequently, there is a shortening of activated partial thromboplastin time and increased thrombin generation. For these reasons, anticoagulant prophylaxis might be considered in patients with Cushing's syndrome with concomitant prothrombotic risk factors. However, caution must be taken as there can be drug interactions that potentiate the effects of blood-thinning medications. Patients should be managed in conjunction with their primary care specialist.

Osteoporosis Corticosteroids are the most common cause of secondary osteoporosis and the first cause in those under the age of 50 years [15]. There is a more rapid effect on bone loss and fracture rates early after the initiation of steroid therapy (within the first 3 months, peaking at 6 months) and then a more prolonged effect related to the dosage and duration of treatment [16]. The increase in fracture risk is not fully assessed by bone mineral density measurements, as bone quality is also altered [16]. Further, osteonecrosis develops in 9–40% of adult patients receiving long-term glucocorticoid therapy [7].

Inflammatory mediators affect osteoclast genesis and thus bone remodeling, which accounts for the initial, more rapid effect of corticosteroids on bone metabolism [16]. At high concentrations there is dramatically decreased bone formation rate, osteoblast numbers, and osteocyte numbers/activity, leading to less bone formation and increased resorption [16]. Further, steroids have other indirect effects that increase fracture rate, such as increased fall risk, and effects on calcium metabolism by decreasing gastrointestinal absorption and increasing renal excretion [16].

The magnitude of bone loss with steroid therapy is variable, and there is no predictor of the individual risk of fracture. However, there is an immediate increase in fracture risk, as early as 3 months after the initiation of therapy, but reverses sharply after discontinuation of GCs [16]. The goal of the specialist should be to limit systemic corticosteroid use as much as possible and consider early adoption of steroid-sparing therapies if there is an anticipated extended course of disease.

Even at low doses of prednisone (2.5–5 mg/day), patients have increased risk of fractures [16]. As such, in all patients treated with systemic corticosteroids, the prevention and treatment of osteoporosis should be addressed [16]. Current international guidelines for the management of corticosteroid-induced osteoporosis suggest following height throughout the course of therapy, minimizing the required dose of steroid, and supplementing any deficiencies in calcium and vitamin D. There is level A evidence that one should recommend calcium intake (including dietary and oral supplementation) of 1200–1500 mg/day and vitamin D supplementation if there is anticipated glucocorticoid use at any dose with duration of ≥3 months [17]. Baseline bone scans should be obtained if prolonged use is expected, especially in those patients with other risk for weak bone, and should be followed serially. Pharmacologic treatment guidelines of osteoporosis exist, such as with bisphosphonates. Physicians regularly using these drugs should be familiar with the most current guidelines. Furthermore, physicians should encourage exercise that can promote bone health.

Diabetes Steroids are the main cause of drug-induced hyperglycemia. They not only exacerbate hyperglycemia in patients with known diabetes mellitus (DM) but also cause DM in patients without documented hyperglycemia before the initiation of GC therapy [18], with increases in glucose levels up to 68% compared to baseline [18]. The reported incidence of DM in patients *without* a prior history of hyperglycemia to steroid use varies between 34.3% and 56% [18].

Only oral corticosteroids have demonstrated an increased risk of diabetes. There is either minimal or no association of incident diabetes with prescribing of GC-containing inhalers, topical preparations, eye drops, or infrequent GC injections [19]. Oral corticosteroids, on the other hand, account for up to 2% of incident cases of diabetes in primary care populations [18].

Factors that have been identified as predictors of developing diabetes are the type of steroid, the dose, the duration of treatment, older age, prior HbA1c, and body mass index [18]. In addition, there are population groups with a greater risk of developing hyperglycemia during treatment with GCs. These patients include those with a history of gestational DM, a family history of diabetes (odds ratio ~10.3), concomitant use of mycophenolate mofetil (odds ratio ~4.8), use of calcineurin inhibitors, abnormal fasting glucose, and impaired glucose tolerance [18].

Mechanistically, GCs provide a substrate for oxidative stress metabolism increasing hepatic glucose production, lipolysis, and proteolysis [4]. They additionally increase glucose intolerance in a similar fashion to that of type 2 DM by increasing insulin resistance, which can be seen in up to 60%–80% depending on the dose and type of steroid used [18]. Steroids induce insulin resistance by directly interfering with signaling cascades, mainly the GLUT4 transporter within skeletal muscle cells (the largest glycogen store in the body where the majority of glucose is deposited) [18]. This results in a 30–50% reduction in insulin-stimulated glucose uptake and a 70% reduction in insulin-stimulated glycogen synthesis [20]. The increase in proteolysis and lipolysis results in small molecule mediators that alter muscle cell signaling, reducing glucose entry and storage of free glucose, further exacerbating insulin resistance-like effects [18, 21].

Prednisone and methylprednisolone are classified as intermediate-acting GCs, with a peak of action 4–6 h following administration. Their effect on glucose levels is primarily during the afternoon and night without affecting fasting glucose when they are administered in a single dose [18]. On the other hand, they cause persistent hyperglycemia when administered in divided doses [18]. The authors favor single daily dose administration, but doses can be divided if patients have other issues that limit tolerance of high doses.

As steroid doses are reduced, their effect on endocrine metabolism returns to baseline and drug-induced diabetes is expected to resolve [4, 18]. However, this is not true in all cases, so follow-up after cessation of steroids is important.

In general, it is recommended that all patients who are started on steroid treatment should have baseline glucose measurements and followed periodically [18]. Patients should be educated on routine daily monitoring if hyperglycemia above 180 mg/dL is identified on more than one occasion in the presence or absence of symptoms associated with hyperglycemia [18, 22].

Since steroid-induced diabetes is detected mainly in the postprandial state, the use of fasting glucose is *not* recommended nor the use of the glucose tolerance curve, as they are not reliable diagnostic methods [18]. If only these measures are used, there is a high possibility of missing some of the hyperglycemic patients. Other studies recommend following postprandial glucose determinations postprandial glycemic level after lunch offers the greatest diagnostic sensitivity, especially when intermediate-acting GCs are administered in a single morning dose, and/or HbA1c levels as screening examinations with long-term steroid use [18]. Coordinating with the primary care provider for this type of follow-up is essential given the significant rates of steroid-induced diabetes.

When selecting the best treatment, the first consideration to make is whether to use oral hypoglycemic drugs or insulin. In patients with fasting glucose levels below 200 mg/dL, without previous diabetes and given low-dose GCs, therapeutic emphasis should focus on exercise, diet therapy, and oral hypoglycemic agents [23]. Insulin is the treatment of choice in patients with persistent hyperglycemia ≥200 mg/dL [23].

Psychological and Sleeping Effects Chief among these is the development of a more labile mood with irritability and bouts of anger that may seem relatively unprovoked. Problems with sleep-onset, staying asleep throughout the night, and early morning awakening are common. Short-term memory is impaired, as is mental calculation [24]. General psychiatric functioning may also deteriorate and can be classically evaluated by history and recall of three objects and serial seven subtractions in the clinic [24]. Additionally worsening of more mild and intermittent depression can occur with the development of severe chronic depression with GC usage [24]. A family history of depression or alcoholism has been reported as a risk factor for the development of corticosteroid affective disorders and is important to screen for [7].

Although the research on psychological effects in the pediatric population is limited, the three most common adverse psychological effects in children on oral and IV corticosteroids are agitation, excitation, and sleep disturbances [25], although decreased mood and tearfulness can also be observed. These effects tend to dissipate as patients taper off corticosteroids and are thought to be more serious at higher doses [25]. Betamethasone was shown to have the most serious psychological side effects in children followed by prednisolone and prednisone [25]. Therefore, it is essential to monitor children's behavior closely while on corticosteroid therapy and consider switching to steroid-sparing medications as a safer alternative.

Obesity Chronic glucocorticoid use induces insulin resistance, as described above, and obesity. These factors are further linked to cardiovascular risk and overall decreased survival [24, 26, 27], as previously explained. Individuals with hypercortisolism have a fourfold higher mortality rate than the general population because of cardiovascular complications, in addition to the associated obesity and insulin resistance [27]. A critical function of steroids is to liberate energy substrates of the body as noted above via enhanced protein breakdown, increased lipolysis, and increased gluconeogenesis, compounded by reduction in glucose utilization, thereby elevating circulating glucose concentrations. Overexposure to steroids eventually alters body composition, which includes expansion of trunk adipose tissue depots [26]. However, the de novo creation of adipose tissue induced by steroids is likely much more complicated and is not well understood, but it is thought that glucocorticoids regulate other factors such as hormones, cytokines, or neuronal signals in tissues other than adipose, which indirectly control adipose tissue functionality and may override the direct effects of lipolysis on adipose tissue [26].

As such, it is important not only to counsel patients on diet and exercise while using corticosteroids but equally important to limit their exposure and move them to steroid-sparing therapies.

Infection Risk The risk of infection is well documented in chronic steroid users. While randomized controlled trials of short-term and lower-dose steroids have generally shown little to no increased risk, observational studies have consistently shown dose-dependent increases in risk for serious infections as well as certain opportunistic infections [28]. As such, those patients on chronic steroid therapy should be appropriately vaccinated and screened regularly to reduce this risk.

Hypercholesterolemia Different studies investigating the lipid profile of GC excess subjects showed dyslipidemia in 37–71% of CS patients [29]. Improvements of dyslipidemia after cure/remission occur, but an adverse lipid profile can persist in approximately 30% of the patients, possibly due to modifications of adipose tissue [30]. Furthermore, other factors such as insulin resistance also play a role, leading to a complex pathophysiology. There are no guidelines on how to follow dyslipidemia with GC use. Baseline cholesterol screening should be performed prior to initiation and followed regularly with chronic use and followed for a period of time after cessation.

Adrenal Suppression Adrenal suppression results from decreased or inadequate cortisol production due to treatment with exogenous GCs. Duration of GC therapy and doses of GC treatment are not reliable predictors of which patients will develop adrenal suppression, as it has been demonstrated after exposure to even 5-day treatments with high-dose GC therapy [7]. It should be noted that inhaled, topical, and intraocular GCs may be absorbed systemically to the degree that they can also cause adrenal suppression [7]. Higher rates of adrenal suppression are associated with long-acting corticosteroids [7]. More importantly, exogenous corticosteroids are associated with a higher rate of adrenal suppression in the pediatric population, and this adrenal suppression is associated with a higher mortality rate [7]. As such, careful attention needs to be given when treating children with corticosteroids.

While no official guidelines exist, clinicians favor tapering steroid therapy to help prevent these effects. Symptoms of adrenal suppression are vague and should be screened as patients are tapered off medications. Typically patients will complain of weakness, dizziness, fatigue, malaise, GI issues, and abdominal pain, as well as morning headaches. These patients may require more gradual tapering or an endocrine evaluation if one cannot wean off corticosteroids.

Myopathy Corticosteroids have direct catabolic effects on skeletal muscles that can lead to reductions in muscle protein synthesis and protein catabolism and, ultimately, muscle weakness. Myopathy generally develops over several weeks to months of GC use [7]. Patients typically present with proximal muscle weakness and atrophy in both the upper and lower extremities. Symptoms generally improve within 3–4 weeks of dose reductions, and usually resolve after discontinuation of GC therapy [7].

Lastly, there are many drug-drug interactions associated with corticosteroids, which are not reviewed here. Prescribing physicians should be familiar with these interactions and review the patient's concomitant medications for potential complications. The patient should be made aware of potential drug conflicts and side effects (see Dosing table, Table 3.3).

In conclusion, while tremendously beneficial in treating inflammatory autoimmune diseases, such as uveitis, glucocorticoid therapy is associated with multiple serious adverse side effects involving many systems of the body, which can increase the risk of death. Thankfully, many of

Table 3.3 Dosing table

Drug type	Route	Formulations	Typical initial dosing	Side effects	Routine monitoring	Routine lab and other testing
Prednisone	Oral	Tablets, syrup	1–2 mg/kg/day	Hyperglycemia Dyslipidemia Obesity Osteoporosis Fluid retention Cushing's syndrome Myopathy Hypertension Psychiatric GI	(1) A directed review of systems at each visit (must specifically ask about mood and ability to sleep) (2) Initial and subsequent BP monitoring at each visit (3) Serial weight and height measurements (4) Spot glucose testing	(1) Baseline and q3month lipid panel (2) Baseline and q3month HgB A1c (3) Baseline Dexa-scan, follow-ups if abnormal or if kept on chronic dosing
Prednisolone	Oral	Tablets, suspension	1–2 mg/kg/day			
Methyl-prednisolone	Oral or intravenous	Tablets, suspension, IV infusion	1–2 mg/kg/day			

these effects can be minimized through judicious use of GCs, careful patient monitoring, and implementation of preventive measures. Patients should be informed about the side effects associated with systemic corticosteroid use and be advised on preventative strategies that may help reduce the risk of these events. Nevertheless, limiting their exposure and moving patients to steroid-sparing therapies remains a priority in chronic uveitis, as the timeline of treatment is on the order of several years.

References

1. Gordon DM. Prednisone and prednisolone in ocular disease. Am J Ophthalmol. 1956;41(4):593–600.
2. Coutinho AE, Chapman KE. The anti-inflammatory and immunosuppressive effects of glucocorticoids, recent developments and mechanistic insights. Mol Cell Endocrinol. 2011;335(1):2–13. https://doi.org/10.1016/j.mce.2010.04.005.
3. Smoak KA, Cidlowski JA. Mechanisms of glucocorticoid receptor signaling during inflammation. Mech Ageing Dev. 2004;125:697–706.
4. Newton R, Holden NS. Separating transrepression and transactivation: a distressing divorce for the glucocorticoid receptor? Mol Pharmacol. 2007;72:799–809.
5. Matyszak MK, Citterio S, Rescigno M, et al. Differential effects of corticosteroids during different stages of dendritic cell maturation. Eur J Immunol. 2000;30:1233–42.
6. Newton R, Seybold J, Kuitert LME, Bergmann M, Barnes PJ. Repression of cyclooxygenase-2 and prostaglandin E2 release by dexamethasone occurs by transcriptional and post-transcriptional mechanisms involving loss of polyadenylated mRNA. J Biol Chem. 1998;273:32312–21.
7. Liu D, Ahmet A, Ward L, et al. A practical guide to the monitoring and management of the complications of systemic corticosteroid therapy. Allergy Asthma Clin Immunol. 2013;9(1):30. https://doi.org/10.1186/1710-1492-9-30.
8. Babu K, Mahendradas P. Medical management of uveitis – current trends. Indian J Ophthalmol. 2013;61(6):277–83. https://doi.org/10.4103/0301-4738.114099.
9. Movahedi M, Costello R, Lunt M, Pye SR, Sergeant JC, Dixon WG. Oral glucocorticoid therapy and all-cause and cause-specific mortality in patients with rheumatoid arthritis: a retrospective cohort study. Eur J Epidemiol. 2016;31(10):1045–55. https://doi.org/10.1007/s10654-016-0167-1.
10. Wasko MC, Dasgupta A, Sears GI, Fries JF, Ward MM. Prednisone use and risk of mortality in patients with rheumatoid arthritis: Moderation by use of disease-modifying anti-rheumatic drugs. Arthritis Care Res. 2016;68(5):706–10. https://doi.org/10.1002/acr.22722.
11. Lewis JD, Scott FI, Brensinger CM, et al. Increased mortality rates with prolonged corticosteroid therapy when compared with antitumor necrosis factor-α-directed therapy for inflammatory bowel disease. Am J Gastroenterol. 2018;113(3):405–17. https://doi.org/10.1038/ajg.2017.479.
12. Waljee AK, Rogers MA, Lin P, Singal AG, Stein JD, Marks RM, Ayanian JZ, Nallamothu BK. Short term use of oral corticosteroids and related harms among adults in the United States: population based cohort study. BMJ. 2017;357:j1415. https://doi.org/10.1136/bmj.j1415.
13. Dekkers OM, Horvath-Puho E, Jorgensen JO, Cannegieter SC, Ehrenstein V, Vandenbroucke JP, Pereira AM, Sorensen HT. Multi-system morbidity and mortality in Cushing's syndrome: a cohort study. J Clin Endocrinol Metab. 2013;98:2277–84.
14. Coelho MC, Santos CV, Vieira Neto L, Gadelha MR. Adverse effects of glucocorticoids: coagulopathy. Eur J Endocrinol. 2015;173:M11–21.
15. Kok C, Sambrook PN. Secondary osteoporosis in patients with an osteoporotic fracture. Best Pract Res Clin Rheumatol. 2009;23:769–79.
16. Briot K, Roux C. Glucocorticoid-induced osteoporosis. RMD Open. 2015;1:e000014. https://doi.org/10.1136/rmdopen-2014-000014.
17. Grossman JM, Gordon R, Ranganath VK, Deal C, Caplan L, Chen W, Curtis JR, Furst DE, McMahaon M, Parker NM, Volkmann E, Saag KG. American College of Rhematology 2010 recommendations for the prevention and treatment of glucocorticoid-induced osteoporosis. Arthritis Care Res. 2010;62(11):1515–26.
18. Tamez-Pérez HE, Quintanilla-Flores DL, Rodríguez-Gutiérrez R, González-González JG, Tamez-Peña AL. Steroid hyperglycemia: prevalence, early detection and therapeutic recommendations: a narrative review. World J Diabetes. 2015;6(8):1073–81. https://doi.org/10.4239/wjd.v6.i8.1073.
19. Gulliford MC, Charlton J, Latinovic R. Risk of diabetes associated with prescribed glucocorticoids in a large population. Diabetes Care. 2006;29:2728–9.
20. Perez A, Jansen-Chaparro S, Saigi I, Bernal-Lopez MR, Miñambres I, Gomez-Huelgas R. Glucocorticoid-induced hyperglycemia. J Diabetes. 2014;6:9–20.
21. Ruzzin J, Wagman AS, Jensen J. Glucocorticoid-induced insulin resistance in skeletal muscles: defects in insulin signalling and the effects of a selective glycogen synthase kinase-3 inhibitor. Diabetologia. 2005;48:2119–30.
22. Trence DL. Management of patients on chronic glucocorticoid therapy: an endocrine perspective. Prim Care. 2003;30:593–605.
23. Hirsch IB, Paauw DS. Diabetes management in special situations. Endocrinol Metab Clin N Am. 1997;26:631–45.

24. Nieman LK. Cushing's syndrome: update on signs, symptoms and biochemical screening. Eur J Endocrinol. 2015;173:M33–8.
25. Drozdowicz LB, Bostwick JM. Psychiatric adverse effects of pediatric corticosteroid use. Mayo Clin Proc. 2014;89(6):817–34.
26. Geer EB, Islam J, Buettner C. Mechanisms of glucocorticoid-induced insulin resistance: focus on adipose tissue function and lipid metabolism. Endocrinol Metab Clin N Am. 2014;43(1):75–102.
27. Etxabe J, Vazquez JA. Morbidity and mortality in Cushing's disease: an epidemiological approach. Clin Endocrinol. 1994;40(4):479–84.
28. Youssef J, Novosad SA, Winthrop KL. Infection risk and safety of corticosteroid use. Rheum Dis Clin N Am. 2016;42(1):157–76.
29. Ferrau F, Korbonits M. Metabolic comorbidities in Cushing's syndrome. Eur J Endocrinol. 2015;173(4):M133–57.

Antimetabolites

4

John A. Gonzales

Pearls

- Antimetabolites are a mainstay of steroid-sparing therapy for noninfectious uveitis, allowing for safe sustained control of inflammation in many patients.
- The SITE study found a 40–70% treatment success rate for antimetabolites.
- Methotrexate 25 mg PO weekly was found to be more effective in uveitis control than mycophenolate 1 g PO BID in a randomized clinical trial.
- For the most part, one should avoid antimetabolites in pregnancy or when trying to conceive.
- Age-appropriate vaccination should be obtained when starting a DMARD, in particular, if a live vaccine is required, then it should preferably be given prior to receiving therapy.

While corticosteroids (whether in topical, oral, parenteral, periocular, or intraocular) are typically the first-line agents to be used in managing noninfectious uveitis, there are indications for the advancement to systemic immunomodulatory therapy. For one, corticosteroids have significant side effects. While many of the side effects of steroids resolve after discontinuation, chronic uveitis requires sustained management, and the use of moderate to high doses of corticosteroids should be avoided. Immunomodulatory agents provide a means to manage uveitis while having a better side effect profile than corticosteroids. Recently, there has been an impressive expansion in the therapeutics available to treat uveitis; some, such as the biologics, have very specific targets in various inflammatory pathways. Nonetheless, antimetabolites are still considered the first-line therapy for corticosteroid-sparing management of uveitis.

Antimetabolites are so named because they have effects with metabolic pathways that are essential in mediating cellular growth and inflammation. Antimetabolites are also known as disease-modifying antirheumatic drugs (DMARDs) in the rheumatology and immunology specialties. Antimetabolites have an even earlier history of being employed as chemotherapy for malignancies and organ transplant rejection prevention.

There is a significant amount of information (mostly in the form of retrospective studies) demonstrating that antimetabolites are effective in managing uveitis as corticosteroid-sparing agents. Past retrospective studies, however, have limitations, which include bias with respect to

J. A. Gonzales (✉)
University of California, San Francisco, Francis I. Proctor Foundation, San Francisco, CA, USA
e-mail: john.gonzales@ucsf.edu

P. Lin, E. Suhler (eds.), *Treatment of Non-infectious Uveitis*,
https://doi.org/10.1007/978-3-030-22827-9_4

indications for using one particular antimetabolite over another (including bias of the treating center or physician), incomplete follow-up, and missing data (including reasons for discontinuing therapy). To date, there has been only one randomized clinical trial evaluating the efficacy of one particular antimetabolite over another for the management of uveitis. One of the burning questions in the uveitis community is what antimetabolite should one turn to first for the management of noninfectious uveitis? Most of the information available to us regarding this question comes in the form of retrospective case series and individual physician experiences. When members of the American Uveitis Society were surveyed about their practice patterns, 92% of respondents used methotrexate as their initial immunomodulatory agent for anterior uveitis, while only 5% used mycophenolate [1]. Other antimetabolites were not routinely used. For intermediate uveitis, 58% of respondents started with methotrexate as their initial corticosteroid-sparing therapy, while 25% relied upon mycophenolate mofetil. Azathioprine was utilized by 3% of respondents in such a scenario. For posterior and panuveitis, 47% of respondents noted they would start with methotrexate, while an increasing number of specialists (27%) would use mycophenolate mofetil. However, when the AUS members were queried as to why they would not prescribe a particular medication, 47% noted that lack of effectiveness was a reason not to prescribe methotrexate, while only 9% considered mycophenolate mofetil to be ineffective. Many members considered mycophenolate mofetil to be prohibitively expensive for a first-line therapeutic. Even among uveitis specialists, practice patterns with respect to the use of antimetabolites varied.

Despite the differences in approach to the management of uveitis, the antimetabolites are a mainstay of therapy. Their use has allowed patients to free themselves of the significant side effects of corticosteroids in addition to manage their inflammation to prevent the sequela of uncontrolled uveitis. Antimetabolites are generally well-tolerated by patients, both young and mature. Undoubtedly, the tolerability and efficacy of the antimetabolites have led to an improvement in patient outcomes for steroid-dependent uveitis.

Azathioprine

Pharmacology and Pharmacokinetics

The chemical, or International Union of Pure and Applied Chemistry (IUPAC), name for azathioprine is 6-[(1-methyl-4-nitro-1H-imidazol-5-yl) sulfanyl]-1H-purine. Its chemical formula is $C_9H_7N_7O_2S$ and the chemical structure for azathioprine is:

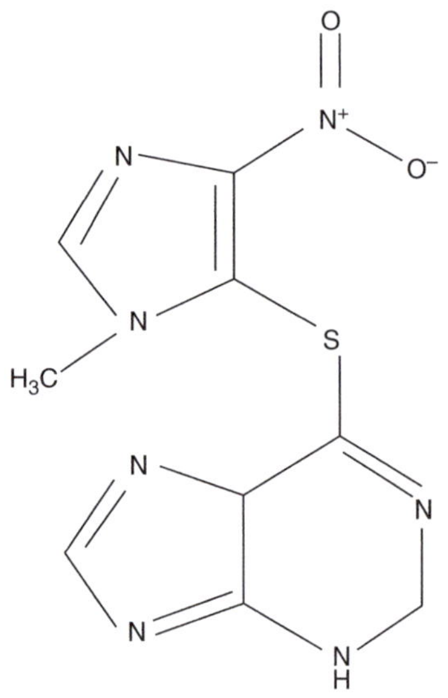

Structure 4.1

Azathioprine is a prodrug (an imidazolyl derivative) of 6-mercaptopurine (6-MP). 6-MP was found to be effective in murine models of lymphoma [2], but was extensively metabolized, so efforts were made to synthesize derivatives with modified metabolism, thereby improving efficacy; azathioprine was the result of this labor [3]. Glutathione S-transferase activity in red blood cells converts approximately 88% of azathioprine to 6-MP [4]. As a purine nucleoside analogue, 6-MP is then metabolized by hypoxanthine guanine phosphoribosyl transferase, resulting in two active metabolites, thioinosinic and thioguanylic acid. The active metabolites then block purine metabolism and halt DNA synthesis. The enzyme thiopurine S-methyltransferase (TPMT) metabolizes 6-MP to the inactive metabolite, 6-methyl-mercaptopurine. TPMP also metabolizes the active metabolites (thioinosinic and thioguanylic acid) of 6-MP. In patients with certain homozygous mutations of *TPMT*, the enzyme is functionally inactive, which can lead to drug toxicity. In patients with heterozygous mutations of *TPMT*, the enzyme is partially functional, and a reduced dose of azathioprine should be used. An assay for homo- or heterozygosity of *TPMT* mutations should be performed prior to instituting therapy with azathioprine. Those that are homozygous for TPMT deficiency should not be considered for azathioprine therapy as bone marrow toxicity with resultant cytopenias can occur early in the commencement of therapy. Heterozygous individuals may be dosed lower than in those homozygous for TPMT mutations. In Han Chinese patients, TPMT mutations are not frequently encountered. However, side effects in this group of patients, particularly leukopenia, may be related to a genotype that leads to higher glutathione S-transferase activity [5].

Azathioprine is absorbed in the stomach and duodenum. Peak plasma levels (ranging from 27% to 83%) [4] are reached within 2 hours of oral administration and taken up into cells with only 30% being protein-bound. Up to 45% of azathioprine is excreted into the urine, while the remainder is converted to 6-MP in red blood cells.

Efficacy

Retrospective Studies

A retrospective study of azathioprine's use in 34 patients with retinal vasculitis from a single center revealed that 56% of eyes exhibited a decrease in ocular inflammation and 64% of eyes either maintained or improved their visual acuities [6]. Relapse of ocular inflammation was also decreased in ten patients who had data available prior to treatment with azathioprine. Patients who did not require an increase in their dose of prednisone were also considered treatment successes.

In the largest retrospective cohort studies evaluating azathioprine's use for treating noninfectious ocular inflammatory diseases involving four uveitis centers, 63% of patients (91 patients) had uveitis [7]. More patients with intermediate uveitis (90.3%) achieved inactive uveitis using the standardization of uveitis nomenclature (SUN) criteria [8] compared to anterior (51.4%) and posterior/panuveitis (74.4%) when treated with azathioprine. Additionally, corticosteroid-sparing control (less than 10 mg PO daily of prednisone) with azathioprine was most frequent in the setting of intermediate uveitis (adjusted hazard ratio 4.75, CI 1.23 to 13.58) compared to anterior uveitis. Posterior/panuveitis had less frequent corticosteroid-sparing control than intermediate uveitis when compared to anterior uveitis (adjusted HR 2.52, CI 0.64 to 9.86).

In the realm of pediatric uveitis, a study of 40 children taking a variety of immunomodulatory agents over 5 years revealed that azathioprine was associated with a 61% improvement in visual acuity, which was lower than mycophenolate mofetil (91% improvement in visual acuity) [9]. Children were also on systemic corticosteroids in conjunction with their immunomodulatory medication.

Placebo-Controlled Trials

The first study assessing azathioprine's efficacy in managing uveitis came in 1969 [10]. Mathews and colleagues enrolled a total of 16 patients with chronic anterior uveitis, and half were randomized by the pharmacist to receive azathioprine 100 mg PO daily or placebo daily and the subjects were followed for 3 months. Interestingly, three patients from the placebo group (who had their data included with the other placebo group subjects) were crossed over to the azathioprine group, and their outcomes were included in the azathioprine group. Statistically speaking, these maneuvers are not typically performed today. The SUN criteria had not been developed during Matthews et al.'s assessment, and they used a scoring system in which a higher score was assigned to less cell and less flare. Additionally, they assessed patients' subjectively reported improvement or worsening of their vision. There was a trend toward improvement in both patient's' reported vision and objective features (visual acuity, cell, and flare), but there was no statistically significant difference between the two groups.

More recently, azathioprine was used in a prospective clinical trial evaluating its efficacy in controlling Behçet's disease-related uveitis in 48 patients compared to placebo [11]. Mean visual acuity remained stable in the azathioprine group compared to a statistically significant decline in vision in the placebo group. Additionally, there were statistically significantly less occurrences of hypopyon uveitis in the azathioprine group compared to the placebo group. Moreover, in 25 patients without ocular disease at enrollment, eight developed newly diagnosed uveitis in the placebo group compared to one in the azathioprine group, a statistically significant difference. In assessing long-term outcomes of the patients randomized to placebo or azathioprine [11], becoming blind and experiencing a two-line drop in visual acuity occurred more frequently in the placebo group compared to the azathioprine group [12].

Comparison with Other Antimetabolites and Immunomodulatory Therapies

A non-randomized trial was conducted utilizing azathioprine or chlorambucil in anterior uveitis [13]. In the 1970s, azathioprine was considered to be a cytotoxic agent by some [14], and the goal of this particular trial was to compare the relative efficacy of these two "cytotoxic" agents for chronic anterior endogenous (noninfectious) uveitis. Of the 25 patients enrolled, 22 received azathioprine, while 3 received chlorambucil. All patients were on doses of prednisone ranging from 10 to 15 mg daily. All but two patients were noted to manifest a response to azathioprine, but this included patients who would, by today's standards, still be considered to have active uveitis. For example, patients with 1+ anterior chamber cell were still considered to be responsive to azathioprine since such patients had exhibited more anterior chamber cell prior to enrollment. While this study did not fit the mold for an RCT, the authors recognized that long-term therapy with azathioprine was essential for preventing relapses of uveitis.

Side Effects

Side effects of azathioprine include gastrointestinal upset and cytopenias due to bone marrow suppression (leukopenia and thrombocytopenia in particular). Testing TPMT enzyme activity is important prior to utilizing azathioprine. Azathioprine is a pregnancy class D medication. As such, there is evidence of human fetal risk. However, several clinical series and a meta-analysis, mostly in the inflammatory bowel literature, demonstrate that thiopurines such as azathioprine and 6-MP can most likely be safely given in pregnancy [15–17]. Since azathioprine is found at very low levels in breast milk, it has been deemed "probably safe" in lactating mothers [18].

Considerations

While azathioprine has been better at controlling inflammation than placebo [11], azathioprine may be the most effective for intermediate uveitis [7]. Compared to mycophenolate mofetil, azathioprine has a slightly longer time to treatment success (4.8 months) but is faster than methotrexate's time (6.5 months). Despite its relatively quick time to treatment success (control of uveitis with prednisone 10 mg PO daily or less), it has a higher rate of side effects and discontinuation [19]. Azathioprine has been combined with T-cell inhibitors and corticosteroids to achieve control of noninfectious uveitis, including serpiginous choroiditis [20] and sympathetic ophthalmia [21–24].

Leflunomide

The chemical name for leflunomide is 5-methyl-N-{4-(trifluoromethyl)phenyl]-1,2-oxazole-4-carboxamide. Its molecular formula is $C_{12}H_9F_3N2O_2$ and its chemical structure is:

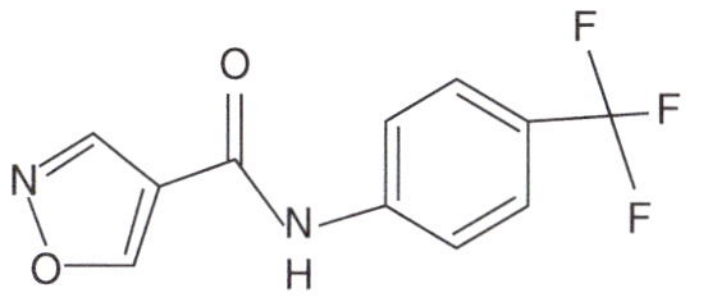

Structure 4.2

Leflunomide is a synthetic isoxazole derivative, which is converted to its active metabolite A77 1726 in the liver. Leflunomide was synthesized during the 1980s and ultimately approved by the FDA for the treatment of rheumatoid arthritis in the 1990s. Leflunomide has been shown to modulate inflammation via antagonizing lymphoproliferation by inhibiting dihydroorotate dehydrogenase, which leads to a reduction in the de novo synthesis of pyrimidines. A lack of pyrimidines results in halting of DNA synthesis and has particular effect on rapidly proliferating cells, including activated CD4+ T cells that are important in mediating inflammation. Specifically, proliferating cells are halted in G_1 phase. Moreover, leflunomide has been shown to have an effect on B-cell autoantibody synthesis [25]. A77 1726 modulates inflammation via other mechanisms as well. For example, it inhibits tyrosine kinase, which is important in mediating the progression of cells from G_0 phase to G_1 phase as well as activating the IL-2 receptor, which is involved in inflammation. Additionally, A77 1726 prevents degradation of IκB, which is the inhibitor of NF-κB [26]. Without activation, NF-κB is unable to translocate into the nucleus to result in transcription of genes that mediate inflammation.

The bioavailability of A77 1726 is not affected by the presence of food in the stomach or intestines. It is extensively bound to plasma proteins and, as a result, its half-life is between 15 to 18 days [26]. Most of leflunomide is eliminated equally in urine and feces. Because of leflunomide's metabolism by the liver and its reliance upon enterohepatic recirculation for its clearance, those with hepatic dysfunction are not ideal candidates for leflunomide. The long half-life of leflunomide means that it can take up to 5 months for it to reach steady-state plasma concentration.

Efficacy

Leflunomide has been shown to be effective at decreasing ocular inflammation in murine models of uveitis [27, 28].

Comparison with Other Antimetabolites

While leflunomide has been used in the treatment of uveitis [29–31], it has been associated with more frequent rates of recurrences compared to methotrexate when used in the chronic anterior uveitis associated with juvenile idiopathic arthritis (JIA) [32]. Others have shown that leflunomide has been effective at managing the chronic anterior uveitis associated with JIA. Molina and colleagues performed a retrospective review of 13 patients with JIA-associated uveitis using leflunomide for at least 7 months [31]. They classified the uveitis response to leflunomide as having no response, improvement, complete remission, and persistent remission. They found that 50% of patients achieved and maintained complete remission, 25% showed improvement, 25% exhibited persistent remission, and 38.5% showed no response to leflunomide. Thus, overall, 61% of the cohort exhibited a favorable response to leflunomide.

Combination with Other Antimetabolites

Leflunomide has been used effectively in combination with methotrexate, particularly in rheumatoid arthritis [33]. While A77 1726 affects pyrimidine synthesis, methotrexate inhibits purine synthesis [34], thereby having a synergistic effect. While antimetabolites are typically used with the biologic infliximab, to prevent human anti-chimeric antibody (HACA) formation, using leflunomide with infliximab is associated with frequent adverse reactions [35]. Use of leflunomide with infliximab is, therefore, not recommended.

Side Effects

Side effects include nausea, diarrhea, rash, and reversible alopecia. Less frequent side effects include hypertension [36], upper respiratory tract infections, and hepatotoxicity. Additionally, there has been an association with increasing total cholesterol and LDL cholesterol with increasing length of time patients take leflunomide.

Other Considerations

Leflunomide has been used as a cheaper alternative treatment in cytomegalovirus (CMV) infection, given that it has been shown to be effective in the treatment of CMV that is resistant to typical antiviral agents [37] (ganciclovir, foscarnet, and cidofovir) in organ transplant recipients [38–40]. Leflunomide affects the maturation of CMV's capsid [41], which is different than the inhibition of viral DNA polymerase that is the mechanism employed by other antivirals.

Methotrexate

The chemical name for methotrexate is N-{4-[[(2,4-diamino-6-pteridinyl)methyl]methylamino]benzoyl]-L-glutamic acid. Its empirical formula is $C_{20}H_{22}N_8O_5$. Its structural formula is:

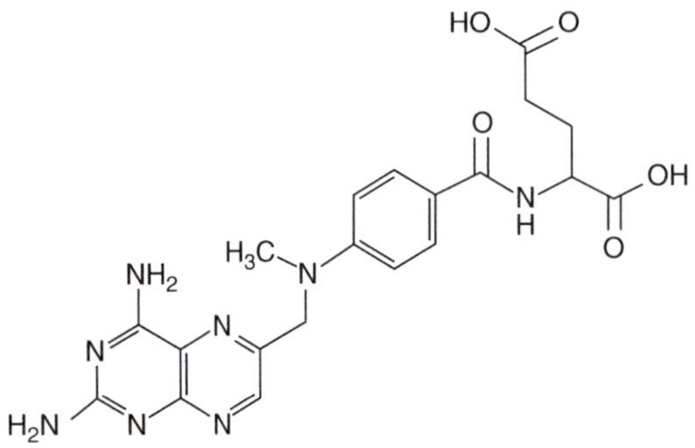

Structure 4.3

Methotrexate is often employed as the first-line corticosteroid-sparing therapy because it is relatively easy to take (once a week by mouth or subcutaneous injection) and relatively well-tolerated. Methotrexate (previously known as amethopterin) is one of the newer antimetabolites, being synthesized in the 1940s. Initially, there was hope that folic acid (a water-soluble B vitamin) and folate conjugates could be used in treating acute leukemia, but the use of these therapeutics actually potentiated the development of this hematologic malignancy. Deficiency in folate, however, was noted to effectively decrease peripheral leukemic cell count [42]. Thus, methotrexate's use started as a chemotherapeutic. Methotrexate is proved to be effective in the 1950s for psoriasis (first-line therapies besides coal tar and ultraviolet light often included arsenic and mercury compounds). Cress and Deaver described a 27-year-old man with psoriatic arthritis [43]. He proved to be recalcitrant to numerous therapies, so methotrexate was commenced and not only did his psoriasis improve, but his arthritis did as well. Methotrexate's use was then extended to rheumatoid arthritis in case reports during the 1960s [44–46]. A pilot study in the treatment of rheumatoid arthritis involving 32 patients demonstrated its efficacy in the majority of subjects [47, 48] and cemented its role not only in the treatment of rheumatoid arthritis but also of other rheumatologic conditions.

The enzyme dihydrofolate reductase (DHFR) has long been an attractive target for antibiotics, chemotherapeutics, and immunosuppressives given its importance in purine (adenine and guanine) and thymidylate synthesis. For example, trimethoprim is an antibiotic that targets bacterial DHFR. Methotrexate, on the other hand, targets mammalian DHFR. Cells that are rapidly growing and dividing, then, utilize DHFR more frequently than cells that are more senescent. In the case of methotrexate, there will be a more profound effect on cancer or inflammatory cells. However, side effects will manifest in other tissues that are not malignant or involved with immune function. For example, the stomach and small intestine epithelium have turnover rates ranging from 2 to 10 days. Neutrophils have turnover rates of 1–5 days and cervical epithelium turns over every 5–6 days. Lymphomas have higher turnover rates [48, 49], so they can be particularly sensitive to folate antagonists.

Pharmacology and Pharmacokinetics

Methotrexate is polyglutamated after entering the cell, which has several functions. One is that it allows for the accumulation of intracellular methotrexate (as the concentration of monoglutamate methotrexate outside of the cell is much lower than that inside) [50]. Additionally, the polyglutamation of methotrexate increases its intracellular life. Finally, polyglutamation enhances methotrexate's enzyme inhibitory potency. Methotrexate inhibits DHFR, an enzyme that reduces dihydrofolic acid to tetrahydrofolic acid, which can be converted to cofactors utilized in one-carbon transfer chemistry (one-carbon units include methyl, methylene, and formate). Tetrahydrofolate is required for the de novo synthesis of purines (important for nucleic acid synthesis) [34], thymidylic acid, and certain amino acids. These molecules are, in turn, required for cell growth and proliferation. Moreover, methotrexate inhibits thymidylate synthase, which is involved in the de novo synthesis of pyrimidines. Since methotrexate primarily enters the cells that make up various tissues, it is minimally bound to plasma proteins. In addition to disrupting purine synthesis, methotrexate exhibits other actions that can be therapeutic. Methotrexate inhibits transmethylation reactions [51, 52], important in metabolism, and inhibits the formation of polyamines [53]. Polyamines play a role in inflammation as seen in the synovial fluid and tissues in patients with rheumatoid arthritis [54]. Additionally, methotrexate promotes adenosine release [55], which can have anti-inflammatory effects [56, 57].

After oral consumption, methotrexate is absorbed from the proximal jejunum, and peak serum levels are attained in 1–2 hours. The bioavailability of methotrexate is approximately 60%–80%. Food does not affect the absorption of methotrexate [58], but it can delay absorption and reduce peak concentration. When administered parenterally (e.g., intramuscularly and subcutaneously), complete absorption occurs and peak serum concentrations are attained in under an hour. The half-life of methotrexate varies from 3 to 10 hours. Methotrexate is eliminated by the renal glomerular filtration and active tubular secretion, so use in those with renal dysfunction should be adjusted according to the creatinine clearance. Delayed drug clearance is a major factor influencing methotrexate toxicity.

Retrospective Studies

In a retrospective cohort study of 384 patients commenced on methotrexate for corticosteroid-sparing monotherapy of ocular inflammation (including uveitis, scleritis, and ocular cicatricial pemphigoid), 66% of patients were able to achieve inactivity of ocular inflammation that was sustained for at least 4 weeks within 1 year of therapy [59]. Approximately 58% of patients were able to achieve corticosteroid-sparing control of inflammation (being on 10 mg or less of daily oral prednisone).

Methotrexate is extensively used in the setting of JIA-associated uveitis. In the past, children with juvenile idiopathic arthritis (JIA)-associated uveitis were noted to achieve control of their ocular inflammation with systemic corticosteroids but also exhibited significant steroid-related side effects. Foster's group performed a retrospective review of children with JIA-associated uveitis from the late 1970s to late 1980s [60]. Of 26 JIA patients, eight used systemic immunomodulatory therapy, including three taking methotrexate with doses ranging from 5 to 15 mg PO weekly and one patient taking both methotrexate and azathioprine. Two of three patients taking methotrexate achieved control of inflammation, while the patient taking both methotrexate and azathioprine did not achieve control. This was a small study but important in demonstrating the use and tolerance of methotrexate in the pediatric uveitis population. In a later retrospective study, Weiss et al. reported that six of seven children requiring advancement to methotrexate due to active uveitis despite topical corticosteroids or occurrence of corticosteroid-related side effect were associated with improvement of uveitis [61]. Later, Foeldvari and Wierk showed that methotrexate was effective in treating JIA-associated uveitis in 84% of their cohort after an average of 4.5 months

[62]. The mean dose of methotrexate used in this cohort was 15.6 mg/m^2. Malik and Pavesio also demonstrated that methotrexate was effective in the management of JIA-associated uveitis in ten children [63]. More recently, Heiligenhaus and colleagues assessed 31 patients with JIA-associated uveitis with 21 (67.7%) achieving control of inflammation (with or without the use of concomitant topical corticosteroids) [64].

If ocular inflammation is not responding to oral methotrexate, consideration should be made, if indicated, for subcutaneous administration. Extrapolating from the rheumatoid arthritis literature [65], and switching from oral administration to subcutaneous administration of methotrexate, may result in more satisfactory control of uveitis.

Methotrexate Resistance

Resistance to methotrexate has been noted in conditions ranging from the rheumatologic (as in rheumatoid arthritis) [66–68] to the ophthalmologic (in the case of primary vitreoretinal lymphoma) [69]. Such resistance mediates lack of control of inflammation or tumor proliferation. Additionally, methotrexate resistance has been suggested to be responsible for the side effects experienced by some patients [70]. Certain mutations in methotrexate transporters and enzymes, such as methylenetetrahydrofolate reductase (MTHFR), may additionally be responsible for methotrexate-related side effects and/or efficacy [71, 72]. In the future, it may become a practice to assess each patient's potential response to different immunomodulatory agents based upon their gene expression of proteins involved in therapeutic responses or via a combination of genetic testing and gene expression analysis.

Side Effects

Methotrexate can be hepatotoxic, causing fibrosis and cirrhosis. For this reason, liver transaminases (including aspartate aminotransferase and alanine aminotransferase) should be routinely monitored. In psoriasis, liver fibrosis and cirrhosis can occur without overt abnormalities in serologically assessed liver transaminases. For this reason, some recommend performing liver biopsies periodically to evaluate for histologic evidence of hepatitis. In the rheumatoid arthritis literature, age when methotrexate was commenced, duration of use, and cumulative dose have been risk factors identified for liver damage [73, 74]. Methotrexate can rarely cause a direct toxic effect to lung parenchymal tissue, characterized by a nonproductive cough and wheezing. Patients should be assessed for pulmonary symptoms while on methotrexate and, should complaints arise, be examined with auscultation of the lungs and consideration for pulmonary radiographic imaging, which can reveal a diffuse interstitial pattern [75]. An ulcerative stomatitis/mucositis can also occur [76]. If gastrointestinal side effects pose difficulty for taking methotrexate orally, consideration should be made to give it subcutaneously. This route is associated with less frequent nausea and has the added benefit of increased bioavailability.

Folic acid or folinic acid (leucovorin) is typically administered to abrogate or abolish the side effects of methotrexate without affecting methotrexate's efficacy [77–79]. Folic acid is typically dosed at 1 mg orally each day. Some specialists will hold folic acid on the day that methotrexate is administered, but there is no data that suggest that taking folic acid on the day of methotrexate administration decreases the efficacy of methotrexate. If side effects continue to persist, then the dose of folic acid may be increased to 3–5 mg daily. Folinic acid may be administered for especially recalcitrant side effects (10 mg orally taken 12 hours after methotrexate administration). Methotrexate is absolutely contraindicated in pregnancy (pregnancy class X) and can induce teratogenic effects and induce fetal death when taken by a pregnant woman. In fact, methotrexate is used in high doses as an abortive medication. Typically, women wishing to conceive are recommended to wait 3 months after cessation of methotrexate. Additionally, men planning to have children should ideally be off of methotrexate for 3 months prior to trying to conceive. Methotrexate can be detected in human breast milk, and breastfeeding should cease if a mother is utilizing methotrexate. Occasionally, fatal opportunistic infections (*Pneumocystis jirovecii* pneumonia) might occur with methotrexate. Caution should be practiced when using methotrexate in patients experiencing an active infection. Additionally, methotrexate can be contraindicated in some patients with immunodeficiencies (whether acquired or primary).

Mycophenolate Mofetil

Mycophenolate mofetil, synthesized in the late 1980s[80], was shown to be effective in preventing organ allograft rejection in animal models [81–83], and this discovery ultimately led to trials involving reversal of human allograft rejection [84]. The chemical name for mycophenolate mofetil is 2-morpholinoethyl (E)-6-(1,3-dihydro-4-hydroxy-6-methoxy-7methyl-3-oxo-5-isobenzofuranyl)-4methyl-4-hexenoate. Its empiric formula is $C_{23}H_{31}NO_7$. Its structural formula is:

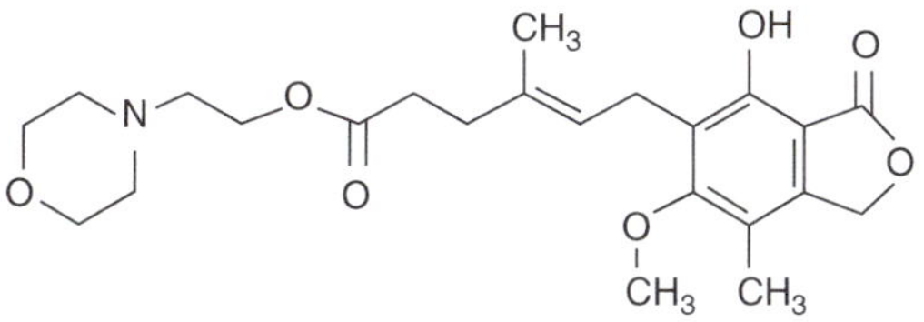

Structure 4.4

Pharmacology and Pharmacokinetics

After oral administration, mycophenolate mofetil is absorbed in the small intestine and metabolized to mycophenolic acid, which then undergoes glucuronidation via glucuronyl transferase to yield the phenolic glucuronide of mycophenolic acid (MPAG). MPAG is converted to mycophenolic acid during enterohepatic recirculation. As the morpholinoethyl ester of mycophenolic acid, mycophenolate mofetil exhibits more bioavailability than mycophenolic acid [80], which ranges up to 94% [85]. Carboxylesterases in the small intestine then convert mycophenolate mofetil to mycophenolic acid [85]. As a noncompetitive and reversible inhibitor of inosine monophosphate dehydrogenase, mycophenolate acid blocks de novo purine synthesis, thereby hindering DNA synthesis and affecting proliferation of lymphocytes. The mean half-life is approximately 18 hours.

While food does not affect the absorption of mycophenolate mofetil, it does result in a lower peak concentration. Thus, it is recommended that mycophenolate be taken on an empty stomach. Mycophenolic acid is 97% bound to serum albumin. Because mycophenolate mofetil is excreted in the urine, renal insufficiency can result in a higher bioavailability, which has the potential to lead to more untoward side effects. Consequently, this medication should be renally dosed. As mycophenolate mofetil is not enteric-coated, it can cause gastrointestinal distress and nausea.

Retrospective Studies

The largest retrospective study involving the use of mycophenolate mofetil in uveitis comes from Siepmann and colleagues in Germany [86]. Of the 106 patients studied, 92 (nearly 87%) experienced less than or equal to one recurrence of uveitis. Follow-up in this cohort ranged from 6 months to 41 months. Visual acuity was particularly well-preserved in patients with anterior and intermediate uveitis (vision was either stable or improved). Only four patients exhibited a lack of control of their uveitis with mycophenolate mofetil. Another study from Germany, involving 60 noninfectious uveitis patients, revealed that corticosteroid-sparing control (defined as ≤10 mg PO daily of prednisolone) of uveitis was achieved in 72% of patients after 1 year of treatment [87]. Relapses, while occurring in 50% of the cohort, exhibited a rate of only 0.23 relapses/year during the treatment period, and most were managed with either increasing the dose of prednisone, mycophenolate, or both. This particular cohort had a large component made up of intermediate uveitis patients (70%), and

32% of these patients failed mycophenolate mofetil due to inefficacy, most often due to uveitic macular edema.

Another large retrospective study involved a cohort of patients from North America at the Wilmer Eye Institute [88]. Fifty-one patients with noninfectious uveitis were included in the study. Most patients achieved control of uveitis with a total daily dose of 2 g. Most patients who did not achieve control with 2 g daily did so with 3 g daily. The median time to treatment success with mycophenolate mofetil 2 g daily was 3.5 months. In those patients requiring 3 g daily, the median time to treatment success was 4.7 months, though this was not statistically different from the lower dosage.

A more recent study involving exclusively Hispanic patients (including 21 with uveitis) revealed that most patients achieved control of ocular inflammation at 6 months after previously failing other immunomodulatory medications [89]. Five patients (23.8%) had active uveitis at 6 month's follow-up. Control of ocular inflammation, in general (patients with uveitis only were not independently assessed though they made up the majority of cases), was achieved with doses of 10 mg PO daily prednisone or less.

Mycophenolate mofetil is not used as frequently as methotrexate for uveitis in children. However, mycophenolate demonstrates effective control of pediatric systemic autoimmune diseases including systemic lupus erythematosus [90]. Mycophenolate is typically dosed in children similar to that used in renal transplantation: 600 mg/m^2 PO BID. In one of the largest retrospective studies evaluating the use of mycophenolate mofetil in the setting of pediatric uveitis of 17 children who were commenced on mycophenolate mofetil, 88% were able to achieve ≤5 mg PO daily of prednisolone [91].. While only 24% of patients during a mean follow-up of 3 years exhibited no relapses, all patients exhibited a reduction in relapses compared to the number experienced prior to starting mycophenolate mofetil.

Mycophenolate mofetil has also been effective in controlling uveitis in patients failing methotrexate. Sobrin and colleagues performed a retrospective review of their patients with noninfectious ocular inflammation failing methotrexate (either due to inefficacy or intolerance) [92]. Approximately half of their patients were able to achieve control of inflammation with mycophenolate. However, the odds of control of uveitis in patients with JIA-associated uveitis were lower than for those patients without this type of ocular inflammation.

Side Effects

The most common side effects of mycophenolate mofetil are gastrointestinal in nature and include gastric pain, diarrhea, and nausea [86]. Fatigue and pruritus are other common side effects. Gastrointestinal bleeding and perforations are rarely encountered. These cases have typically occurred in the organ transplantation literature. Additionally, infections involving opportunistic organisms as well as herpetic viral infections are more frequent in azathioprine, but again, these have been encountered in organ transplant patients. There is an increased risk of malignancy, particularly skin cancers, in transplant patients taking mycophenolate mofetil. However, the Systemic Immunosuppressive Therapy for Eye (SITE) diseases retrospective cohort study showed no increased risk of cancer (skin or otherwise) in uveitis patients taking most immunosuppressive agents, including antimetabolites and calcineurin inhibitors [93].

Fetal loss and congenital malformations are noted with mycophenolate. Consequently, contraception must be practiced while taking mycophenolate mofetil. Additionally, patients taking oral contraceptives should be made aware that mycophenolate mofetil can decrease the serum levels of contraceptive hormones with a theoretically reduced efficacy of the contraceptive.

Considerations

The use of proton pump inhibitors (PPI) for peptic ulcer disease and gastroesophageal reflux disease decreases both the serum concentration and bioavailability of mycophenolate mofetil. Patients who are on a PPI and who are to commence mycophenolate mofetil for their uveitis management should consider switching to a histamine-2 receptor antagonist (e.g., famotidine).

Mycophenolic Acid

The chemical name for mycophenolic acid is (4E)-6-(4-hydroxy-6methoxy-7-methyl-3-oxo-1,3-dihydro-2-benzofuran-5-y)-4-methylhex-4-enoic acid. Its chemical structure is:

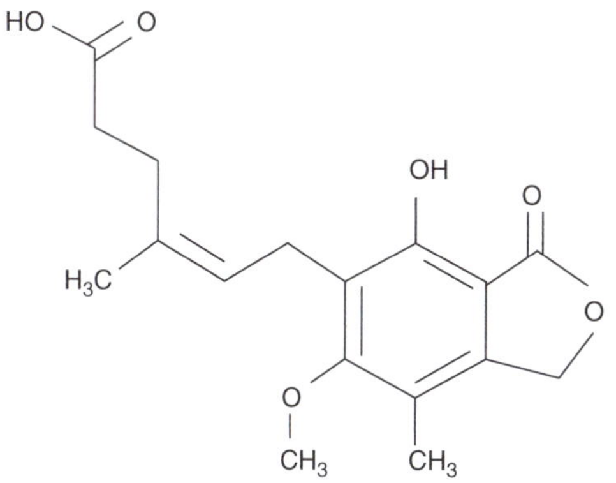

Structure 4.5

Mycophenolic acid was originally recognized to have antibiotic properties. *Penicillium brevicompactum*, a mold (recall that the Greek root word "myco" means fungus), was noted to secrete a substance (mycophenolic acid) that inhibited the growth of *Staphylococcus aureus*. Bartolomeo Gosio, an Italian physician, is credited with this discovery [94]. Gosio was looking to implicate different molds as a cause of niacin deficiency (pellagra).

Pharmacology and Pharmacokinetics

After oral consumption, mycophenolic acid is absorbed into the small intestine. Because mycophenolic acid is enteric-coated, it often exhibits better gastrointestinal tolerability than mycophenolate mofetil [95]. Mycophenolic acid inhibits inosine 5′-monophosphate dehydrogenase. After oral consumption, the bioavailability of mycophenolic acid is 72%. As noted for mycophenolate mofetil (which is converted to mycophenolic acid), 97% of mycophenolic acid is bound to albumin. Mycophenolic acid's mechanism of action, metabolism, and excretion is the same as that for mycophenolate mofetil.

Use in Uveitis

Mycophenolic acid has been suggested as a possible therapy for intraocular use, but this continues to be entirely experimental and is not being utilized in humans. However, toxicity of human retinal pigment epithelium and Müller cells was not seen for doses of mycophenolic acid at 50 μg/mL or less [96].

There is a Phase 3 clinical trial aimed at determining the efficacy, safety, and tolerability of mycophenolic acid in patients with intermediate uveitis (ClinicalTrials.gov Identifier NCT01092533).

Sulfasalazine

While sulfasalazine is not an antimetabolite, it bears mentioning since it has certainly been used as a DMARD in rheumatology and has been used occasionally in the treatment of uveitis. The IUPAC name for sulfasalazine is 2-hydroxy-5-[[4-(2-pyridinylsulfamoyl)phenyl]diazenyl]benzoic acid. Its molecular formula is $C_{18}H_{14}N_4O_5S$ and its chemical structure is:

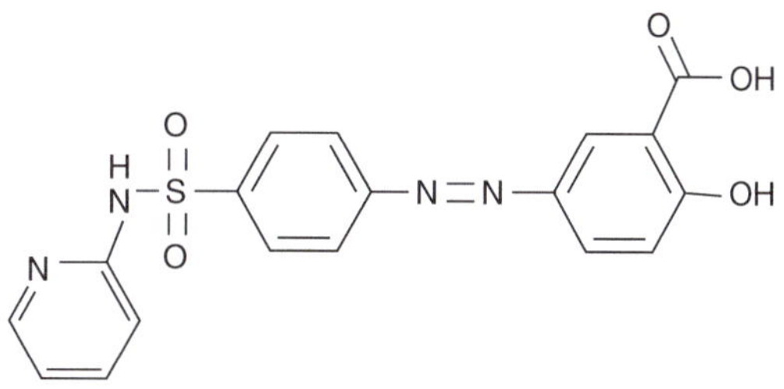

Structure 4.6

Pharmacology and Pharmacokinetics

Sulfasalazine is either absorbed in the upper gastrointestinal system (up to 30% of the intact drug) or is cleaved into sulfapyridine and 5-amino salicylate by colonic bacteria. The cleavage products are thought to be involved in inhibiting folate absorption and metabolism [97–99]. Additionally, sulfasalazine and 5-amino salicylate inhibit in vitro leukocyte motility [100].

Placebo-Controlled Trials

In a small placebo-controlled trial, 22 patients with ankylosing spondylitis-associated recurrent anterior uveitis were randomized either to sulfasalazine (10 patients) or placebo (12 patients) and followed for 3 years. Uveitis activity was assessed by fluorophotometry. The number of recurrences was less than one for each year in the patients taking sulfasalazine (with the highest number of mean recurrences during year two with 0.6 +/− 0.84 recurrences). In the placebo group, the number of recurrences was significantly higher (with the highest recurrences occurring during the first year of follow-up at 1.33 +/− 1.23 recurrences, $p = 0.016$). Additionally, the formation of posterior synechiae was less frequently encountered in the sulfasalazine group [101]. While this study was and continues to be useful, uveitis activity is no longer graded in this fashion, and generalizability to the current definition of meaningful control of uveitis is unknown.

Prospective Studies

Ten patients with recurrent anterior uveitis were commenced on sulfasalazine and followed for 1 year [102]. In the year prior to the institution of sulfasalazine, there was a mean of 3.4 flares, significantly more than while on the DMARD (less than 1 flare), representing a statistically significant difference.

Retrospective Studies

In a study of chronic uveitis, four Taiwanese children with JIA or ankylosing spondylitis were placed on sulfasalazine due to failing to taper off of steroid drops as well as exhibiting a lack of uveitis control with oral nonsteroidal anti-inflammatory drugs. Two children with JIA-associated uveitis and the child with ankylosing spondylitis-associated uveitis showed improvement in their anterior chamber cell and visual acuity afterward. The medication was tolerated well by all four children [103].

Side Effects

Common side effects include gastrointestinal discomfort and rash. Stevens-Johnson syndrome and neutropenia are less frequent but serious side effects.

See Table 4.1 for dosing of antimetabolites.

General Considerations with the Antimetabolites

In a large retrospective study in which patients with noninfectious ocular inflammatory diseases were assessed, three of the most commonly used antimetabolites to control ocular inflammation (including uveitis) were assessed [19]. The median time to treatment success (on $\leq$10 mg prednisone PO daily) with methotrexate (oral and subcutaneous routes were included) was 6.5 months compared to that of mycophenolate mofetil (4 months) and azathioprine (4.8 months). It was noted that methotrexate was frequently started at a low dose and increased over time, whereas mycophenolate mofetil and azathioprine were typically started at more therapeutic doses. After 6 months of therapy, the proportion of all ocular inflammation patients achieving treatment success with mycophenolate was 70% compared to 42% of those on methotrexate and 48% of those taking azathioprine. Methotrexate seems to manage ocular inflammation in association with sarcoidosis. Even low-

Table 4.1 Antimetabolites dosing table

Name	Year discovered or synthesized	Mechanism of action	Typical adult starting dose	Maximum adult dose	Typical pediatric starting dose	Maximum pediatric dose	Lab monitoring
Azathioprine	1957	Acts as a purine nucleoside analogue → block purine synthesis → prevent DNA synthesis	1 mg/kg/day PO divided daily or BID	2.5 to 4 mg/kg/day divided daily or BID	1 mg/kg/day PO divided daily or BID	2.5 mg/kg/day divided daily or BID	CBC/creatinine/LFTs at baseline, then monthly. Consider genotyping for TPMT *or* starting low dose and following creatinine before increasing
Leflunomide	1991	Inhibits dihydroorotate dehydrogenase → inhibits pyrimidine synthesis → prevent DNA synthesis	100 mg PO daily × 3 days, then 10 mg PO QOD to 20 mg PO daily	20 mg PO daily	Not applicable	Not applicable	CBC/LFTs at baseline, monthly × 6 months, then q6–8 weeks
Methotrexate	1947	Inhibits dihyrdrofolate reductase → inhibits purine base synthesis → prevent DNA synthesis	7.5 to 15 mg PO/IM weekly	25 mg PO/IM weekly	For 2–16 years old: 5 to15 mg/m2 PO/IM weekly	For 2–16 years old: 30 mg/m^2 PO/IM weekly	CBC/BUN/creatinine/LFTs/pregnancy test at baseline, then monthly × 6 months, then q4–8 weeks
Mycophenolate mofetil	1990	Inhibits inosine monophosphate → purine synthesis → prevent DNA synthesis	500 mg PO BID	1000 mg to 1500 mg PO BID	600 mg/m2 PO BID	1000 mg PO BID	CBC/BUN/creatinine/pregnancy test at baseline, then weekly × 4 weeks, then q14 days × 8 weeks, then monthly
Mycophenolic acid	1893	Inhibits inosine monophosphate → purine synthesis → prevent DNA synthesis	360 mg to 540 mg PO BID	720 mg PO BID	Greater than 5 years old BSA = 1.19 m^2 to 1.58 m^2: 360 to 540 mg PO BID Greater than 5 years old and BSA > 1.58 m^2: 360 to 540 mg PO BID	Greater than 5 years old BSA = 1.19 m^2 to 1.58 m^2: 540 to 720 mg PO BID Greater than 5 years old and BSA > 1.58 m^2: 540 to 720 mg PO BID	CBC/BUN/creatinine/pregnancy test at baseline, then weekly × 4 weeks, then q14 days × 8 weeks, then monthly
Sulfasalazine (not an antimetabolite, but a synthetic salicylate)	1942	Inhibits folate absorption and NF-κB activation → reduction in inflammation	0.5 g to 1 g PO q 6–8 hours	4 g to 6 g PO daily (divided q12 hours)	6 years old: 10–50 mg/kg/day PO divided BID	2 g/day PO divided BID	CBC/BUN/creatinine/LFTs at baseline, then q2 weeks × 3 months, then monthly × 3 months, then q3 months

TPMT thiopurine methyltransferase, *BSA* body surface area (m^2) = $\sqrt{[(\text{weight in kilograms} \times \text{height in centimeters})/3600\ \text{cm kg/m}^4]}$, *IM* intramuscular (also subcutaneous), *NF-κB* nuclear factor kappa-light-chain-enhancer of activated B-cells

dose oral methotrexate (12.5 mg weekly) has been shown to result in stability or decrease in inflammation in sarcoid-related uveitis in the overwhelming majority of patients studied [104]. While these results are intriguing, there still remains the issue of determining the best antimetabolite to use as the first-line therapy for corticosteroid-sparing control of uveitis in general. To address this important issue, Acharya and colleagues compared oral methotrexate and mycophenolate mofetil (two of the most commonly used antimetabolites) for initial corticosteroid-sparing control of noninfectious intermediate, posterior, and panuveitis. While past retrospective studies have suggested that mycophenolate mofetil may be more effective in the management of uveitis, Acharya's RCT found that a higher proportion of those randomized to methotrexate achieved control of their uveitis compared to those randomized to mycophenolate mofetil [105]. Control of uveitis was defined as less than 1+ anterior chamber cell or vitreous haze or inactive retinal or choroidal lesions. However, while the maximum dose of methotrexate was used (25 mg PO weekly), the maximum dose for mycophenolate mofetil in the trial was 1 g PO BID rather than the higher maximum dose of 1.5 g PO BID. To address this issue, Acharya is currently conducting a National Eye Institute-sponsored randomized controlled trial, which is powered to detect a smaller difference (20%) between the two randomization groups and utilizing the typical maximum doses of these medications. The data gathered from this pivotal study will provide uveitis specialists with much needed evidence to support the initial use of either methotrexate or mycophenolate mofetil as initial corticosteroid-sparing therapy.

Contraception should be practiced while on antimetabolites (particularly with methotrexate and mycophenolate mofetil). Developing fetuses with their rapid cell turnover are especially vulnerable to the effects of antimetabolites that affect nucleic acid synthesis. In fact, high-dose methotrexate is utilized as an abortive agent. It is recommended in both men and women wishing to become pregnant to discontinue using it and wait at least 3 months prior to conceiving. Azathioprine, however, is considered safe to continue during conception and during pregnancy.

Antimetabolites can be used in conjunction with other immunomodulatory agents, particularly from other classes such as the T-cell inhibitors (e.g., cyclosporine [106, 107]) or with biologics. In the case of biologics, antimetabolites may help decrease the frequency of developing antibodies (e.g., human anti-chimeric antibodies (HACAs)) against monoclonal antibodies (e.g., rituximab, infliximab, adalimumab).

Much of the information regarding cancer and systemic immunomodulatory therapy with antimetabolites comes from the transplant literature. For example, renal transplant patients on azathioprine have 50- to 100-fold increase in the relative risk of malignancy. However, it has been noted that rheumatoid arthritis carries a background risk of cancer development compared to patients without rheumatoid arthritis. Rheumatoid arthritis patients have been noted to have a fivefold increase in cancer compared to the general population. Azathioprine-treated RA patients have a tenfold increase in cancer compared to the general population [108]. The most common neoplasias include squamous cell carcinoma of the skin, non-Hodgkin's lymphoma, and Kaposi's sarcoma [109].

In a retrospective cohort study evaluating nearly 8000 patients with ocular inflammatory diseases (1155 patients with uveitis), the antimetabolites were not associated with an increased risk in overall mortality and were not associated with an increased risk in cancer-related mortality [93]. Conveying this information to patients or the parents of patients can do much to mollify their concerns about starting antimetabolite therapy. Oftentimes in uveitis, escalation to systemic immunomodulatory therapy must be made, and the knowledge that these medications are not only effective, but also safe, can do much to treat the mind *and* body of the person in the uveitis specialist's examination chair.

References

1. Esterberg E, Acharya NR. Corticosteroid-sparing therapy: practice patterns among uveitis specialists. J Ophthalmic Inflamm Infect. 2012;2(1):21–8.
2. Elion GB, Hitchings GH, Vanderwerff H. Antagonists of nucleic acid derivatives. VI. Purines. J Biol Chem. 1951;192(2):505–18.

3. Lecture EGBN. The purine path to chemotherapy. Biosci Rep. 1989;9(5):509–29.
4. Hoffmann M, Rychlewski J, Chrzanowska M, Hermann T. Mechanism of activation of an immunosuppressive drug: azathioprine. Quantum chemical study on the reaction of azathioprine with cysteine. J Am Chem Soc. 2001;123(26):6404–9.
5. Liu H, Ding L, Zhang F, et al. The impact of glutathione S-transferase genotype and phenotype on the adverse drug reactions to azathioprine in patients with inflammatory bowel diseases. J Pharmacol Sci. 2015;129(2):95–100.
6. Greenwood AJ, Stanford MR, Graham EM. The role of azathioprine in the management of retinal vasculitis. Eye (Lond). 1998;12(Pt 5):783–8.
7. Pasadhika S, Kempen JH, Newcomb CW, et al. Azathioprine for ocular inflammatory diseases. Am J Ophthalmol. 2009;148(4):500–9.e502
8. Jabs DA, Nussenblatt RB, Rosenbaum JT. Standardization of uveitis nomenclature for reporting clinical data. Results of the First International Workshop. Am J Ophthalmol. 2005;140(3):509–16.
9. Schatz CS, Uzel JL, Leininger L, Danner S, Terzic J, Fischbach M. Immunosuppressants used in a steroid-sparing strategy for childhood uveitis. J Pediatr Ophthalmol Strabismus. 2007;44(1):28–34.
10. Mathews JD, Crawford BA, Bignell JL, Mackay IR. Azathioprine in active chronic iridocyclitis. A double-blind controlled trial. Br J Ophthalmol. 1969;53(5):327–30.
11. Yazici H, Pazarli H, Barnes CG, et al. A controlled trial of azathioprine in Behcet's syndrome. N Engl J Med. 1990;322(5):281–5.
12. Hamuryudan V, Ozyazgan Y, Hizli N, et al. Azathioprine in Behcet's syndrome: effects on long-term prognosis. Arthritis Rheum. 1997;40(4):769–74.
13. Andrasch RH, Pirofsky B, Burns RP. Immunosuppressive therapy for severe chronic uveitis. Arch Ophthalmol (Chicago, Ill: 1960). 1978;96(2): 247–51.
14. Cytotoxic drugs in treatment of nonmalignant diseases. Ann Intern Med. 1972;76(4):619–42.
15. Casanova MJ, Chaparro M, Domenech E, et al. Safety of thiopurines and anti-TNF-alpha drugs during pregnancy in patients with inflammatory bowel disease. Am J Gastroenterol. 2013;108(3):433–40.
16. Cleary BJ, Kallen B. Early pregnancy azathioprine use and pregnancy outcomes. Birth Defects Res A Clin Mol Teratol. 2009;85(7):647–54.
17. Mozaffari S, Abdolghaffari AH, Nikfar S, Abdollahi M. Pregnancy outcomes in women with inflammatory bowel disease following exposure to thiopurines and antitumor necrosis factor drugs: a systematic review with meta-analysis. Hum Exp Toxicol. 2015;34(5):445–59.
18. Nielsen OH, Maxwell C, Hendel J. IBD medications during pregnancy and lactation. Nat Rev Gastroenterol Hepatol. 2014;11(2):116–27.
19. Galor A, Jabs DA, Leder HA, et al. Comparison of antimetabolite drugs as corticosteroid-sparing therapy for noninfectious ocular inflammation. Ophthalmology. 2008;115(10):1826–32.
20. Hooper PL, Kaplan HJ. Triple agent immunosuppression in serpiginous choroiditis. Ophthalmology. 1991;98(6):944–51; discussion 951-942
21. Moore CE. Sympathetic ophthalmitis treated with azathioprine. Br J Ophthalmol. 1968;52(9):688–90.
22. Hakin KN, Pearson RV, Lightman SL. Sympathetic ophthalmia: visual results with modern immunosuppressive therapy. Eye (Lond). 1992;6(Pt 5):453–5.
23. Hellmund K, Fruhauf A, Seiler T, Naumann GO. Sympathetic ophthalmia 50 years after penetrating injury. A case report. Klinische Monatsblatter fur Augenheilkunde. 1998;213(3):182–5.
24. Sisk RA, Davis JL, Dubovy SR, Smiddy WE. Sympathetic ophthalmia following vitrectomy for endophthalmitis after intravitreal bevacizumab. Ocul Immunol Inflamm. 2008;16(5):236–8.
25. Siemasko KF, Chong AS, Williams JW, Bremer EG, Finnegan A. Regulation of B cell function by the immunosuppressive agent leflunomide. Transplantation. 1996;61(4):635–42.
26. Manna SK, Aggarwal BB. Immunosuppressive leflunomide metabolite (A77 1726) blocks TNF-dependent nuclear factor-kappa B activation and gene expression. J Immunol. 1999;162(4):2095–102.
27. Robertson SM, Lang LS. Leflunomide: inhibition of S-antigen induced autoimmune uveitis in Lewis rats. Agents Actions. 1994;42(3–4):167–72.
28. Fang CB, Zhou DX, Zhan SX, et al. Amelioration of experimental autoimmune uveitis by leflunomide in Lewis rats. PLoS One. 2013;8(4):e62071.
29. Wang J, Xie QB, Zhao Y, Liu Y. Flare up of rheumatoid arthritis associated with Vogt-Koyanagi-Harada syndrome treated with leflunomide. Int J Ophthalmol. 2014;7(5):909–11.
30. Steigerwalt RD Jr, Bacci S, Valesini G. Severe uveitis successfully treated with leflunomide. Retin Cases Brief Rep. 2007;1(1):54–5.
31. Molina C, Modesto C, Martin-Begue N, Arnal C. Leflunomide, a valid and safe drug for the treatment of chronic anterior uveitis associated with juvenile idiopathic arthritis. Clin Rheumatol. 2013;32(11):1673–5.
32. Bichler J, Benseler SM, Krumrey-Langkammerer M, Haas JP, Hugle B. Leflunomide is associated with a higher flare rate compared to methotrexate in the treatment of chronic uveitis in juvenile idiopathic arthritis. Scand J Rheumatol. 2015;44(4):280–3.
33. Kremer JM, Genovese MC, Cannon GW, et al. Concomitant leflunomide therapy in patients with active rheumatoid arthritis despite stable doses of methotrexate. A randomized, double-blind, placebo-controlled trial. Ann Intern Med. 2002;137(9): 726–33.
34. Fairbanks LD, Ruckemann K, Qiu Y, et al. Methotrexate inhibits the first committed step of purine biosynthesis in mitogen-stimulated human T-lymphocytes: a metabolic basis for efficacy in rheumatoid arthritis? Biochem J. 1999;342 (. Pt 1:143–52.

35. Kiely PD, Johnson DM. Infliximab and leflunomide combination therapy in rheumatoid arthritis: an open-label study. Rheumatology (Oxford). 2002;41(6):631–7.
36. Nurmohamed MT, van Halm VP, Dijkmans BA. Cardiovascular risk profile of antirheumatic agents in patients with osteoarthritis and rheumatoid arthritis. Drugs. 2002;62(11):1599–609.
37. Erice A. Resistance of human cytomegalovirus to antiviral drugs. Clin Microbiol Rev. 1999;12(2):286–97.
38. Andrassy J, Illner WD, Rentsch M, Jaeger G, Jauch KW, Fischereder M. Leflunomide: a treatment option for ganciclovir-resistant cytomegalovirus infection after renal transplantation. NDT Plus. 2009;2(2):149–51.
39. Chon WJ, Kadambi PV, Xu C, et al. Use of leflunomide in renal transplant recipients with ganciclovir-resistant/refractory cytomegalovirus infection: a case series from the University of Chicago. Case Rep Nephrol Dial. 2015;5(1):96–105.
40. Verkaik NJ, Hoek RA, van Bergeijk H, et al. Leflunomide as part of the treatment for multidrug-resistant cytomegalovirus disease after lung transplantation: case report and review of the literature. Transpl Infect Dis. 2013;15(6):E243–9.
41. Waldman WJ, Knight DA, Blinder L, et al. Inhibition of cytomegalovirus in vitro and in vivo by the experimental immunosuppressive agent leflunomide. Intervirology. 1999;42(5–6):412–8.
42. Heinle RW, Welch AD. Experiments with pteroylglutamic acid and pteroylglutamic acid deficiency in human leukemia. J Clin Invest. 1948;27(4):539.
43. Cress RH, Deaver NL. Methotrexate in the management of severe psoriasis and arthritis: report of a Case. South Med J. 1964;57:1088–90.
44. Enderlin M. Experiences with antimetabolite therapy of malignant forms of progressive chronic polyarthritis. Helv Med Acta Suppl. 1966;46:171.
45. Gross D, Enderlin M, Fehr K. Immunosuppressive therapy of progredient chronic polyarthritis using antimetabolites and cytostatics. Schweiz Med Wochenschr. 1967;97(40):1301–10.
46. Fosdick WM. Cytotoxic therapy in rheumatoid arthritis. Med Clin North Am. 1968;52(3):747–57.
47. Wilke WS, Calabrese LH, Scherbel AL. Methotrexate in the treatment of rheumatoid arthritis; pilot study. Cleve Clin Q. 1980;47(4):305–9.
48. Hall PA, Levison DA. Review: assessment of cell proliferation in histological material. J Clin Pathol. 1990;43(3):184–92.
49. Spina D, Leoncini L, Del Vecchio MT, et al. Low versus high cell turnover in diffusely growing non-Hodgkin's lymphomas. J Pathol. 1995;177(4):335–41.
50. Day RO, Furst DE, van Riel PLCM, Bresnihan B. Antirheumatic therapy: actions and outcomes. Basel/Boston/Berlin: Birhäuser Verlag; 2005. ISBN 3-7643-6595-1.
51. Jurgensen CH, Huber BE, Zimmerman TP, Wolberg G. 3-deazaadenosine inhibits leukocyte adhesion and ICAM-1 biosynthesis in tumor necrosis factor-stimulated human endothelial cells. J Immunol. 1990;144(2):653–61.
52. Jurgensen CH, Wolberg G, Zimmerman TP. Inhibition of neutrophil adherence to endothelial cells by 3-deazaadenosine. Agents Actions. 1989;27(3–4):398–400.
53. Nesher G, Moore TL. The in vitro effects of methotrexate on peripheral blood mononuclear cells. Modulation by methyl donors and spermidine. Arthritis Rheum. 1990;33(7):954–9.
54. Yukioka K, Wakitani S, Yukioka M, et al. Polyamine levels in synovial tissues and synovial fluids of patients with rheumatoid arthritis. J Rheumatol. 1992;19(5):689–92.
55. Morabito L, Montesinos MC, Schreibman DM, et al. Methotrexate and sulfasalazine promote adenosine release by a mechanism that requires ecto-5′-nucleotidase-mediated conversion of adenine nucleotides. J Clin Invest. 1998;101(2):295–300.
56. Cronstein BN, Rosenstein ED, Kramer SB, Weissmann G, Hirschhorn R. Adenosine; a physiologic modulator of superoxide anion generation by human neutrophils. Adenosine acts via an A2 receptor on human neutrophils. J Immunol. 1985;135(2):1366–71.
57. Cronstein BN, Daguma L, Nichols D, Hutchison AJ, Williams M. The adenosine/neutrophil paradox resolved: human neutrophils possess both A1 and A2 receptors that promote chemotaxis and inhibit O2 generation, respectively. J Clin Invest. 1990;85(4):1150–7.
58. Jundt JW, Browne BA, Fiocco GP, Steele AD, Mock D. A comparison of low dose methotrexate bioavailability: oral solution, oral tablet, subcutaneous and intramuscular dosing. J Rheumatol. 1993;20(11):1845–9.
59. Gangaputra S, Newcomb CW, Liesegang TL, et al. Methotrexate for ocular inflammatory diseases. Ophthalmology. 2009;116(11):2188–2198.e2181.
60. Hemady RK, Baer JC, Foster CS. Immunosuppressive drugs in the management of progressive, corticosteroid-resistant uveitis associated with juvenile rheumatoid arthritis. Int Ophthalmol Clin. 1992;32(1):241–52.
61. Weiss AH, Wallace CA, Sherry DD. Methotrexate for resistant chronic uveitis in children with juvenile rheumatoid arthritis. J Pediatr. 1998;133(2):266–8.
62. Foeldvari I, Wierk A. Methotrexate is an effective treatment for chronic uveitis associated with juvenile idiopathic arthritis. J Rheumatol. 2005;32(2):362–5.
63. Malik AR, Pavesio C. The use of low dose methotrexate in children with chronic anterior and intermediate uveitis. Br J Ophthalmol. 2005;89(7):806–8.
64. Heiligenhaus A, Mingels A, Heinz C, Ganser G. Methotrexate for uveitis associated with juvenile idiopathic arthritis: value and requirement for additional anti-inflammatory medication. Eur J Ophthalmol. 2007;17(5):743–8.
65. Herman RA, Veng-Pedersen P, Hoffman J, Koehnke R, Furst DE. Pharmacokinetics of low-dose methotrexate in rheumatoid arthritis patients. J Pharm Sci. 1989;78(2):165–71.

66. Prasad S, Tripathi D, Rai MK, Aggarwal S, Mittal B, Agarwal V. Multidrug resistance protein-1 expression, function and polymorphisms in patients with rheumatoid arthritis not responding to methotrexate. Int J Rheum Dis. 2014;17(8):878–86.
67. Wessels JA, van der Kooij SM, le Cessie S, et al. A clinical pharmacogenetic model to predict the efficacy of methotrexate monotherapy in recent-onset rheumatoid arthritis. Arthritis Rheum. 2007;56(6):1765–75.
68. Wessels JA, Kooloos WM, De Jonge R, et al. Relationship between genetic variants in the adenosine pathway and outcome of methotrexate treatment in patients with recent-onset rheumatoid arthritis. Arthritis Rheum. 2006;54(9):2830–9.
69. Sen HN, Chan CC, Byrnes G, Fariss RN, Nussenblatt RB, Buggage RR. Intravitreal methotrexate resistance in a patient with primary intraocular lymphoma. Ocul Immunol Inflamm. 2008;16(1):29–33.
70. Micsik T, Lorincz A, Gal J, Schwab R, Petak I. MDR-1 and MRP-1 activity in peripheral blood leukocytes of rheumatoid arthritis patients. Diagn Pathol. 2015;10(1):216.
71. Saleh MM, Irshaid YM, Mustafa KN. Methylene tetrahydrofolate reductase genotypes frequencies: association with toxicity and response to methotrexate in rheumatoid arthritis patients. Int J Clin Pharmacol Ther. 2015;53(2):154–62.
72. Fisher MC, Cronstein BN. Metaanalysis of methylenetetrahydrofolate reductase (MTHFR) polymorphisms affecting methotrexate toxicity. J Rheumatol. 2009;36(3):539–45.
73. Sotoudehmanesh R, Anvari B, Akhlaghi M, Shahraeeni S, Kolahdoozan S. Methotrexate hepatotoxicity in patients with rheumatoid arthritis. Middle East J Digest Dis. 2010;2(2):104–9.
74. Sakthiswary R, Chan GY, Koh ET, Leong KP, Thong BY. Methotrexate-associated nonalcoholic fatty liver disease with transaminitis in rheumatoid arthritis. ScientificWorldJournal. 2014;2014:823763.
75. Jakubovic BD, Donovan A, Webster PM, Shear NH. Methotrexate-induced pulmonary toxicity. Can Respir J. 2013;20(3):153–5.
76. Troeltzsch M, von Blohn G, Kriegelstein S, et al. Oral mucositis in patients receiving low-dose methotrexate therapy for rheumatoid arthritis: report of 2 cases and literature review. Oral Surg Oral Med Oral Pathol Oral Radiol. 2013;115(5):e28–33.
77. Morgan SL, Baggott JE, Vaughn WH, et al. Supplementation with folic acid during methotrexate therapy for rheumatoid arthritis. A double-blind, placebo-controlled trial. Ann Intern Med. 1994;121(11):833–41.
78. Morgan SL, Baggott JE, Vaughn WH, et al. The effect of folic acid supplementation on the toxicity of low-dose methotrexate in patients with rheumatoid arthritis. Arthritis Rheum. 1990;33(1):9–18.
79. Shea B, Swinden MV, Ghogomu ET, et al. Folic acid and folinic acid for reducing side effects in patients receiving methotrexate for rheumatoid arthritis. J Rheumatol. 2014;41(6):1049–60.
80. Lee WA, Gu L, Miksztal AR, Chu N, Leung K, Nelson PH. Bioavailability improvement of mycophenolic acid through amino ester derivatization. Pharm Res. 1990;7(2):161–6.
81. Morris RE, Hoyt EG, Murphy MP, Eugui EM, Allison AC. Mycophenolic acid morpholinoethylester (RS-61443) is a new immunosuppressant that prevents and halts heart allograft rejection by selective inhibition of T- and B-cell purine synthesis. Transplant Proc. 1990;22(4):1659–62.
82. Platz KP, Sollinger HW, Hullett DA, Eckhoff DE, Eugui EM, Allison AC. RS-61443 – a new, potent immunosuppressive agent. Transplantation. 1991;51(1):27–31.
83. Platz KP, Bechstein WO, Eckhoff DE, Suzuki Y, Sollinger HW. RS-61443 reverses acute allograft rejection in dogs. Surgery. 1991;110(4):736–40; discussion 740–731
84. Sollinger HW, Deierhoi MH, Belzer FO, Diethelm AG, Kauffman RS. RS-61443 – a phase I clinical trial and pilot rescue study. Transplantation. 1992;53(2):428–32.
85. Staatz CE, Tett SE. Clinical pharmacokinetics and pharmacodynamics of mycophenolate in solid organ transplant recipients. Clin Pharmacokinet. 2007;46(1):13–58.
86. Siepmann K, Huber M, Stubiger N, Deuter C, Zierhut M. Mycophenolate mofetil is a highly effective and safe immunosuppressive agent for the treatment of uveitis : a retrospective analysis of 106 patients. Graefes Arch Clin Exp Ophthalmol. 2006;244(7):788–94.
87. Doycheva D, Zierhut M, Blumenstock G, Stuebiger N, Deuter C. Long-term results of therapy with mycophenolate mofetil in chronic non-infectious uveitis. Graefes Arch Clin Exp Ophthalmol. 2011;249(8):1235–43.
88. Thorne JE, Jabs DA, Qazi FA, Nguyen QD, Kempen JH, Dunn JP. Mycophenolate mofetil therapy for inflammatory eye disease. Ophthalmology. 2005;112(8):1472–7.
89. Cuchacovich M, Solanes F, Perez C, et al. Mycophenolate Mofetil therapy in refractory inflammatory eye disease. J Ocul Pharmacol Ther. 2016;32(1):55–61.
90. Filler G, Hansen M, LeBlanc C, et al. Pharmacokinetics of mycophenolate mofetil for autoimmune disease in children. Pediatr Nephrol (Berlin, Germany). 2003;18(5):445–9.
91. Doycheva D, Deuter C, Stuebiger N, Biester S, Zierhut M. Mycophenolate mofetil in the treatment of uveitis in children. Br J Ophthalmol. 2007;91(2):180–4.
92. Sobrin L, Christen W, Foster CS. Mycophenolate mofetil after methotrexate failure or intolerance in the treatment of scleritis and uveitis. Ophthalmology. 2008;115(8):1416–1421, 1421.e1411.
93. Kempen JH, Daniel E, Dunn JP, et al. Overall and cancer related mortality among patients with ocular inflammation treated with immunosuppressive drugs: retrospective cohort study. BMJ (Clinical research ed). 2009;339:b2480.

94. Bentley R. Mycophenolic acid: a one hundred year odyssey from antibiotic to immunosuppressant. Chem Rev. 2000;100(10):3801–26.
95. Doycheva D, Jagle H, Zierhut M, et al. Mycophenolic acid in the treatment of birdshot chorioretinopathy: long-term follow-up. Br J Ophthalmol. 2015;99(1):87–91.
96. Zacharias LC, Damico FM, Kenney MC, et al. In vitro evidence for mycophenolic acid dose-related cytotoxicity in human retinal cells. Retina (Philadelphia, Pa). 2013;33(10):2155–61.
97. Franklin JL, Rosenberg HH. Impaired folic acid absorption in inflammatory bowel disease: effects of salicylazosulfapyridine (Azulfidine). Gastroenterology. 1973;64(4):517–25.
98. Selhub J, Dhar GJ, Rosenberg IH. Inhibition of folate enzymes by sulfasalazine. J Clin Invest. 1978;61(1):221–4.
99. Baum CL, Selhub J, Rosenberg IH. Antifolate actions of sulfasalazine on intact lymphocytes. J Lab Clin Med. 1981;97(6):779–84.
100. Rhodes JM, Jewell DP. Motility of neutrophils and monocytes in Crohn's disease and ulcerative colitis. Gut. 1983;24(1):73–7.
101. Benitez-Del-Castillo JM, Garcia-Sanchez J, Iradier T, Banares A. Sulfasalazine in the prevention of anterior uveitis associated with ankylosing spondylitis. Eye (Lond). 2000;14(Pt 3A):340–3.
102. Munoz-Fernandez S, Hidalgo V, Fernandez-Melon J, et al. Sulfasalazine reduces the number of flares of acute anterior uveitis over a one-year period. J Rheumatol. 2003;30(6):1277–9.
103. Huang JL, Hung IJ, Hsieh KH. Sulphasalazine therapy in chronic uveitis of children with chronic arthritis. Asian Pac J Allergy Immunol. 1997;15(2):71–5.
104. Dev S, McCallum RM, Jaffe GJ. Methotrexate treatment for sarcoid-associated panuveitis. Ophthalmology. 1999;106(1):111–8.
105. Rathinam SR, Babu M, Thundikandy R, et al. A randomized clinical trial comparing methotrexate and mycophenolate mofetil for noninfectious uveitis. Ophthalmology. 2014;121(10):1863–70.
106. Kaklamani VG, Kaklamanis PG. Treatment of Behcet's disease – an update. Semin Arthritis Rheum. 2001;30(5):299–312.
107. Arcinue CA, Radwan A, Lebanan MO, Foster CS. Comparison of two different combination immunosuppressive therapies in the treatment of Vogt-Koyonagi-Harada syndrome. Ocul Immunol Inflamm. 2013;21(1):47–52.
108. Silman AJ, Petrie J, Hazleman B, Evans SJ. Lymphoproliferative cancer and other malignancy in patients with rheumatoid arthritis treated with azathioprine: a 20 year follow up study. Ann Rheum Dis. 1988;47(12):988–92.
109. Penn I. Cancers complicating organ transplantation. N Engl J Med. 1990;323(25):1767–9.

Suggested Reading

Antirheumatic therapy: actions and outcomes. In: Day RO, Furst DE, van Riel PLCM, Bresnihan B, editors. Progress in inflammation research. ISBN 3-7643-6595-1. Basel/Boston/Berlin: Birhäuser Verlag. UCSF ID RM 405 A64; 2005.

Cronstein BN, Bertino JR, editors. Milestones in Drug Therapy. Methotrexate. Basel/Boston/Berlin: Birkhäuser Verlag; 2000. RM 666 M52 M48 2000.

Rainsford KD, editor. CRC anti-inflammatory and antirheumatic drugs volume III. Boca Raton: CRC Press; 1985. 33431. RM405 A58 1985.

T Cell Inhibitors

5

Russell W. Read

Pearls

- T cell inhibitors can be effective therapy to treat noninfectious uveitis, but, due to potential side effects, are commonly used at slightly lower doses as adjunctive therapy with other immunosuppressive agents.
- Cyclosporine does not have an effect on primed T cells and, thus, is most likely to be effective given systemically, although some studies show promise when given through a local route as well.
- Tacrolimus appears to be a useful agent for the treatment of uveitis with at least equal efficacy to cyclosporine with a more favorable side effect profile.

Introduction

Uveitis is not a single disease, but rather encompasses an entire category of diseases, the common thread of which is an inflammatory attack on the inner eye. New-onset disease occurs in approximately 52 of each 100,000 individuals in the United States per year with a prevalence of 112 per 100,00 at any one time [1]. Uveitis is a major cause of human visual morbidity [2, 3] and is estimated to be responsible for 5 to 20% of the blindness in the United States [4, 5]. This loss of vision places a large social, physical, and economic burden on the United States and other countries and emphasizes the need for safe effective treatments to reduce the level of inflammation and thus potential complications and visual loss. However, because uveitis is not a single disease, the underlying inflammatory pathophysiology encompasses multiple potential processes, including trauma, infection, and autoimmunity. While at the midpoint of the last century the vast majority of uveitis cases were assumed to be of an infectious etiology such as syphilis or tuberculosis [6], at present greater than 85% of cases are assumed to be autoimmune in nature [7]. It is in the situation of autoimmune uveitis – and therefore the majority of cases –that T cell inhibitors may have utility.

Rationale for Use in Autoimmune Uveitis

There is abundant evidence – both from experimental models and clinical studies – that T cells are involved and important in the autoimmune form of uveitis. While a comprehensive review of

R. W. Read (✉)
Uveitis and Ocular Inflammatory Diseases Service, Department of Ophthalmology and Visual Sciences, University of Alabama at Birmingham, Birmingham, AL, USA
e-mail: rread@uabmc.edu

P. Lin, E. Suhler (eds.), *Treatment of Non-infectious Uveitis*,
https://doi.org/10.1007/978-3-030-22827-9_5

the immunologic mechanisms underlying autoimmune uveitis and the intricate role therein of T cells is beyond the scope of this chapter, an understanding of basic adaptive immune responses is helpful to understand why T cell inhibitors are useful in uveitis. For a more complete review, the reader is directed to several excellent papers that cover this topic [8–10]. In brief, phagocytic cells are constantly engulfing material from throughout the body. Following this phagocytosis of antigen, these cells, termed antigen-presenting cells, process the material and travel to draining lymph nodes where the processed antigen is presented in the context of other cell surface molecules to T cells in residence. If the processed antigen is presented to a T cell with a receptor specific to its structure, in concert with appropriate additional signals required, then those antigen-specific T cells are primed and partially activated. It is during this phase that the production and release of the proinflammatory cytokine interleukin (IL)-2 is crucial. Depending in part on the antigen and immunologic environment in which the presentation is made, differing subtypes of T cells result which vary in the profile of cytokines produced and cell surface markers expressed. The primed T cells proliferate in the lymph node and are released into the circulation. As they traffic throughout the body, if they are again presented with their specific antigen in a peripheral location, they become fully activated and orchestrate an immune attack in that tissue. If that tissue is contained within the eye, then uveitis develops. And in fact, various animal models of uveitis have been used to explore these immune processes leading to ocular autoimmune inflammation. The most widely studied model is experimental autoimmune uveitis (EAU), induced with retinal antigens such as S-antigen [11] or interphotoreceptor retinoid-binding protein (IRBP) [12]. Studies in these models have clearly shown the critical role of organ-specific T cell-mediated autoimmunity [7, 13–15]. There is empirical evidence that T cell inhibition is effective in the control of autoimmune uveitis, again both from experimental models and clinical studies [16–26]. In addition, clinical studies have shown the presence of activated T cells in the peripheral circulation [27–29] and intraocular fluids [30] of humans with uveitis. Further, there is evidence of T cell autoimmunity via their reaction ex vivo to uveitis-associated antigen [31]. Based on existing evidence then, inhibition of the processes T cells utilize to mediate uveitis should therefore be viable as a therapeutic intervention.

Specific Agents

The term "T cell inhibitor" potentially encompasses a wide variety of therapeutic agents with disparate mechanisms of action that by definition result in the inhibition of some action of T cells. That multiple mechanisms of action could result in inhibition of T cell function underscores their (and in fact the entire immune system's) physiological complexity and highlights why such agents should not be expected to have universal efficacy in a condition as varied as "uveitis." This chapter shall include within its scope agents traditionally categorized as T cell inhibitors and leave more recent therapeutic agents in the biologics category to other chapters. The traditional T cell inhibitors act on molecules within the T cell cytoplasm. These traditional agents include the calcineurin inhibitors cyclosporine and tacrolimus and the inhibitors of the "mammalian target of rapamycin" or mTOR, sirolimus and everolimus. Details on the specific agents discussed below are summarized in Table 5.1.

Calcineurin Inhibitors

Calcineurin is a phosphatase that, in the setting of increased cytoplasmic calcium induced by engagement of the T cell receptor with antigen, dephosphorylates – and thus activates – the T cell-specific transcription factor *nuclear factor of activated T cells* (NF-AT) [32]. Dephosphorylated NF-AT enters the T cell nucleus and participates in the regulation of multiple cytokines, primarily among these IL-2 (Fig. 5.1), which as described above is crucial for the priming and activation of T cells after exposure to their specific antigen in the lymph node. But in addition to IL-2, NF-AT

Table 5.1 T cell inhibitors in clinical use

Agent	Baseline evaluation	Dosage range	Monitoring	Side effects
Cyclosporine	Serum creatinine, BUN, CBC, serum magnesium, potassium, uric acid, lipids, screening for latent tuberculosis	Orally 2.5–5 mg/kg/day divided into two doses	Serum creatinine, BUN, blood pressure, CBC, uric acid, potassium, lipids, and magnesium every 2 weeks during the first 3 months of therapy and then monthly if stable	Nephrotoxicity, hypertension, hyperglycemia, liver dysfunction, hyperkalemia, altered mental status, seizures, hirsutism, lymphoma, skin cancers, progressive multifocal leukoencephalopathy, seizures, posterior reversible encephalopathy syndrome
Tacrolimus	Same as for cyclosporine	Orally 0.03–0.08 mg/kg/day divided into two doses	Same as for cyclosporine	Nephrotoxicity, neurotoxicity, hyperglycemia, hypertension, hyperkalemia, and gastrointestinal complaints
Sirolimus	Same as for cyclosporine	Oral loading dose of 6 mg followed by 1–4 mg once daily consistently with or without food	Drug trough levels, otherwise same as for cyclosporine	Myelosuppression (especially thrombocytopenia), hepatotoxicity, diarrhea, hypertriglyceridemia, pneumonitis, hemolytic-uremic syndrome, and headache. Renal toxicity is less common
Everolimus	Same as for cyclosporine	Orally 0.75 mg two times per day, adjusted to obtain trough serum levels of 3–8 ng/ml (total daily dosage of 2.5 mg)	Drug trough levels, otherwise same as for cyclosporine	As a derivative, side effects are similar to sirolimus

also regulates IL-4, interferon gamma, and tumor necrosis factor alpha [33], all cytokines that are also involved in uveitis [34–36]. The inhibition of calcineurin-mediated dephosphorylation of NF-AT therefore inhibits the activation of NF-AT, decreasing the activation of T cells and production of proinflammatory cytokines. It has been increasingly realized that, in addition to its effect on T cells, NF-AT is also involved in innate immunity, acting on myeloid cells, including granulocytes and dendritic cells, promoting inflammation, regulating adaptive immunity, and affecting these mediators of early immune responses [37]. Therefore, inhibition of calcineurin appears to influence both innate and adaptive immune responses to produce an immunosuppressive effect.

Cyclosporine A

Cyclosporine (cyclosporin A, CSA) is a lipophilic cyclic polypeptide isolated from the fungus *Beauveria nivea* [38]. Cyclosporine achieves its immunosuppressive effects by complexing with the cytoplasmic protein cyclophilin-1. The resulting cyclosporine-cyclophilin complex inhibits calcineurin, the function of which is described above. This inhibits T cell activation by interfering at an early stage in antigen receptor-induced differentiation. As suggested above, studies in vitro have shown that cyclosporine inhibits gene transcription of not only IL-2 but also other factors produced by antigen-stimulated T cells [33]. It is important to note that cyclosporine does not have an effect on these cytokines in already primed T cells nor does it block interaction with antigen. This mechanism of action would be therefore expected to limit the effectiveness of cyclosporine to that achieved by actions on T cells in the periphery that have yet to be primed and therefore only achievable by systemic administration. However, there have been efforts to use cyclosporine locally in order to reduce systemic side effects (discussed later). He and colleagues showed that microspheres

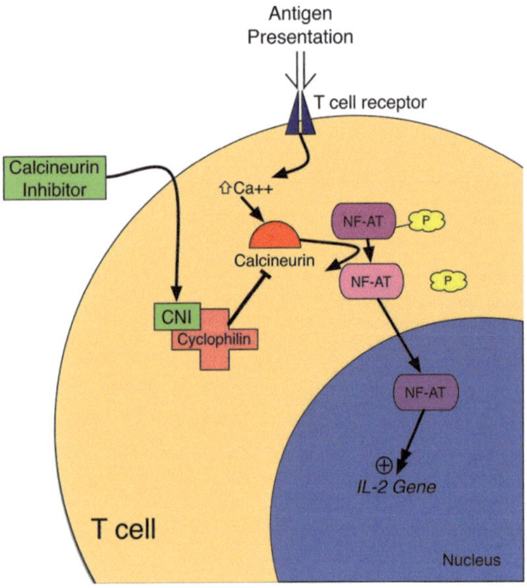

Fig. 5.1 Mechanism of action of calcineurin inhibitors. T cell engagement with processed antigen results in an increase in intracellular calcium which stimulates calcineurin via calmodulin. Calcineurin dephosphorylates the transcription factor nuclear factor of activated T cells (NF-AT) which then translocates to the nucleus and activates target genes, especially interleukin (IL)-2, resulting in the priming and activation of previously naive T cells. Calcineurin inhibitors function by binding to a cytoplasmic protein, either cyclophilin (illustrated here) or FK-binding protein, collectively termed immunophilins. The drug-immunophilin complex blocks the phosphatase activity of calcineurin so that NF-AT is not dephosphorylated and downstream activation of proinflammatory genes is inhibited. This inhibition prevents the production of IL-2 and IL-2 receptors by T cells and thus inhibits priming and proliferation of antigen-specific T cells

loaded with cyclosporine could be safely and effectively delivered intravitreally [39]. Others have used intravitreal cyclosporine implants in animal models and equine uveitis, showing a reduction in uveitis severity [40–44]. It is possible that the effectiveness of locally administered cyclosporine is carried out via the agent's effects on non-T cell innate inflammatory cells, as described in the calcineurin inhibitor section above, or it is also possible that there are yet to be understood effects of calcineurin inhibition on already primed and activated T cells acting in the periphery that modulate their proinflammatory activity. Despite this possibility, a recent literature search shows no reports on the use of intravitreal cyclosporine in human uveitis. A topical form of cyclosporine is commercially available as a 0.05% concentration and has been studied in anterior uveitis. Prabhu and coworkers found that cyclosporine 0.05% instituted during a flare-up of acute recurrent anterior uveitis concurrent with traditional treatment with corticosteroids reduced the frequency and duration of subsequent flare-ups following discontinuation of the traditional agent [45]. However, the study is limited by a small number of patients, retrospective nature, and possible regression to the mean as an explanation for reduced flares. The frequency of administration of cyclosporine 0.05% was not detailed. A study of topical cyclosporine in experimental uveitis using a different formulation than what is commercially available suggested effectiveness in anterior uveitis but not posterior disease [46].

Based on the above data, cyclosporine is typically used in uveitis as an oral agent, though it is available as an intravenous formulation as well. Orally, it is slowly, erratically, and incompletely absorbed with large variations in bioavailability between individuals. Complicating this further, there are multiple formulations of cyclosporine, each with a different bioavailability, therefore caution must be exercised if a switch from one formulation to another is required. The microemulsion formulation improves consistency and bioavailability, and unless other considerations overrule, it should probably be the default formulation used and the brand name agent specified, as even the same formulation from different generic drug manufacturers could have different bioavailabilities.

The clinical usefulness of cyclosporine has been limited by its toxicities, which are numerous and include nephrotoxicity, hypertension, hyperglycemia, liver dysfunction, hyperkalemia, altered mental status, seizures, and hirsutism [47]. Lymphoma and other malignancies (especially skin cancers) have been observed at a higher rate in transplant recipients receiving cyclosporine. Patients should be cautioned regarding ultraviolet light exposure while on cyclosporine. A particularly devastating complication of cyclosporine (as well as other immunosuppressive regimens) is the development of progressive multifocal leukoencephalopathy due to JC virus infection that may have serious outcomes. In addition, neurologic toxicity in the form of seizures and posterior reversible encephalopathy syndrome (PRES) has been described both in post-marketing reports and in the literature [47, 48]. Manifestations of PRES can include impaired consciousness, convulsions, visual disturbances (including blindness), loss of motor function, movement disorders, and psychiatric disturbances. White matter changes have been detected on neuroimaging. The condition has typically been reversible upon discontinuation of cyclosporine [47].

Initial publications on cyclosporine in uveitis used up to 10 mg/kg/day, which produced a significantly higher rate of these adverse effects [18]. Currently, typical starting dosages are 2.5–5 mg/kg/day divided into two doses (1.25–2.5 mg/kg per dose) [49]. Cyclosporine use in uveitis is off-label. For rheumatoid arthritis, the manufacturer recommends an initial dose of cyclosporine microemulsion of 2.5 mg/kg/day total, divided into two daily doses. If tolerated (including serum creatinine less than 30% above baseline) but with a need for additional immunosuppression, the dose may be increased by 0.5–0.75 mg/kg/day after 8 weeks and again after 12 weeks to a maximum of 4 mg/kg/day. Again per the manufacturer for rheumatoid arthritis, if no benefit is seen by 16 weeks, therapy should be discontinued. These recommendations seem reasonable for uveitis as well. Prior to therapy initiation, baseline evaluations should include serum creatinine, BUN, CBC, serum magnesium, potassium, uric acid, and lipids. Screening for latent tuberculosis should be included as well. Once therapy is begun, the manufacturer recommends monitoring of serum creatinine, BUN, blood pressure, CBC, uric acid, potassium, lipids, and magnesium every 2 weeks during the first 3 months of therapy and then monthly if stable. A rise of creatinine 25% above the pretreatment level should prompt retesting within 2 weeks with a dose reduction of 25%–50% if it remains persistently elevated. A single increase of 50% above pretreatment level should prompt an immediate 25%–50% dose reduction. If a return of serum creatinine to within 25% of baseline is not achieved after two dose modifications, then the drug should be discontinued. Persistent hypertension should prompt dosage reductions in a similar manner as with serum creatinine monitoring. The importance of regular and careful monitoring of cyclosporine effects on renal function cannot be overemphasized. The risk of nephrotoxicity increases with higher doses and with prolonged therapy and may result in permanent structural kidney damage and persistent renal dysfunction [47].

The absorbed drug is primarily metabolized by the cytochrome P450 3A enzyme system in the liver resulting in the possibility of multiple drug interactions [50]. Agents that increase cyclosporine levels through competition for metabolism include antifungal azoles (ketoconazole, voriconazole, itraconazole, osaconazole, fluconazole, clotrimazole), protease inhibitors (except tipranavir), macrolide antibiotics (erythromycin and clarithromycin, but not azithromycin), calcium channel blockers (diltiazem, verapamil, and nicardipine but not nifedipine or amlodipine), and grapefruit juice [51, 52]. Conversely, agents that activate the cytochrome P450 system and therefore decrease cyclosporine levels include rifampin, anti-seizure medications (carbamazepine, phenobarbital, and phenytoin), and St. John's wort [51, 52]. If patients are on these agents concurrently, then careful attention to drug levels and toxicity and careful counseling to avoid sudden changes in dosages are needed. Grapefruit juice, for example, may increase cyclosporine bioavailability by as much as 62% [50]. Because of these factors, cyclosporine dosing must be individualized. In addition to the monitoring of renal function, blood pressure, and electrolytes outlined previously, routine monitoring of trough blood levels is common in cyclosporine's use post transplantation [47, 53–55]. It has been suggested that monitoring of trough levels is useful in uveitis patients as well [56]. Trough levels obtained just before the morning dose (T0) are desired to be between 125 and 225 ng/ml, as measured by a monoclonal-specific radioimmunoassay [56]. A study in uveitis patients of the utility of monitoring trough levels

6 hours (T6) after the morning dose with cyclosporine dose adjustments to achieve a T6 level of 150–250 ng/ml showed that using this protocol, eight of eight patients with chronic, bilateral, severe, noninfectious uveitis (two idiopathic panuveitis, two idiopathic retinal vasculitis, two multifocal choroiditis, one HLA-B27-related uveitis, and one Behcet disease) improved clinically. The mean dose of cyclosporine was 3.9 ± 1.4 mg/kg/day. The initial and final serum creatinine, potassium, magnesium, and uric acid serum levels and systolic/diastolic blood pressure measurements were not statistically different, and there was no change in the creatinine clearance, glomerular filtration rate, or the effective renal plasma flow performed before starting T6 monitoring and at 13 ± 8 months of follow-up [56].

Keeping all the above in mind, cyclosporine may be used safely and effectively in the treatment of uveitis. Cyclosporine may be used alone or in combination with other immunosuppressants. A number of studies, both prospective and retrospective, have been conducted on the use of cyclosporine in uveitis, mostly Behcet disease, Vogt-Koyanagi-Harada disease, and serpiginous choroidopathy [19, 57–62]. Dosages used vary by the era in which the study was conducted, with earlier studies using much higher doses than more recent studies. Overall, the recommendations given above for dosage and monitoring are the same regardless of the uveitic syndrome one is treating. As with all immunosuppressives, cyclosporine is not universally effective. A recent paper reported that in 59 patients with widely varying uveitic syndromes, the most common being Behcet in 32%, treated with cyclosporine at a mean starting dose of 4.2 mg/kg/day and a mean maintenance dose of 3.2 mg/kg/day, cyclosporine was judged effective in 85% and oral steroid dosage was reduced in 73% (by half or more in 51%). However, adverse effects were almost universal, including peripheral paresthesias in 70%, fatigue in 67%, systemic hypertension in 27%, and elevated serum creatinine leading to dose reduction in 30%. Cyclosporine needed to be discontinued in 35%, being intolerable in 20% and ineffective in 15% [63].

In summary, cyclosporine is a reasonably effective immunosuppressive in the treatment of noninfectious uveitis. Treatment should be avoided in patients with preexisting kidney disease or poorly controlled hypertension. Initial starting doses should be low (~2.5 mg/kg/day) and careful monitoring for adverse effects must be carried out.

Tacrolimus

Tacrolimus (FK 506) is a macrolide antibiotic with immunosuppressant activity produced by *Streptomyces tsukubaensis*. The mechanism of action of tacrolimus is very similar to cyclosporine, despite not being chemically related. Tacrolimus binds to the immunophilin FK-binding protein (FKBP) rather than cyclophilin, which is the target of cyclosporine. The tacrolimus-FKBP complex inhibits calcineurin just as cyclosporine-cyclophilin does, resulting in the same effects on NF-AT. Tacrolimus is 10–100 times more potent than cyclosporine in inhibiting immune responses [64].

Tacrolimus can be administered orally or intravenously and is metabolized primarily by cytochrome P450 enzymes in the liver, resulting in the potential for drug interactions just as with cyclosporine, and therefore these will not be detailed again. The toxic effects of tacrolimus are also similar to those of cyclosporine, including nephrotoxicity, neurotoxicity, hyperglycemia, hypertension, hyperkalemia, and gastrointestinal complaints, and, again, will not be detailed.

Tacrolimus has been shown to be effective in experimental uveitis [65–70]. Clinical studies in uveitis have also demonstrated its efficacy [71–75]. Murphy and colleagues [76] performed a randomized prospective unmasked trial of tacrolimus versus cyclosporine in 37 patients with noninfectious uveitis requiring second-line immunosuppression. Patients received either tacrolimus (0.03–0.08 mg/kg daily) or cyclosporine (2.5–5.0 mg/kg daily) with doses adjusted based on clinical response and blood drug levels. Target whole blood trough levels were 8–12 ng/L for tacrolimus and 100–225 ng/L for cyclosporine, although the protocol allowed trough levels below these ranges if the uveitis was under control. Diagnoses included a variety of conditions, including idiopathic disease, Behcet disease, sarcoidosis, sympathetic ophthalmia, and choroidal inflammations. Approximately two thirds of patients in each group responded to treatment. A significantly higher number of cyclosporine-treated patients experienced adverse effects compared to tacrolimus-treated patients. One third of patients on tacrolimus had no adverse effects, while only 6% (1 patient) in the cyclosporine group had no adverse effects. Perhaps most significantly, it appeared that equal effectiveness could be achieved with a dose of tacrolimus than was used in the study. Since calcineurin inhibitor toxicity is dose dependent, tacrolimus appears to have a superior therapeutic index compared to cyclosporine [76].

In summary, tacrolimus appears to be a useful agent for the treatment of uveitis with at least equal efficacy to cyclosporine with a more favorable side effect profile. Patients can be started at doses ranging from 0.03 to 0.08 mg/kg daily (divided into two doses). Other than dosage, which is significantly lower for tacrolimus compared to cyclosporine due to tacrolimus' greater potency, the monitoring requirements, drug interactions, and cautions for tacrolimus do not differ from those of cyclosporine, and the reader should review that section of this chapter.

Molecular Target of Rapamycin Inhibitors

Sirolimus (rapamycin) and its metabolite everolimus constitute a different group of immunosuppressives from the calcineurin inhibitors but which still have T cell inhibitor effects. Their mechanism of action differs in that they bind the circulating immunophilin FK506-binding protein 12, the resulting complex then blocking the "molecular target of rapamycin" (mTOR). mTOR is a key component of a complex intracellular signaling pathway involved in cellular processes such as cell growth and proliferation, angiogenesis, and metabolism. Thus, blockade of mTOR leads to inhibition of interleukin-driven T cell proliferation. mTOR inhibitors may also inhibit B cell proliferation and immunoglobulin production [50]. Toxicities of the mTOR inhibitors can include profound myelosuppression (especially thrombocytopenia), hepatotoxicity, diarrhea, hypertriglyceridemia, pneumonitis, and headache. Renal toxicity is less common with mTOR inhibitors, but there appears to be an increased incidence of hemolytic-uremic syndrome. The mTOR inhibitors are metabolized by the cytochrome P450 3A4 system as with the calcineurin inhibitors; thus the same caveats and monitoring parameters exist, as detailed previously.

Sirolimus

Sirolimus (also known as rapamycin) is a macrocyclic lactone produced by *Streptomyces hygroscopicus* [77]. Sirolimus suppresses cytokine-driven (IL-2, IL-4, and IL-15) T cell proliferation, inhibiting the progression from the G1 to the S phase of the cell cycle. Sirolimus also inhibits antibody production. Sirolimus suppresses immune-mediated events associated with a number of experimental models, including systemic lupus erythematosus, collagen-induced arthritis, autoimmune type I diabetes, autoimmune myocarditis, experimental allergic encephalomyelitis, graft-versus-host disease, and, most pertinent to the current text, autoimmune uveoretinitis [77–79], as well as in patients with uveitis [80]. This appears to be dose related, as another group found that while sirolimus at high doses reduced the severity of experimental autoimmune uveitis, low doses actually caused an exacerbation of disease severity [81]. Thus, dosing in the use of sirolimus may be critical to achieve the desired effect of uveitis control while avoiding paradoxical worsening of disease and also to avoid any dose-related adverse side effects. In addition to its anti-inflammatory actions, sirolimus has been shown to have antiangiogenic actions in murine models of choroidal neovascularization and retinal hypoxia [82].

Sirolimus is commercially available as an oral drug. It is rapidly but incompletely absorbed, and elimination is similar to that of cyclosporine and tacrolimus, being a substrate for both cytochrome P450 3A and P-glycoprotein with the attendant risk of significant drug and food interactions. Details of these risks are reviewed in the preceding sections. For organ transplant rejection prevention, it is administered once daily consistently either with or without food. Loading doses are common but not standardized for use in uveitis. Monitoring of blood trough levels is recommended by the manufacturer when used in transplant rejection prevention, but whether these levels are appropriate for monitoring in uveitis is unknown [77].

In uveitis, sirolimus has been used both systemically and locally. Shanmuganathan and colleagues [83] performed an open-label study in eight patients with noninfectious uveitis not controlled with at least two immunosuppresants. Dosing of sirolimus consisted of a loading dose of 6 mg followed by initially 2 mg per day (but increased to 4 mg per day initial dose later in the study due to a slower than desired achievement of desired drug levels) with escalation based on drug trough levels, though the authors did not state what their target trough level was. Five of the eight (63%) patients were considered to be successes. Those patients that had adverse effects did so at high blood trough levels (> 25 ng/ml) emphasizing again the need for dose optimization. Phillips and Wroblewski [84] looked retrospectively at eight patients treated with sirolimus at doses between 1 and 4 mg per day and found half had successful control of disease, but in three of those four only in combination with methotrexate. Nussenblatt et al. [85] reported a single case of punctate inner choroidopathy complicated by choroidal neovascularization successfully treated with sirolimus with minimal adverse effects (only a slight rise in serum cholesterol). This case highlights the antiangiogenic properties of sirolimus. Because of a relatively high rate of systemic side effects, sirolimus has been studied as a locally administered agent in uveitis as well, using both subconjunctival and intravitreal routes of administration. Douglas and coworkers [86] found no evidence of ocular toxicity in normal horses after subconjunctival or intravitreal injections of sirolimus. Sen et al. [87] performed a prospective nonrandomized open-label pilot study of subconjunctival sirolimus in chronic anterior uveitis. Five patients received a single subconjunctival injection of 1320 μg of sirolimus. Three of the five showed at least a two-step decrease in disease activity scoring, and the other two showed a one-step decrease, all without serious adverse events. Mudumba and colleagues [88] studied a single intravitreal injection of sirolimus in rabbits and humans and found good tolerability with only "minor" lenticular changes. Nguyen and coworkers [89] performed a prospective, randomized, open-label study of sirolimus subconjunctival and intravitreal administration. They found both routes to be well tolerated and showed moderate efficacy in reducing vitreous flare measurements. The same group [90] reported 1 year data from the study. They found continued tolerance to the local injections (both subconjunctival and intravitreal). A reduction in vitreous haze of two steps or more was found in 70% of patients who had active uveitis at study onset, and 88% of patients with inactive disease at study onset did not demonstrate worsening. No statistical differences were found in efficacy between the two routes at the 1 year time point. These formulations are not commercially available and studies are ongoing. A phase 3 randomized controlled trial comparing two doses of intravitreal sirolimus (440 μg and 880 μg) to an active control (44 μg) published in December 2016 demonstrated that only the low dose (440 μg) met the primary endpoint of vitreous haze 0 at 5 months after 3 injections. Best corrected visual acuity did not significantly improve compared to the control group, although there was a mean gain of 10.5 letters at 5 months in the 440 μg group in a post hoc analysis of patients with baseline <20/100 visual acuity. Elevated intraocular pressure occurred at a rate of 16.1%, and cataracts occurred at a rate of 6.3% in the 440 μg sirolimus group [91].

In summary, sirolimus shows efficacy in the treatment of noninfectious uveitis both systemically and by local delivery. Systemic use may have a tighter therapeutic index than desired, and if additional clinical trials end up successful, local delivery may be a superior approach with good efficacy.

Everolimus

Everolimus is a derivative of sirolimus and few studies of everolimus in uveitis exist. Hennig and colleagues [92] tested the efficacy and immunological effects of everolimus on experimental autoimmune uveoretinitis (EAU) in B10. RIII mice. Everolimus was administered orally at 5 mg/kg/d either 2 days before or 14 days after EAU induction. Histopathologically graded uveitis scores were significantly reduced compared to sham-treated mice. Delayed-type hypersensitivity, humoral immune responses, proliferation of splenocytes, and intraocular levels of Th1, Th2, and Th17 cytokines were impaired after everolimus treatment. Heiligenhaus and coworkers [93] then performed a prospective, open-label, nonrandomized, phase II pilot study of everolimus in 12 patients. These patients with noninfectious anterior and intermediate uveitis, or panuveitis, had been under at least 3 months of treatment with a combination of topical and systemic corticosteroids and cyclosporine and still had active disease. Patients were treated with oral everolimus 0.75 mg two times per day, adjusted from week 1 to obtain trough serum levels in the range of 3–8 ng/ml, reaching total daily dosages of up to 2.5 mg. Corticosteroids and cyclosporine were continued until quiescence was achieved, and then each was tapered per a standardized protocol. At month 3 following the addition of everolimus, uveitis was inactive in all patients. By 12 months, uveitis had recurred in four patients after tapering or withdrawing cyclosporine. The authors report that it was possible to achieve a 50% reduction in the dose of systemic corticosteroid or cyclosporine. After withdrawing everolimus at the prescribed time point of 12 months, uveitis recurred in 50% within 1 month. No serious adverse effects were reported.

In summary, everolimus, as a metabolite of sirolimus, would logically have similar efficacy to its parent compound. No studies are in publication regarding the use of everolimus in uveitis either as sole therapy or in combination with only corticosteroids; thus it is difficult at this point to determine where in the uveitis treatment paradigm everolimus should fall, but it appears to be moderately effective as an adjunct to ongoing cyclosporine therapy.

Conclusions

The T cell has been shown by decades of research to be one of the key drivers of autoimmune uveitis. Multiple agents that interfere with T cell functions exist, but all are hampered by significant drug and food interactions that must be considered when adding these agents to a preexisting medication regimen. Systemic administration has shown moderate effectiveness in control of uveitic disease. Local delivery has been explored for the oldest member of the family, cyclosporine, but has not resulted in commercially available formulations for local use. Sirolimus is currently under study as a locally administered therapy and may increase the utility of this therapeutic class in uveitis.

References

1. Gritz DC, Wong IG. Incidence and prevalence of uveitis in Northern California; the Northern California Epidemiology of Uveitis Study. Ophthalmology. 2004;111(3):491–500; discussion.
2. Henderly DE, Genstler AJ, Smith RE, Rao NA. Changing patterns of uveitis. Am J Ophthalmol. 1987;103(2):131–6.
3. National Advisory Eye Council. Vision research, a national plan: 1999–2003. Bethesda: National Eye Institute; 1998. p. 98–4120.
4. Research to Prevent Blindness. Glossary of common eye diseases: uveitis [Internet]. Research to Prevent Blindness, Inc. Available from: http://www.rpbusa.org/hc2/commondisorders.asp.
5. Durrani OM, Meads CA, Murray PI. Uveitis: a potentially blinding disease. Ophthalmologica. 2004;218(4):223–36.
6. Guyton JS, Woods AC. Etiology of uveitis: a clinical study of 562 cases. Arch Ophthalmol. 1941;26:983–1018.
7. Gery I, Nussenblatt RB. Immunologic basis of uveitis. In: Pepose JS, Holland GN, Wilhelmus KR, editors. Ocular infection & immunity. St. Louis: Mosby; 1996. p. 141–56.
8. Caspi RR. A look at autoimmunity and inflammation in the eye. J Clin Invest. 2010;120(9):3073–83.
9. Caspi R. Mechanisms underlying autoimmune uveitis. Drug Discovery Today Dis Mech. 2006;3(2):199–206.

10. Dick AD. Experimental approaches to specific immunotherapies in autoimmune disease: future treatment of endogenous posterior uveitis? Br J Ophthalmol. 1995;79(1):81–8.
11. Caspi RR, Roberge FG, Chan CC, Wiggert B, Chader GJ, Rozenszajn LA, et al. A new model of autoimmune disease. Experimental autoimmune uveoretinitis induced in mice with two different retinal antigens. J Immunol. 1988;140(5):1490–5.
12. Avichezer D, Silver PB, Chan CC, Wiggert B, Caspi RR. Identification of a new epitope of human IRBP that induces autoimmune uveoretinitis in mice of the H-2b haplotype. Invest Ophthalmol Vis Sci. 2000;41(1):127–31.
13. Prendergast RA, Iliff CE, Coskuncan NM, Caspi RR, Sartani G, Tarrant TK, et al. T cell traffic and the inflammatory response in experimental autoimmune uveoretinitis. Invest Ophthalmol Vis Sci. 1998;39(5):754–62.
14. Caspi RR, Roberge FG, McAllister CG, el-Saied M, Kuwabara T, Gery I, et al. T cell lines mediating experimental autoimmune uveoretinitis (EAU) in the rat. J Immunol. 1986;136(3):928–33.
15. Mochizuki M, Kuwabara T, McAllister C, Nussenblatt RB, Gery I. Adoptive transfer of experimental autoimmune uveoretinitis in rats. Immunopathogenic mechanisms and histologic features. Invest Ophthalmol Vis Sci. 1985;26(1):1–9.
16. Nussenblatt RB, Rodrigues MM, Wacker WB, Cevario SJ, Salinas-Carmona MC, Gery I. Cyclosporin a. Inhibition of experimental autoimmune uveitis in Lewis rats. J Clin Invest. 1981;67(4):1228–31.
17. Nussenblatt RB, Rodrigues MM, Salinas-Carmona MC, Gery I, Cevario S, Wacker W. Modulation of experimental autoimmune uveitis with cyclosporin A. Arch Ophthalmol. 1982;100(7):1146–9.
18. Nussenblatt RB, Palestine AG, Chan CC. Cyclosporin A therapy in the treatment of intraocular inflammatory disease resistant to systemic corticosteroids and cytotoxic agents. Am J Ophthalmol. 1983;96(3):275–82.
19. Nussenblatt RB, Palestine AG, Rook AH, Scher I, Wacker WB, Gery I. Treatment of intraocular inflammatory disease with cyclosporin A. Lancet. 1983;2(8344):235–8.
20. Nussenblatt RB, Salinas-Carmona M, Waksman BH, Gery I. Cyclosporin A: alterations of the cellular immune response in S-antigen-induced experimental autoimmune uveitis. Int Arch Allergy Appl Immunol. 1983;70(4):289–94.
21. Graham EM, Sanders MD, James DG, Hamblin A, Kasp Grochowska E, Dumonde D. Cyclosporin A in the treatment of posterior uveitis. Trans Ophthalmol Soc U K. 1985;104(Pt 2):146–51.
22. Le Hoang P, Fontaine M, Khalaf A, Travers C, Saraux H, Coscas G, et al. Treatment of noninfectious posterior uveitis with a new immunomodulator, cyclosporin A: initial results. Bull Soc Ophtalmol Fr. 1985;85(8–9):873–6.
23. Nussenblatt RB, Dinning WJ, Fujikawa LS, Chan CC, Palestine AG. Local cyclosporine therapy for experimental autoimmune uveitis in rats. Arch Ophthalmol. 1985;103(10):1559–62.
24. Nussenblatt RB, Palestine AG, Chan CC. Cyclosporine therapy for uveitis: long-term followup. J Ocul Pharmacol. 1985;1(4):369–82.
25. Nussenblatt RB, Palestine AG, Chan CC. Proposed immune mechanisms in uveitis and their modulation. Int Ophthalmol Clin. 1985;25(2):81–93.
26. Nussenblatt RB, Scher I. Effects of cyclosporine on T-cell subsets in experimental autoimmune uveitis. Invest Ophthalmol Vis Sci. 1985;26(1):10–4.
27. Deschenes J, Char DH, Kaleta S. Activated T lymphocytes in uveitis. Br J Ophthalmol. 1988;72(2):83–7.
28. Dick AD, Cheng YF, Purdie AT, Liversidge J, Forrester JV. Immunocytochemical analysis of blood lymphocytes in uveitis. Eye (Lond). 1992;6 (. Pt 6:643–7.
29. Feron EJ, Calder VL, Lightman SL. Distribution of IL-2R and CD45Ro expression on CD4+ and CD8+ T-lymphocytes in the peripheral blood of patients with posterior uveitis. Curr Eye Res. 1992;11 Suppl:167–72.
30. Liversidge J, Dick A, Cheng YF, Scott GB, Forrester JV. Retinal antigen specific lymphocytes, TCR-gamma delta T cells and CD5+ B cells cultured from the vitreous in acute sympathetic ophthalmitis. Autoimmunity. 1993;15(4):257–66.
31. de Smet MD, Yamamoto JH, Mochizuki M, Gery I, Singh VK, Shinohara T, et al. Cellular immune responses of patients with uveitis to retinal antigens and their fragments. Am J Ophthalmol. 1990;110(2):135–42.
32. Guaguere E, Steffan J, Olivry T. Cyclosporin A: a new drug in the field of canine dermatology. Vet Dermatol. 2004;15(2):61–74.
33. Taylor AL, Watson CJ, Bradley JA. Immunosuppressive agents in solid organ transplantation: Mechanisms of action and therapeutic efficacy. Crit Rev Oncol Hematol. 2005;56(1):23–46.
34. Chen W, Zhao B, Jiang R, Zhang R, Wang Y, Wu H, et al. Cytokine expression profile in aqueous humor and sera of patients with acute anterior uveitis. Curr Mol Med. 2015;15(6):543–9.
35. Zhao R, Zhou H, Su SB. A critical role for interleukin-1beta in the progression of autoimmune diseases. Int Immunopharmacol. 2013;17(3):658–69.
36. Horai R, Caspi RR. Cytokines in autoimmune uveitis. J Interf Cytokine Res. 2011;31(10):733–44.
37. Fric J, Zelante T, Wong AY, Mertes A, Yu HB, Ricciardi-Castagnoli P. NFAT control of innate immunity. Blood. 2012;120(7):1380–9.
38. Forsythe P, Paterson S. Ciclosporin 10 years on: indications and efficacy. Vet Rec. 2014;174(Suppl 2):13–21.
39. He Y, Liu Y, Liu Y, Wang J, Zhang X, Lu W, et al. Cyclosporine-loaded microspheres for treatment of uveitis: in vitro characterization and in vivo pharmacokinetic study. Invest Ophthalmol Vis Sci. 2006;47(9):3983–8.
40. Gilger BC, Malok E, Stewart T, Horohov D, Ashton P, Smith T, et al. Effect of an intravitreal cyclospo-

rine implant on experimental uveitis in horses. Vet Immunol Immunopathol. 2000;76(3–4):239–55.
41. Enyedi LB, Pearson PA, Ashton P, Jaffe GJ. An intravitreal device providing sustained release of cyclosporine and dexamethasone. Curr Eye Res. 1996;15(5):549–57.
42. Pearson PA, Jaffe GJ, Martin DF, Cordahi GJ, Grossniklaus H, Schmeisser ET, et al. Evaluation of a delivery system providing long-term release of cyclosporine. Arch Ophthalmol. 1996;114(3):311–7.
43. Jaffe GJ, Yang CS, Wang XC, Cousins SW, Gallemore RP, Ashton P. Intravitreal sustained-release cyclosporine in the treatment of experimental uveitis. Ophthalmology. 1998;105(1):46–56.
44. Gilger BC, Malok E, Stewart T, Ashton P, Smith T, Jaffe GJ, et al. Long-term effect on the equine eye of an intravitreal device used for sustained release of cyclosporine A. Vet Ophthalmol. 2000;3(2–3):105–10.
45. Prabhu SS, Shtein RM, Michelotti MM, Cooney TM. Topical cyclosporine A 0.05% for recurrent anterior uveitis. Br J Ophthalmol. 2016;100(3):345–7.
46. Sasamoto Y, Hirose S, Ohno S, Onoe K, Matsuda H. Topical application of ciclosporin ophthalmic solution containing alpha-cyclodextrin in experimental uveitis. Ophthalmologica. 1991;203(3):118–25.
47. Neoral [package insert]. East Hanover: Novartis Pharmaceuticals Corporation; 2015.
48. Tagami M, Azumi A. Cyclosporine-associated leukoencephalopathy in a case of sympathetic ophthalmitis. Case Rep Ophthalmol. 2016;7(1):61–6.
49. Jabs DA, Rosenbaum JT, Foster CS, Holland GN, Jaffe GJ, Louie JS, et al. Guidelines for the use of immunosuppressive drugs in patients with ocular inflammatory disorders: recommendations of an expert panel. Am J Ophthalmol. 2000;130(4):492–513.
50. Katzung BG, Anthony JT. Basic & clinical pharmacology. 13th ed. New York: McGraw-Hill Education; 2015.
51. Lien YH. Top 10 things primary care physicians should know about maintenance immunosuppression for transplant recipients. Am J Med. 2016;129(6): 568–72.
52. Manitpisitkul W, McCann E, Lee S, Weir MR. Drug interactions in transplant patients: what everyone should know. Curr Opin Nephrol Hypertens. 2009;18(5):404–11.
53. Armstrong AW, Aldredge L, Yamauchi PS. Managing patients with psoriasis in the busy clinic: practical tips for health care practitioners. J Cutan Med Surg. 2016;20(3):196–206.
54. McShane AJ, Bunch DR, Wang S. Therapeutic drug monitoring of immunosuppressants by liquid chromatography-mass spectrometry. Clin Chim Acta. 2016;454:1–5.
55. Mika A, Stepnowski P. Current methods of the analysis of immunosuppressive agents in clinical materials: a review. J Pharm Biomed Anal. 2016;127:207.
56. Rocha G, Deschênes J, Cantarovich M. Cyclosporine monitoring with levels 6 hours after the morning dose in patients with noninfectious uveitis. Ophthalmology. 1997;104(2):245–51.
57. Agarwal M, Ganesh SK, Biswas J. Triple agent immunosuppressive therapy in Vogt-Koyanagi-Harada syndrome. Ocul Immunol Inflamm. 2006;14(6): 333–9.
58. Hooper PL, Kaplan HJ. Triple agent immunosuppression in serpiginous choroiditis. Ophthalmology. 1991;98(6):944–51; discussion 51–2
59. Pascalis L, Pia G, Aresu G, Frongia T, Barca L. Combined cyclosporin A-steroid-MTX treatment in endogenous non-infectious uveitis. J Autoimmun. 1993;6(4):467–80.
60. Nussenblatt RB, Palestine AG, Chan CC, Stevens G Jr, Mellow SD, Green SB. Randomized, double-masked study of cyclosporine compared to prednisolone in the treatment of endogenous uveitis. Am J Ophthalmol. 1991;112(2):138–46.
61. Secchi AG, De Rosa C, Pivetti-Pezzi P, Rossi A, De Molfetta V, Tognon S, et al. Open noncontrolled multicenter long-term trial with ciclosporin in endogenous non-infectious uveitis. Ophthalmologica. 1991;202(4):217–24.
62. Secchi AG, Tognon MS, Maselli C. Cyclosporine-A in the treatment of serpiginous choroiditis. Int Ophthalmol. 1990;14(5–6):395–9.
63. Mathews D, Mathews J, Jones NP. Low-dose cyclosporine treatment for sight-threatening uveitis: efficacy, toxicity, and tolerance. Indian J Ophthalmol. 2010;58(1):55–8.
64. Peters DH, Fitton A, Plosker GL, Faulds D. Tacrolimus. A review of its pharmacology, and therapeutic potential in hepatic and renal transplantation. Drugs. 1993;46(4):746–94.
65. Fujino Y, Mochizuki M, Chan CC, Raber J, Kotake S, Gery I, et al. FK506 treatment of S-antigen induced uveitis in primates. Curr Eye Res. 1991;10(7): 679–90.
66. Fujino Y, Chan CC, de Smet MD, Hikita N, Gery I, Mochizuki M, et al. FK 506 treatment of experimental autoimmune uveoretinitis in primates. Transplant Proc. 1991;23(6):3335–8.
67. Mochizuki M, Kawashima H. Effects of FK506, 15-deoxyspergualin, and cyclosporine on experimental autoimmune uveoretinitis in the rat. Autoimmunity. 1990;8(1):37–41.
68. Kawashima H, Mochizuki M. Effects of a new immunosuppressive agent, FK 506, on the efferent limb of the immune responses. Exp Eye Res. 1990;51(5):565–72.
69. Kawashima H, Fujino Y, Mochizuki M. Antigen-specific suppressor cells induced by FK506 in experimental autoimmune uveoretinitis in the rat. Invest Ophthalmol Vis Sci. 1990;31(12):2500–7.
70. Kawashima H, Fujino Y, Mochizuki M. Effects of a new immunosuppressive agent, FK506, on experimental autoimmune uveoretinitis in rats. Invest Ophthalmol Vis Sci. 1988;29(8):1265–71.

71. Sloper CM, Powell RJ, Dua HS. Tacrolimus (FK506) in the treatment of posterior uveitis refractory to cyclosporine. Ophthalmology. 1999;106(4):723–8.
72. Ishioka M, Ohno S, Nakamura S, Isobe K, Watanabe N, Ishigatsubo Y, et al. FK506 treatment of noninfectious uveitis. Am J Ophthalmol. 1994;118(6):723–9.
73. Mochizuki M, Masuda K, Sakane T, Ito K, Kogure M, Sugino N, et al. A clinical trial of FK506 in refractory uveitis. Am J Ophthalmol. 1993;115(6):763–9.
74. Mochizuki M, Ikeda E, Shirao M, Fujito S, Yoshimura K, Shimada N. Preclinical and clinical study of FK506 in uveitis. Curr Eye Res. 1992;11 Suppl:87–95.
75. Mochizuki M, Masuda K, Sakane T, Inaba G, Ito K, Kogure M, et al. A multicenter clinical open trial of FK 506 in refractory uveitis, including Behcet's disease. Japanese FK 506 Study Group on Refractory Uveitis. Transplant Proc. 1991;23(6):3343–6.
76. Murphy CC, Greiner K, Plskova J, Duncan L, Frost NA, Forrester JV, et al. Cyclosporine vs tacrolimus therapy for posterior and intermediate uveitis. Arch Ophthalmol. 2005;123(5):634–41.
77. Rapamune [package insert]. Philadelphia: Wyeth Pharmaceuticals Inc; 2015.
78. Roberge FG, Xu D, Chan CC, de Smet MD, Nussenblatt RB, Chen H. Treatment of autoimmune uveoretinitis in the rat with rapamycin, an inhibitor of lymphocyte growth factor signal transduction. Curr Eye Res. 1993;12(2):197–203.
79. Ikeda E, Hikita N, Eto K, Mochizuki M. Tacrolimus-rapamycin combination therapy for experimental autoimmune uveoretinitis. Jpn J Ophthalmol. 1997;41(6):396–402.
80. Yang K, Wen J, Liu X, Kijlstra A, Chen L, Chi W, et al. Inhibitory effect of rapamycin and dexamethasone on production of IL-17 and IFN-gamma in Vogt-Koyanagi-Harada patients. Br J Ophthalmol. 2009;93(2):249–53.
81. Zhang Z, Wu X, Duan J, Hinrichs D, Wegmann K, Zhang GL, et al. Low dose rapamycin exacerbates autoimmune experimental uveitis. PLoS One. 2012;7(5):e36589.
82. Dejneka NS, Kuroki AM, Fosnot J, Tang W, Tolentino MJ, Bennett J. Systemic rapamycin inhibits retinal and choroidal neovascularization in mice. Mol Vis. 2004;10:964–72.
83. Shanmuganathan VA, Casely EM, Raj D, Powell RJ, Joseph A, Amoaku WM, et al. The efficacy of sirolimus in the treatment of patients with refractory uveitis. Br J Ophthalmol. 2005;89(6):666–9.
84. Phillips BN, Wroblewski KJ. A retrospective review of oral low-dose sirolimus (rapamycin) for the treatment of active uveitis. J Ophthalmic Inflamm Infect. 2011;1(1):29–34.
85. Nussenblatt RB, Coleman H, Jirawuthiworavong G, Davuluri G, Potapova N, Dahr SS, et al. The treatment of multifocal choroiditis associated choroidal neovascularization with sirolimus (rapamycin). Acta Ophthalmol Scand. 2007;85(2):230–1.
86. Douglas LC, Yi NY, Davis JL, Salmon JH, Gilger BC. Ocular toxicity and distribution of subconjunctival and intravitreal rapamycin in horses. J Vet Pharmacol Ther. 2008;31(6):511–6.
87. Sen HN, Larson TA, Meleth AD, Smith WM, Nussenblatt RB. Subconjunctival sirolimus for the treatment of chronic active anterior uveitis: results of a pilot trial. Am J Ophthalmol. 2012;153(6):1038–42.
88. Mudumba S, Bezwada P, Takanaga H, Hosoi K, Tsuboi T, Ueda K, et al. Tolerability and pharmacokinetics of intravitreal sirolimus. J Ocul Pharmacol Ther. 2012;28(5):507–14.
89. Nguyen QD, Ibrahim MA, Watters A, Bittencourt M, Yohannan J, Sepah YJ, et al. Ocular tolerability and efficacy of intravitreal and subconjunctival injections of sirolimus in patients with non-infectious uveitis: primary 6-month results of the SAVE Study. J Ophthalmic Inflamm Infect. 2013;3(1):32.
90. Ibrahim MA, Sepah YJ, Watters A, Bittencourt M, Vigil EM, Do DV, et al. One-year outcomes of the SAVE Study: Sirolimus as a Therapeutic Approach for UVEitis. Transl Vis Sci Technol. 2015;4(2):4.
91. Nguyen QD, Merrill PT, Clark WL, et al. Intravitreal Sirolimus for Noninfectious Uveitis: A Phase III Sirolimus Study Assessing Double-masked Uveitis Treatment (SAKURA). Ophthalmology. 2016 Nov;123(11):2413–23.
92. Hennig M, Bauer D, Wasmuth S, Busch M, Walscheid K, Thanos S, et al. Everolimus improves experimental autoimmune uveoretinitis. Exp Eye Res. 2012;105:43–52.
93. Heiligenhaus A, Zurek-Imhoff B, Roesel M, Hennig M, Rammrath D, Heinz C. Everolimus for the treatment of uveitis refractory to cyclosporine A: a pilot study. Graefes Arch Clin Exp Ophthalmol. 2013;251(1):143–52.

Alkylating Agents

6

Debra A. Goldstein and Kara C. LaMattina

Pearls

- Cyclophosphamide has high oral bioavailability, and there is some evidence that daily oral therapy is more effective for uveitis than pulse monthly IV therapy.
- Risks of cyclophosphamide include myelosuppression, hematologic malignancy, sterility, hemorrhagic cystitis, and subsequent bladder cancer.
- Chlorambucil carries similar risks to cyclophosphamide, but does not increase the risk of bladder cancer.
- While the risks of malignancy and sterility have been well established in the literature, alkylating agents remain a valuable treatment option for select patients with sight-threatening ocular inflammation and are among the few agents that can potentially induce drug-free remission.

Introduction

After sulfur mustard gas was observed to cause aplasia of the bone marrow and lymphoid tissue during World War I, scientists sought to harness it in the treatment of malignancies. Gilman and Philips first described such research in 1946, when they used intravenous nitrogen mustards in patients with lymphoma [1]. Since that time, various analogues have been derived from this gas in the pursuit of less toxic antineoplastic agents. These intermediates function by alkylating reactive amines, oxygens, or phosphates on DNA. Nitrogen mustard derivatives possess a 2-chlorethyl side chain, which covalently bonds to various targets, including the N7 of guanine in DNA. This reaction creates instability and strand breakage. As nitrogen mustards are bifunctional, a second 2-chlorethyl side chain can also lead to cross-linking by alkylation of a second guanine residue, causing cessation of the cell cycle. If cells are unable to repair the alkylated DNA, they ultimately undergo apoptosis [2].

While these drugs were originally pioneered for oncologic purposes, they have been utilized in life-threatening rheumatologic conditions and subsequently in sight-threatening ocular disease. Nitrogen mustard was first described as a treatment for intractable uveitis by Roda in 1951. Roda presented a paper at the Ophthalmological Society of Madrid describing its use in the treatment of recurrent idiopathic uveitis refractory to other available therapies, showing that the patient had recovery of visual acuity with improvement in pain and redness [3]. Use

D. A. Goldstein (✉)
Department of Ophthalmology, Northwestern University Feinberg School of Medicine, Chicago, IL, USA

K. C. LaMattina
Department of Ophthalmology, Boston University School of Medicine, Boston, MA, USA

P. Lin, E. Suhler (eds.), *Treatment of Non-infectious Uveitis*,
https://doi.org/10.1007/978-3-030-22827-9_6

of such agents is limited to severe disease given the accompanying risks of malignancy and infertility.

Cyclophosphamide

Pharmacokinetics

Cyclophosphamide undergoes metabolic activation in the liver by cytochrome P450 2B, where it is oxidized into 4-hydroxycyclophosphamide and aldophosphamide. The 4-hydroxy intermediate is oxidized by aldehyde oxidase to inactive metabolites. Aldophosphamide spontaneously cleaves into acrolein and phosphoramide mustard and oxidizes into carboxyphosphamide. Phosphoramide mustard is the antineoplastic metabolite, while adverse effects of hemorrhagic cystitis and bladder cancer are largely attributed to acrolein [2]. Studies have shown that cyclophosphamide decreases the number of B and T cells while also reducing lymphocyte proliferation, antibody production, and development of delayed-type hypersensitivity reactions [4, 5]. It has a half-life of 2–8 hours and is excreted by the kidneys [6].

Dosage and Administration

Cyclophosphamide has high oral bioavailability [7]. Standard dosing of cyclophosphamide is 1–3 mg/kg/day orally over 12 months. If toxic effects are observed, such as mild leukopenia, it is generally decreased by 25–50 mg. In 1982, Dinant and colleagues first proposed intravenous (IV) pulsation of cyclophosphamide in the treatment of lupus nephritis [8]. Eleven years later, Eiser et al. showed that IV pulsation had comparable efficacy with less renal toxicity than oral regimens in patients with lupus nephritis [9]. Pulse therapy is administered at 1 g/m^2 every 3–4 weeks until disease in quiescent or the leukocyte count falls below 2500 cells/μl.

Efficacy in Ocular Inflammation

In 1978, Jampol and colleagues described the use of cyclophosphamide in three patients who had intractable scleritis with progressive thinning of the sclera despite oral corticosteroids. Patients received 75–150 mg/day of cyclophosphamide over a period of 9 months to 2 years with control of inflammation [10]. A report from 2000 found cyclophosphamide useful for control of scleritis (most commonly necrotizing scleritis) in 16 patients who were started on 2 mg/kg/day for failure to control inflammation or unacceptable side effects from systemic prednisone. Inflammation was successfully controlled with a median maximum dose of 150 mg/kg/day (range 100–250 mg/kg/day) with a median duration of therapy of 48.5 weeks (range, 12–235 weeks.) [11]

The Systemic Immunosuppressive Therapy for Eye Diseases (SITE) group published data in 2010 on a multicenter retrospective cohort of 215 patients treated with cyclophosphamide. The most common indication for treatment was mucous membrane pemphigoid (45.6%) followed by scleritis (22.3%) and uveitis (20.4%). After 6 months of treatment, 43%, 53.3%, and 50.2% of patients, respectively, were deemed inactive. The percent of patients achieving quiescence improved to 68.7%, 82.2%, and 81.3%, respectively, at 12 months. Persistent inflammation led to discontinuation of therapy in 9.7% of patients. A secondary outcome of steroid-sparing success (defined as inflammation control with 10 mg/day of prednisone or less) was achieved by 30.1% of patients at 6 months and 61.2% of patients at 12 months. No statistically significant differences were detected between oral and IV administration in time-to-control of inflammation or in steroid-sparing success, though daily oral administration did show a tendency toward higher success in inflammation control than monthly pulse IV therapy [12].

In a retrospective case series by Durrani and colleagues, pulse IV cyclophosphamide was described in 38 patients. The most common indications for treatment were panuveitis with retinal vasculitis (15.8%) and ocular cicatricial pemphigoid (15.8%) with rheumatoid arthritis being the most common etiology of inflammation (18%). Starting with a mean dose of 968 mg, and subsequent doses ranging from 500 to 1500 mg, patients received a mean cumulative dose of 10.2 g over 14 months. Twenty-one patients (55%) had resolution of inflammation, while nine patients (24%) had worsening of inflammation during treatment. Systemic corticosteroids were discontinued in 9 of 22 patients and tapered to a mean dose of 12.5 mg daily in the remaining 13. Visual acuity improved by two or more Snellen lines in eight patients (21%) and worsened in five (13%) [13].

A study out of Birmingham investigated the use of 15 mg/kg pulsed IV cyclophosphamide used concurrently with 10 mg/kg IV methylprednisone at intervals of 0, 2, 4, 7, 10, and 13 weeks (with a total of up to nine pulses, depending on clinical response). Twenty-six patients with refractory scleritis, sclerokeratitis, or noninfectious uveitis received a median of six pulses over three months. At 6 months, 33% of affected eyes were quiescent, improving to 49% of eyes at 12 months. Nineteen eyes (44%) failed treatment at both 6 and 12 months. Median visual acuity at baseline was 0.5 LogMAR, with 19% and 16% of eyes improving by halving the visual angle at 6 and 12 months, respectively [14].

Akpek et al. reported on the use of alkylating agents (both cyclophosphamide and chlorambucil) in the treatment of eight patients with serpiginous choroiditis. Treated with 2 mg/kg/day of oral cyclophosphosphamide for a mean 26.5 months, two patients achieved drug-free remission off of treatment for more than 90 months and two became quiescent with treatment. Visual acuity stabilized or improved in all patients [15].

Adverse Events

Bone marrow suppression is a common adverse effect of cyclophosphamide treatment, with 18.1–37.5% of patients reported to develop significant leukopenia and 3.8% developing significant thrombocytopenia [11, 12, 14]. Infections are a secondary effect of this immunosuppression, with one study showing 3% of patients developing opportunistic infections and another showing that 25% of patients developed infection with herpes zoster virus [12, 15]. Anywhere from 7.7–43% of patients develop hemorrhagic cystitis with treatment, a concerning side effect as it portends a higher risk of bladder cancer [11, 12, 16]. Hemorrhagic cystitis is more common during oral administration, as IV cyclophosphamide is typically co-administered with 2-mercaptoethanesulfonate, which binds acrolein in the urine and limits bladder toxicity [2]. Other minor adverse effects include fatigue, nausea, headache, and diarrhea [13].

A study of 158 patients with systemic granulomatosis with polyangiitis (GPA, previously known as Wegener granulomatosis) treated with 2 mg/kg/day of cyclophosphamide found that 43% of patients developed cystitis with 2.8% developing bladder cancer. Three patients (2%) developed myelodysplasia a mean of 8.1 years after treatment, and two patients (1.3%) developed lymphoma a mean of 5.1 years after treatment. Seventy-three patients had infections at a rate of 0.11 infections per patient year, with pneumonia and skin infections accounting for 39% and 26% of all serious infections, respectively. Hair loss affected 17% of patients. Sixteen women (57%) developed amenorrhea or other signs of premature ovarian failure [16].

While sterility is a concern with any chemotherapeutic agent, studies have shown that the use of concurrent gonadotropin-releasing hormone agonists (GnRH-a) can preserve ovarian function. In one study by Blumenfeld and colleagues, all four patients receiving cyclophosphamide for lymphoma with concurrent GnRH-a therapy resumed normal menstrual function after treatment, while only four of ten age-matched patients receiving cyclophosphamide alone did so [17]. A subsequent study investigating the same treatment in patients with lupus supported these results, with seven patients who received concurrent GnRH-a having normal function, whereas four of the eight patients receiving cyclophosphamide alone experienced premature ovarian failure [18]. The risk of developing amenorrhea and premature ovarian failure has been shown to increase with both age and mean cumulative dose of cyclophosphamide [19, 20].

Sterility in male patients is of equal concern. Meistrich and colleagues showed that all 11 men whose sperm counts were monitored during treatment with cyclophosphamide for Ewing and soft tissue sarcomas developed azoospermia. While 80% of patients had improvement in sperm counts after cessation of treatment, only 40% returned to normospermic levels after 5 years [21].

A retrospective series of 75 patients with a variety of autoimmune diseases, most commonly systemic lupus erythematosus (SLE) and vasculitis, who had received pulsed IV cyclophosphamide, found infection to be the most common adverse event, affecting 28% of patients and resulting in hospitalization in 10%. Alopecia and stomatitis were each observed in 2.7% of patients, with no patient suffering from hemorrhagic cystitis. None of the 25 female patients suffered from amenorrhea. Five patients (6.7%) were diagnosed with malignancies between 5 and 14 months after the start of treatment [22].

As malignancy is the most serious adverse effect of cyclophosphamide, much research has been done to assess the risks of secondary malignancies and their effects on survival. One such study followed 119 patients treated with cyclophosphamide for rheumatoid arthritis, with a mean follow-up of 13.1 years. When compared to a control group of matched rheumatoid arthritis patients, investigators found that a significantly higher percentage of patients in the treatment group developed malignancies than in the control group (31% and 21%, respectively, $p < 0.05$). Only the treatment group developed bladder cancer ($p < 0.001$). Patients who developed malignancy in the treatment group received a mean cumulative dose of 79.0 g of cyclophosphamide, while those who did not develop cancer received a mean cumulative dose of 41.2 g. The mean duration of treatment was also higher in those patients who developed malignancy (45.6 months vs 24. 8 months, $p < 0.001$). There was no statistically significant difference in the mean age at death, although malignancy was the cause of death for more patients in the treatment group than the control group (20% versus 13%, $p < 0.001$) [23].

Monitoring

Given the risk of bone marrow suppression and urotoxicity, it is recommended that complete blood count, platelet count, and urinalysis with microscopy be checked weekly until dosing is stable and monthly for the duration of treatment. Treatment is interrupted in cases of severe bone marrow suppression (less than 2500 white blood cells/μL) and may be resumed at a lower dose when counts recover. While prophylaxis with hyperhydration or sodium-2 mercaptoethanesulfonate may reduce its likelihood, any evidence of hematuria warrants consideration of discontinuation of treatment given the association with bladder cancer.

Contraindications

Cyclophosphamide is contraindicated in pregnancy as it has been shown to have teratogenic effects. It was associated with the absence of thumbs, cleft palate, low-set ears, and eye anomalies (including bilateral blepharophimosis and unilateral microphthalmos) in an infant exposed during the first trimester [24]. In mouse studies, cyclophosphamide exposure in utero is associated with synostoses, both poly- and oligodactyly, and lethality depending on the stage of exposure [25].

Chlorambucil

Pharmacokinetics

Chlorambucil is well absorbed by the GI tract and subsequently metabolized by the liver to its primary metabolite, phenylacetic acid [26]. It has a half-life of approximately 1.5 hours and is excreted renally.

Dosage and Administration

Chlorambucil is well tolerated orally, with minimal gastrointestinal discomfort. Traditionally, it was given at a dosage of 0.1–0.2 mg/kg once a day (generally a dose of 6–12 mg) for a year after disease control was achieved. Studies, such as that by Palmer and colleagues, which showed that the damage chlorambucil inflicts on chromosomes is both cumulative and dose-dependent, support limiting both the duration and total dosage of this therapy [27]. This finding has led to some researchers advocating the use of short-term, high-dose therapy. In this regimen, chlorambucil is administered at 2 mg daily for a week with escalation by 2 mg/day each week. The dose is increased incrementally until bone marrow suppression (white blood cell count less than 2400 cells/μL or platelet count less than 100–125,000 cells/μL) is achieved, which typically takes 3 to 6 months. An attempt is made during this therapy to taper patients off of all other steroid and nonsteroid immunomodulatory therapy [28–30].

Efficacy in Ocular Inflammation

Mamo and colleagues first reported the use of chlorambucil in the treatment of ocular Behçet disease in 1970. Eleven patients treated with 0.1–0.2 mg/kg/day of chlorambucil showed cessation of disease progression, control of active inflammation, and maintenance of vision in all cases over a mean 7 months of follow-up. All patients initially treated with topical and systemic corticosteroids were able to discontinue these treatments [31]. Using an initial dose of 10 to 15 mg daily for 1 to 2 months, followed by an adjusted maintenance dose for 6 to 8 months, Abdalla et al. found that chlorambucil was effective in obtaining quiescence after 6 to 11 months without recurrence off of treatment, when followed for a total of 40 months in four cases of posterior uveitis and three cases of neuroretinitis, although there was only partial improvement in one of three cases of iridocyclitis [32]. Shortly thereafter, the Proctor Foundation published their experience with 31 patients treated with chlorambucil for a variety of etiologies, most commonly Behçet disease and sympathetic ophthalmia (16.1% each). Patients were started at 2 mg of chlorambucil daily, increasing to a maximal dose of 22 mg/day depending on response to therapy as well as toxicity. Patients were treated for a mean 28.8 weeks (range 4–188 weeks). They reported improvement in ten patients (32.3%), with the remainder showing minimal or no improvement [33]. Elliott and Ballinger reported seven patients with Behçet disease treated with 0.1–0.2 mg/kg/day of chlorambucil, all of whom had improvement of inflammation, with four achieving remission off of therapy for greater than 36 months of follow-up [34].

A report from the Massachusetts Eye and Ear Infirmary described 28 patients, 26 of whom were female, treated with chlorambucil for a variety of etiologies. Patients were started on a dose of 0.1 mg/kg/day and titrated up to a median dose of 8 mg/day (range 4–22 mg/day), which was administered over a mean 12 months (range 4–166 months). Nineteen patients (68%) maintained improvement in inflammation even after cessation of treatment, while four patients (14%) had improvement in inflammation with relapse after cessation of treatment, which necessitated using alternative systemic therapies. Two patients (7%) showed no improvement in ocular inflammation, and three patients (11%) showed no improvement in systemic inflammation during treatment with chlorambucil. Seven patients had to discontinue treatment due to adverse effects. Nineteen of 28 patients (68%) initially taking systemic corticosteroids were able to discontinue this treatment, with 9 patients (32%) still requiring chronic low doses [35].

Tessler and Jennings reported their results with high-dose, short-term chlorambucil therapy in patients with sympathetic ophthalmia (SO) and Behçet disease. Starting at 2 mg daily, treatment was increased by 2 mg/day each week with a goal of inducing leukopenia below $2.4\text{x}10^9$/l, a platelet count below $100\text{x}10^9$/l, or remission of inflammation ($\leq$1+ flare, $\leq$ occasional cells, no active fundus lesions). Twelve patients were included, six with SO and six with Behçet disease. They found that induction of bone marrow suppression to the target level, when causing a 6-week depression in blood counts, was followed by a sustained remission off of therapy. Mean cumulative dose of chlorambucil in patients with SO was 0.85 ± 0.48 g and in patients with Behçet disease 2.18 ± 1.10 g, with mean duration of treatment 11.2 ± 3.2 weeks and 22.8 ± 9 weeks, respectively. Final visual acuities ranged from 20/20 to 20/400 in eyes with SO (those with less than 20/25 had subretinal neovascularization in the macula) and 20/50 or better in all patients with Behçet disease [28]. A subsequent study also from the University of Illinois at Chicago employing the same treatment protocol included 53 patients who were treated for a mean of 16 weeks (with only four patients receiving more than 26 weeks of therapy) followed for a mean 4.3 years (range, 6 months to 24 years). The mean cumulative dose was 1.416 g (range 0.392–5.2 g,) with 23 patients receiving more than 1.5 g of chlorambucil. At last follow-up, 77% of patients were in remission without need for systemic treatment. The remainder of patients had recurrence requiring treatment with systemic corticosteroids and/or immunosuppressive treatment. The majority of patients (88.6%) had an improvement in vision by at least two Snellen lines, with six patients (11%) worsening in vision by an average of two lines. Thirty-eight of the 49 patients (78%) on oral corticosteroids at the start of chlorambucil therapy were able to discontinue this during treatment [29].

Patel and colleagues used the same protocol of short-term, high-dose chlorambucil therapy in the treatment of 16 patients with SO. Patients received a mean cumulative dose of 1.466 g (range 0.518–2.002 g) over a mean 14.5 weeks (range 12–19 weeks). Best-corrected visual acuity (BCVA) in the sympathizing eye improved by two lines or more in nine patients (56%) and worsened in none. All patients achieved control of inflammation and were able to be tapered off of systemic corticosteroids. Only four patients (16%) had recurrence of inflammation after discontinuation of chlorambucil, three of whom were controlled with topical therapy alone and the fourth of whom required short-term systemic corticosteroids. Ninety-three percent of patients achieved drug-free remission for greater than 5 years.

A study of chlorambucil use in patients with Behçet disease from Turkey reported on 44 patients followed over 51.4 ± 32.5 months. The mean duration of chlorambucil use was 22.4 ± 5 weeks with a mean total dose of 1.637 ± 0.429 g. Researchers observed a decrease in the mean frequency of flares from 4.9 ± 2.3 per year to 0.9 ± 1.4 per year with treatment ($p < 0.0001$). BCVA improved in 32.9% of patients and decreased in 34.2%. The majority of patients (68.2%) experienced quiescence of longer than 1 year on treatment, with 31.8% still in remission during the 14–86 months follow-up after cessation of chlorambucil. Eighteen patients (40.9%) were switched to an alternative immunosuppressant due to treatment failure [36].

In Akpek's study on alkylating agents in the treatment of serpiginous choroiditis, five patients were treated with chlorambucil. All patients achieved quiescence with a mean of 4.3 months of treatment. Four patients had improvement in visual acuity, ranging from 1 to 7 Snellen lines, with no patients experiencing a decline in vision [15].

Adverse Events

Leukopenia is one of the most common adverse effects of chlorambucil, affecting anywhere from 5.9 to 28.6% of patients [32, 36, 37]. Thrombocytopenia is reportedly less common, affecting 3.8–7.1% [29, 37]. Infections, including both minor infections such as oral mycosis and more serious infections such as bronchopneumonia, affect anywhere from 6.3 to 14.3% of patients [30, 37]. Herpes zoster virus infection has been reported in 11.3–28.6% of patients [29, 34].

Other minor adverse effects include drug rashes [32], mild hair loss [36], gastric pain [36], nausea and vomiting [15, 30], elevated liver transaminases [30], and muscle cramps and pain [30].

Sterility is a concern for both men and women treated with chlorambucil. Amenorrhea is reported to affect 14.3–26% of women [29, 37]. Blumenfeld and colleagues reported their results on the preservation of ovarian function in a single patient treated with chlorambucil and concurrent GnRH-a, while a patient who received chlorambucil alone suffered premature ovarian failure [18]. In a study of prepubescent boys who had received a mean cumulative dose of 1.476 g of chlorambucil for nephrotic syndrome, significant effects were found in gonadal development. Four patients (19%) and nine patients (42.9%) were below average in penis size and testicular size, respectively. Seventeen patients (81.0%) developed azoospermia, and this was universal in patients who received greater than 25 mg/kg of chlorambucil [38]. Goldstein and colleagues found that 3.8% of patients treated with chlorambucil reported testicular atrophy with another 7.7% reporting erectile dysfunction [29].

The most concerning adverse event associated with chlorambucil use is malignancy. Reeves showed significant increases in chromosomal aberrations in patients with uveitis who had been treated with chlorambucil, a finding which persisted in some patients many years after the completion of therapy [39]. The chromosomal damage from chlorambucil has been shown to be both dose- and duration-dependent [27]. A study on the use of chlorambucil in the treatment of chronic lymphocytic leukemia suggested that the risk of treatment-related malignancy is highest between 5 and 10 years after the initiation of treatment [40]. A follow-up study of the 53 uveitis patients treated with chlorambucil at the University of Illinois found that after an average of 8.9 years of clinical follow-up and 14.2 years of mortality data, no patients died of cancer. Two cases of cancer were reported; one patient developed renal cell carcinoma, but he had two siblings who also had renal cell carcinoma. One patient with a family history of colon cancer developed colon cancer. Neither patient died of their malignancy [41]. It has been postulated that the lower risk of malignancy with the high-dose, short-term protocol is due to the induction of apoptosis from high-dose administration of chlorambucil, while lower doses are more likely to lead to DNA instability and mutagenesis [30].

Monitoring

The risk of bone marrow suppression has led to the recommendation that complete blood counts be monitored weekly until dosage is stabilized and monthly thereafter until cessation of therapy. With high-dose, short-term therapy, CBC is monitored weekly.

Contraindications

As with cyclophosphamide, pregnancy is contraindicated with chlorambucil use. It has been associated with renal agenesis in humans, limb defects in mice and rats, decreased weight and length in mice and rats, and syndactyly and encephalocele in rats [42–44].

Conclusion

While the risks of malignancy and sterility have been well established in the literature, alkylating agents remain a valuable treatment option for select patients with sight-threatening ocular inflammation. The success of biologic agents, with their safer side effect profile, has made the latter class a more appealing choice in the management of refractory uveitis. Patients with severe or refractory disease, however, may still benefit from the use of alkylating agents, which are one of the only classes of drugs that have been shown to result in long-term drug-free remission. TNF inhibitors have not yet been shown to induce prolonged drug-free remission, although studies have suggested such success with interferon-α [45, 46] [see Table 6.1 for Alkylating Agents Dosing Table].

Table 6.1 Alkylating agents dosing table

	Route	Dosage	Side effects	Lab monitoring
Cyclophosphamide				
Standard	IV/oral	1–3 mg/kg/day for 1 year	Bone marrow suppression, infection, sterility, hemorrhagic cystitis, malignancy	CBC, UA (weekly until dosing stable and then monthly for duration of treatment)
Pulse	IV	1 g/m^2 every 3–4 weeks until leukocytes <2500 cells/μl		CBC weekly until leukocytes <2500 cells/μl
Chlorambucil				
Standard	Oral	0.1–0.2 mg/kg/day for 1 year	Bone marrow suppression, infection, sterility, malignancy	CBC (weekly until dosing stable and then monthly for duration of treatment)
Short-term, high-dose	Oral	2 mg daily for 1 week with escalation of 2 mg/day/week until leukocytes <2400 cells/μl or platelets <125,000 (ad units)		CBC weekly while on therapy, continued until counts recover

CBC complete blood count, *UA* urinalysis

References

1. Gilman A, Philips FS. The biological actions and therapeutic applications of the B-chloroethyl amines and sulfides. Science. 1946;103(2675):409–15.
2. Goodman LS, Brunton LL, Chabner B, Knollmann BC. Goodman & Gilman's the pharmacological basis of therapeutics. 12th ed. New York: McGraw-Hill; 2011. xvi, 2084 p.
3. Roda E. Uveitis treated with nitrogen mustard. Am J Ophthalmol. 1952;35(1):114.
4. Lacki JK, Schochat T, Sobieska M, Leszczynski P, Wiktorowicz K, Mackiewicz U, et al. Immunological studies in patients with rheumatoid arthritis treated with methotrexate or cyclophosphamide. Z Rheumatol. 1994;53(2):76–82.
5. Fauci AS, Wolff SM, Johnson JS. Effect of cyclophosphamide upon the immune response in Wegener's granulomatosis. N Engl J Med. 1971;285(27):1493–6.
6. Bagley CM Jr, Bostick FW, DeVita VT Jr. Clinical pharmacology of cyclophosphamide. Cancer Res. 1973;33(2):226–33.
7. Katzung BG, Trevor AJ. Basic & clinical pharmacology. New York: McGraw-Hill Education LLC; 2015. Available from: http://hdl.library.upenn.edu/1017.12/1492976 Connect to full text.
8. Dinant HJ, Decker JL, Klippel JH, Balow JE, Plotz PH, Steinberg AD. Alternative modes of cyclophosphamide and azathioprine therapy in lupus nephritis. Ann Intern Med. 1982;96(6 Pt 1):728–36.
9. Eiser AR, Grishman E, Dreznin S. Intravenous pulse cyclophosphamide in the treatment of type IV lupus nephritis. Clin Nephrol. 1993;40(3):155–9.
10. Jampol LM, West C, Goldberg MF. Therapy of scleritis with cytotoxic agents. Am J Ophthalmol. 1978;86(2):266–71.
11. Jabs DA, Mudun A, Dunn JP, Marsh MJ. Episcleritis and scleritis: clinical features and treatment results. Am J Ophthalmol. 2000;130(4):469–76.
12. Pujari SS, Kempen JH, Newcomb CW, Gangaputra S, Daniel E, Suhler EB, et al. Cyclophosphamide for ocular inflammatory diseases. Ophthalmology. 2010;117(2):356–65.
13. Durrani K, Papaliodis GN, Foster CS. Pulse IV cyclophosphamide in ocular inflammatory disease: efficacy and short-term safety. Ophthalmology. 2004;111(5):960–5.
14. Khan IJ, Barry RJ, Amissah-Arthur KN, Carruthers D, Elamanchi SR, Situnayake D, et al. Ten-year experience of pulsed intravenous cyclophosphamide and methylprednisolone protocol (PICM protocol) in severe ocular inflammatory disease. Br J Ophthalmol. 2013;97(9):1118–22.
15. Akpek EK, Jabs DA, Tessler HH, Joondeph BC, Foster CS. Successful treatment of serpiginous choroiditis with alkylating agents. Ophthalmology. 2002;109(8):1506–13.
16. Hoffman GS, Kerr GS, Leavitt RY, Hallahan CW, Lebovics RS, Travis WD, et al. Wegener granulomatosis: an analysis of 158 patients. Ann Intern Med. 1992;116(6):488–98.
17. Blumenfeld Z, Avivi I, Linn S, Epelbaum R, Ben-Shahar M, Haim N. Prevention of irreversible chemotherapy-induced ovarian damage in young women with lymphoma by a gonadotrophin-releasing hormone agonist in parallel to chemotherapy. Hum Reprod. 1996;11(8):1620–6.
18. Blumenfeld Z, Shapiro D, Shteinberg M, Avivi I, Nahir M. Preservation of fertility and ovarian function and minimizing gonadotoxicity in young women with systemic lupus erythematosus treated by chemotherapy. Lupus. 2000;9(6):401–5.
19. Koyama H, Wada T, Nishizawa Y, Iwanaga T, Aoki Y. Cyclophosphamide-induced ovarian failure and its therapeutic significance in patients with breast cancer. Cancer. 1977;39(4):1403–9.
20. Mok CC, Lau CS, Wong RW. Risk factors for ovarian failure in patients with systemic lupus erythematosus receiving cyclophosphamide therapy. Arthritis Rheum. 1998;41(5):831–7.
21. Meistrich ML, Wilson G, Brown BW, da Cunha MF, Lipshultz LI. Impact of cyclophosphamide on long-term reduction in sperm count in men treated with combination chemotherapy for Ewing and soft tissue sarcomas. Cancer. 1992;70(11):2703–12.
22. Martin F, Lauwerys B, Lefebvre C, Devogelaer JP, Houssiau FA. Side-effects of intravenous cyclophosphamide pulse therapy. Lupus. 1997;6(3):254–7.
23. Radis CD, Kahl LE, Baker GL, Wasko MC, Cash JM, Gallatin A, et al. Effects of cyclophosphamide on the development of malignancy and on long-term survival of patients with rheumatoid arthritis. A 20-year followup study. Arthritis Rheum. 1995;38(8):1120–7.
24. Kirshon B, Wasserstrum N, Willis R, Herman GE, McCabe ER. Teratogenic effects of first-trimester cyclophosphamide therapy. Obstet Gynecol. 1988;72(3 Pt 2):462–4.
25. Gebhardt DO. The embryo lethal and teratogenic effects of cyclophosphamide on mouse embryos. Teratology. 1970;3(3):273–7.
26. McLean A, Newell D, Baker G, Connors T. The metabolism of chlorambucil. Biochem Pharmacol. 1980;29(14):2039–47.
27. Palmer RG, Dore CJ, Denman AM. Chlorambucil-induced chromosome damage to human lymphocytes is dose-dependent and cumulative. Lancet. 1984;1(8371):246–9.
28. Tessler HH, Jennings T. High-dose short-term chlorambucil for intractable sympathetic ophthalmia and Behcet's disease. Br J Ophthalmol. 1990;74(6):353–7.
29. Goldstein DA, Fontanilla FA, Kaul S, Sahin O, Tessler HH. Long-term follow-up of patients treated with short-term high-dose chlorambucil for sight-threatening ocular inflammation. Ophthalmology. 2002;109(2):370–7.
30. Patel SS, Dodds EM, Echandi LV, Couto CA, Schlaen A, Tessler HH, et al. Long-term, drug-free remission of sympathetic ophthalmia with high-dose,

short-term chlorambucil therapy. Ophthalmology. 2014;121(2):596–602.
31. Mamo JG, Azzam SA. Treatment of Behcet's disease with chlorambucil. Arch Ophthalmol. 1970;84(4):446–50.
32. Abdalla MI, el DBN. Long-lasting remission of Behcet's disease after chlorambucil therapy. Br J Ophthalmol. 1973;57(9):706–11.
33. Godfrey WA, Epstein WV, O'Connor GR, Kimura SJ, Hogan MJ, Nozik RA. The use of chlorambucil in intractable idiopathic uveitis. Am J Ophthalmol. 1974;78(3):415–28.
34. Elliott JH, Ballinger WH. Behcet's syndrome: treatment with chlorambucil. Trans Am Ophthalmol Soc. 1984;82:264–81.
35. Miserocchi E, Baltatzis S, Ekong A, Roque M, Foster CS. Efficacy and safety of chlorambucil in intractable noninfectious uveitis: the Massachusetts Eye and Ear Infirmary experience. Ophthalmology. 2002;109(1):137–42.
36. Mudun BA, Ergen A, Ipcioglu SU, Burumcek EY, Durlu Y, Arslan MO. Short-term chlorambucil for refractory uveitis in Behcet's disease. Ocul Immunol Inflamm. 2001;9(4):219–29.
37. O'Duffy JD, Robertson DM, Goldstein NP. Chlorambucil in the treatment of uveitis and meningoencephalitis of Behcet's disease. Am J Med. 1984;76(1):75–84.
38. Guesry P, Lenoir G, Broyer M. Gonadal effects of chlorambucil given to prepubertal and pubertal boys for nephrotic syndrome. J Pediatr. 1978;92(2):299–303.
39. Reeves BR, Casey G, Harris H, Dinning WJ. Long-term cytogenetic follow-up study of patients with uveitis treated with chlorambucil. Carcinogenesis. 1985;6(11):1615–9.
40. Morrison VA, Rai KR, Peterson BL, Kolitz JE, Elias L, Appelbaum FR, et al. Therapy-related myeloid leukemias are observed in patients with chronic lymphocytic leukemia after treatment with fludarabine and chlorambucil: results of an intergroup study, cancer and leukemia group B 9011. J Clin Oncol. 2002;20(18):3878–84.
41. Birnbaum AD, Oh F, Sahin O, Little DM, Tessler HH, Goldstein DA. Chlorambucil and malignancy. Ophthalmology. 2010;117(7):1466–e1.
42. Shotton D, Monie IW. Possible teratogenic effect of chlorambucil on a human fetus. JAMA. 1963;186:74–5.
43. Salder TW, Kochhar DM. Teratogenic effects of chlorambucil on in vivo and in vitro organogenesis in mice. Teratology. 1975;12(1):71–8.
44. Murphy ML. A comparison of the teratogenic effects of five polyfunctional alkylating agents on the rat fetus. Pediatrics. 1959;23(1 Part 2): 231–44.
45. Diwo E, Gueudry J, Saadoun D, Weschler B, LeHoang P, Bodaghi B. Long-term efficacy of interferon in severe uveitis associated with Behcet disease. Ocul Immunol Inflamm. 2017;25(1):76–84.
46. Deuter C, Stubiger N, Zierhut M. Interferon-alpha therapy in noninfectious uveitis. Dev Ophthalmol. 2012;51:90–7.

Biologics Targeting Tumor Necrosis Factor

7

Laura J. Kopplin and Amde Selassie Shifera

Pearls

- There are five commercially available TNF inhibitors available for the treatment of inflammatory eye disease: monoclonal antibodies (infliximab, adalimumab, golilumab and certolizumab) and decocy receptors (etanercept).
- Adalimumab is the only FDA-approved TNF inhibitor for the treatment of non-infectious intermediate posterior and panuveitis in adult patients and in pediatric patients 2 years or older.
- There is extensive experience with the use of infliximab and adalimumab for treatment of uveitis and other types of ocular inflammation; less experience exists for the other monoclonal antibodies.
- Etanercept has demonstrated less effectiveness for the treatment of uveitis and other types of ocular inflammation than monoclonal antibody therapy.
- Prior to use of TNF inhibitors, tuberculosis must be ruled out and treated if present.
- TNF inhibitors are contraindicated with severe heart failure, with demyelinating disease, or in the presence of active infection.
- Patients with intermediate uveitis or unexplained neurologic symptoms should be screened for multiple sclerosis prior to initiation of treatment with TNF blockers.

Introduction

Tumor necrosis factor (TNF), also referred to as TNFα, is a pleiotropic cytokine that plays a key role in inflammation. Targeting TNF has been shown to control inflammation in a number of immune-mediated systemic and ocular inflammatory diseases. Increased TNF levels have been demonstrated in the aqueous humor and peripheral blood of various animal models of uveitis and in patients with uveitis [1–3]. The strongest evidence for the role of TNF in uveitis

L. J. Kopplin
Department of Ophthalmology and Visual Sciences, University of Wisconsin – Madison, Madison, WI, USA
e-mail: ljkopplin@wisc.edu

A. S. Shifera (✉)
Division of Ocular Immunology, Wilmer Eye Institute, Johns Hopkins University School of Medicine, Baltimore, MD, USA

P. Lin, E. Suhler (eds.), *Treatment of Non-infectious Uveitis*,
https://doi.org/10.1007/978-3-030-22827-9_7

comes from the robust and sustained response of a number of entities of noninfectious uveitis to TNF inhibitors [4]. The TNF inhibitors currently in clinical use belong to the category of biologic drugs. The biologics that target TNF belong to two groups: monoclonal antibodies that neutralize TNF (infliximab, adalimumab, golimumab, or certolizumab) and decoy receptors that bind TNF (etanercept) (Table 7.1). There is strong clinical evidence for the efficacy and safety of infliximab and adalimumab in the treatment of various types of noninfectious uveitis, whereas etanercept appears to be ineffective and is not recommended for use in the treatment of uveitis. At this writing, there is very limited data on the utility of golimumab or certolizumab in the treatment of uveitis.

Tumor Necrosis Factor (TNF)

TNF is a cytokine that was initially discovered as a protein that exhibited cytotoxicity on a number of murine and human transformed cell lines and

Table 7.1 Currently available biologics that target TNF

Category	Drug	FDA-approved indications	Route of administration	Dosing	Therapeutic monitoring
Neutralizing antibodies	Infliximab	Crohn's disease Rheumatoid arthritis Ulcerative colitis Ankylosing spondylitis Psoriatic arthritis Plaque psoriasis	Intravenous infusion	Crohn's disease: 5 mg/kg at 0, 2, and 6 weeks and then every 8 weeks. 10 mg/kg in adults with initial response who later lose their response Ulcerative colitis, psoriatic arthritis, plaque psoriasis: 5 mg/kg at 0, 2, and 6 weeks and then every 8 weeks Rheumatoid arthritis: 3–10 mg/kg at 0, 2, and 6 weeks and then every 4–8 weeks Ankylosing spondylitis: 5 mg/kg at 0, 2, and 6 weeks and then every 6 weeks	Prior to initiation of treatment: Tuberculosis screening Hepatitis B serology Baseline complete blood count, hepatic function and renal function testing Consider screening brain MRI to assess for any demyelinating diseases in patients with intermediate uveitis After initiation of treatment: Repeat complete blood count, hepatic function and renal function testing 4–6 weeks after starting therapy and following any significant dose modifications Interval complete blood count, hepatic function and renal function testing every 3–6 months in absence of other immunosuppressive therapy or hepatic/renal risk factors

Table 7.1 (continued)

Category	Drug	FDA-approved indications	Route of administration	Dosing	Therapeutic monitoring
	Adalimumab	Noninfectious intermediate uveitis, posterior uveitis, and panuveitis Rheumatoid arthritis Ulcerative colitis Crohn's disease Psoriatic arthritis Plaque psoriasis Ankylosing spondylitis Juvenile idiopathic arthritis Hidradenitis suppurativa	Subcutaneous injection	Noninfectious intermediate, posterior and panuveitis in adult patients Initial dose: 80 mg 40 mg every other week starting 1 week after initial dose Rheumatoid arthritis, psoriatic arthritis, ankylosing spondylitis: 40 mg every other week. May increase dose to 40 mg every week in patients with rheumatoid arthritis not on methotrexate Juvenile idiopathic arthritis or noninfectious intermediate uveitis, posterior uveitis, and panuveitis in pediatric patients 2 years or older: 10 kg to <15 kg: 10 mg every other week 15 kg to <30 kg: 20 mg every other week ≥30 kg: 40 mg every other week Adult Crohn's disease and Ulcerative colitis: Initial dose: 160 mg Day 15: 80 mg Day 29: start 40 mg every other week Pediatric Crohn's disease: 17 kg to <40 kg: Initial dose: 80 mg Day 15: 40 mg Day 29: start 20 mg every other week ≥40 kg: Initial dose: 160 mg Day 15: 80 mg Day 29: start 40 mg every other week Plaque psoriasis Initial dose: 80 mg 40 mg every other week starting 1 week after initial dose Hidradenitis suppurativa: 60 kg or more Initial dose: 160 mg Day 15: 80 mg Day 29: start 40 mg every week <60 kg Initial dose: 80 mg Day 8 and then every other week: 40 mg	

(continued)

Table 7.1 (continued)

Category	Drug	FDA-approved indications	Route of administration	Dosing	Therapeutic monitoring
	Golimumab	Rheumatoid arthritis Psoriatic arthritis Ankylosing spondylitis Ulcerative colitis	Subcutaneous injection	Rheumatoid arthritis, psoriatic arthritis, and ankylosing spondylitis: 50 mg monthly Ulcerative colitis: Initial dose: 200 mg Day 15: start 100 mg every 4 weeks	
	Certolizumab	Crohn's disease Rheumatoid arthritis Psoriatic arthritis Ankylosing spondylitis Non-radiographic axial ankylosing spondyloarthritis Plaque psoriasis	Subcutaneous injection	Crohn's disease: Initial dose: 400 mg Day 15: 400 mg Day 29: 400 mg, if response continue 400 mg every 4 weeks Rheumatoid arthritis, psoriatic arthritis, ankylosing spondylitis and non-radiographic ankylosing spondyloarthritis: Initial dose: 400 mg Day 15: 400 mg Day 29: 400 mg and then 200 mg every other week or 400 mg every 4 weeks Plaque psoriasis: 400 mg every other week	
Decoy receptors	Etanercept	Rheumatoid arthritis Polyarticular juvenile idiopathic arthritis Psoriatic arthritis Ankylosing spondylitis Plaque psoriasis	Subcutaneous injection	Rheumatoid arthritis, psoriatic arthritis, ankylosing spondylitis: 50 mg weekly Adult plaque psoriasis: 50 mg twice weekly for 3 months and then 50 mg weekly Pediatric plaque psoriasis and polyarticular juvenile idiopathic arthritis: 0.8 mg/kg weekly, maximum dose 50 mg weekly	

that induced necrosis of tumors in some murine tumor models [5]. Subsequently, TNF was shown to be a pleiotropic cytokine with both physiological and pathological roles that are executed via autocrine and/or paracrine interactions [6]. TNF is primarily produced by activated macrophages, although several other cell types synthesize the protein in smaller amounts. It is secreted as a transmembrane homotrimeric protein, from which a soluble homotrimeric form is released after cleavage that is catalyzed by the TNF converting enzyme [5].

The functional form of TNF is the TNF homotrimer, either in a membrane-bound form or as a soluble protein. The TNF homotrimer exerts its effects on target cells by binding to and activating TNF receptors (TNFR) expressed on the surfaces of those cells. There are two types of TNF receptors, named TNFR1 (p55) and TNFR2 (p75) [5]. TNFR1 is widely expressed throughout the body in a constitutive manner, while TNFR2 is typically expressed in cells of the immune system in a highly regulated manner [5]. TNFR1 is the key mediator of TNF responses in most tissues, whereas TNRF2 appears to be the major receptor in the lymphoid system [5]. Both receptors can bind both the soluble and the membrane forms of TNF, but only the membrane form can cause full activation of TNFR2, while TNFR1 can be fully activated by either soluble or membrane-bound TNF. Activation of TNFR in turn leads to the activation of intracellular signaling pathways that result in cellular responses by directly modulating cellular processes or by altering the expression of target genes.

One of the major functions of TNF is that of being a key mediator of inflammation. TNF is produced in large quantities at tissue sites where there is a trigger of inflammation such as an infectious pathogen or an autoimmune reaction [7]. The mechanisms by which TNF induces inflammation include the upregulation of cell adhesion molecules on the endothelial cells of nearby blood vessels, thus facilitating the migration of neutrophils and monocytes to sites of inflammation [6]. Additionally, TNF promotes inflammation by activating CD4 T cells that respond by activating multiple signaling pathways and secreting a number of cytokines, including interferon γ and lymphotoxin α. It is important, however, to note that apart from TNF, other cytokines such as IL-1 and IL-6 also have potent proinflammatory activities and can promote inflammation in the absence of TNF.

The Role of TNF in Noninfectious Uveitis

The pathogenesis of the majority of uveitis cases seen in clinical practice does not appear to involve an infectious pathogen and is believed to be immune-mediated with innate and/or adaptive immune mechanisms playing a role in the induction of the inflammatory processes [8]. There is a substantial amount of evidence from both experimental and clinical observations that supports the involvement of TNF in the pathogenesis of noninfectious uveitis. In the endotoxin-induced rat model of uveitis in which acute anterior uveitis is induced by a footpad injection of lipopolysaccharide (LPS), the level of TNF in the aqueous humor showed an early rise 4 hours after LPS injection with another larger increase at 22 hours after LPS injection concomitant with maximal uveitis [1]. In addition, the level of TNF in the peripheral blood was increased to a maximum level 2 hours after LPS injection with another smaller increase occurring at 18–20 hours after injection. Increased TNF activity has also been demonstrated in the experimental autoimmune uveitis model [9]. In addition, intravitreal injection of TNF in rats and rabbits has been shown to induce acute uveitis, characterized by increase in aqueous humor protein content and infiltration of the anterior chamber with polymorphonuclear leukocytes [10, 11].

In patients with active uveitis, increased levels of TNF have been demonstrated in the aqueous humor and in peripheral blood. In a study of 23 patients with active uveitis and 16 controls, analysis of aqueous humor and peripheral blood specimens showed significantly higher levels of TNF in the aqueous humor and peripheral blood of patients with active uveitis compared to controls [2]. In addition, a significant association was found between the serum levels of TNF and recurrent uveitis. In a prospective study involving 43 patients with ocular Behçet's disease, the serum levels of TNF were found to be significantly higher in the 20 patients who had active posterior uveitis compared to the 23 patients who did not have active ocular inflammation at the time of the study [3]. In addition, the robust response of various forms of noninfectious uveitis to TNF inhibitors supports the importance of TNF in the pathogenesis of this disease [4].

Infliximab

Infliximab (Remicade, Janssen Biotech, Horsham, PA) is a chimeric IgG1κ monoclonal antibody against human TNF produced using recombinant DNA technology. The immunoglobulin molecule is composed of human constant regions and murine variable regions. It binds to both soluble and membrane-bound TNF and prevents it from binding to TNF receptors. Infliximab was first approved by the Food and Drug Administration (FDA) in 1998 for the treatment of Crohn's disease. Subsequently, infliximab was also approved for the treatment of rheumatoid arthritis, ulcerative colitis, ankylosing spondylitis, psoriatic arthritis, and plaque psoriasis. Infliximab is administered by intravenous infusion over a period not less than 2 hours. It is given as a loading regimen at 0, 2, and 6 weeks followed by maintenance doses given typically every 8 weeks, though the interval may be reduced to 4–6 weeks for more refractory disease. The typical starting dose is 3–5 mg/kg, but in adult patients with Crohn's disease, the dose can be increased to 10 mg/kg in those who lose their response to the initial lower dose. In rheumatoid arthritis, the recommended dose is 3 mg/kg in conjunction with methotrexate, but the dose can be increased to up to 10 mg/kg and can also be given every 4 weeks.

Initial reports on the use of infliximab in the treatment of ocular inflammation appeared in 2001 [12]. One of those early reports involved a retrospective case series in which two patients, one with panuveitis and the other with rheumatoid arthritis-associated scleritis, were treated with infliximab and had their inflammation controlled. In another report during the same year, five patients with panuveitis secondary to Behçet's disease who were each given a single infusion of infliximab at the time of a relapse experienced remission of ocular inflammation within 24 hours, with complete suppression evident in all five patients within 7 days of the infusion [13]. Since the initial reports in 2001, several case series have documented the efficacy of infliximab in Behçet's disease [14–19]. In addition, a number of case reports, case series, and a few non-comparative prospective trials have been published documenting the efficacy of infliximab in the treatment of HLA-B27-associated anterior uveitis [20–22], juvenile idiopathic arthritis (JIA)-associated anterior uveitis [23–26], sarcoid uveitis [16, 27–29], uveitis secondary to Crohn's disease [27, 30–32], Vogt-Koyanagi-Harada (VKH) disease [27], birdshot chorioretinitis [27], idiopathic posterior uveitis [17], or scleritis [25]. The remission of inflammation that is achieved with infliximab appears to be sustained (Fig. 7.1). In a prospective study of patients with posterior uveitis secondary to Behçet's disease, 9 of 12 patients achieved complete remission at the 12-month follow-up with no relapse during the treatment period [33]. One prospective trial of infliximab for refractory uveitis of various types found that in initial responders, 60% retained effectiveness at 2 years [34].

Some attempts have been made to use infliximab via intravitreal administration, but the results have been mixed. One study suggested the benefit of intravitreal infliximab in the treatment of acute attacks of uveitis secondary to Behçet's disease with improvement of vision, retinitis, and vasculitis up to 1 month after injection, although

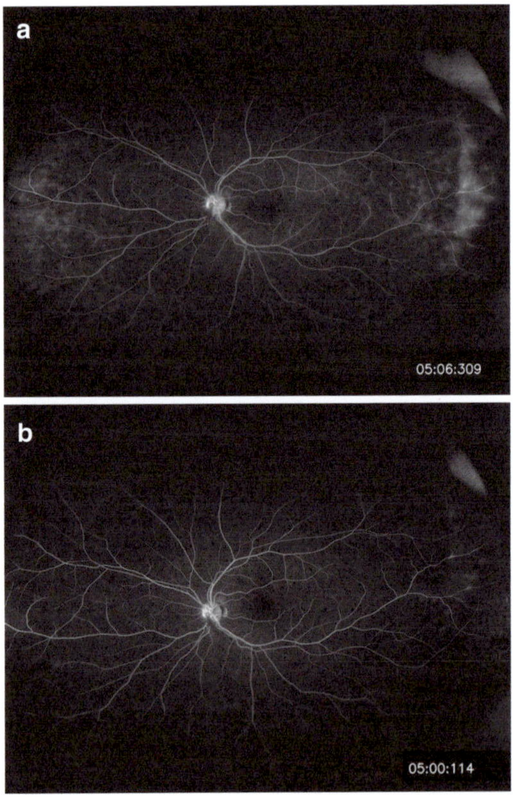

Fig. 7.1 Reduction of retinal vasculitis after infliximab therapy. Fluorescein angiography of the left eye of a 27-year-old female with idiopathic intermediate uveitis and retinal vasculitis is shown. Before the initiation of infliximab, the patient had significant vascular leakage (**a**). After the three loading infusions of infliximab, the patient demonstrated marked improvement in vascular leakage (**b**)

cystoid macular edema (CME) was more resistant to intravitreal treatment [35]. On the other hand, intravitreal infliximab used in patients with diabetic macular edema or choroidal neovascularization secondary to age-related macular degeneration was implicated as being possibly retinotoxic and inflammatory, in addition to lacking in efficacy in achieving an improvement in those non-uveitic conditions [36, 37].

Adalimumab

Adalimumab (Humira, AbbVie Inc., North Chicago, IL) is a recombinant human monoclonal IgG1κ antibody specific for TNF. It can bind both the soluble and membrane forms of TNF. Adalimumab was initially approved by the FDA in 2002 for the treatment of rheumatoid arthritis. Subsequently, it was approved for the treatment of ulcerative colitis, Crohn's disease, psoriatic arthritis, plaque psoriasis, ankylosing spondylitis, JIA, and hidradenitis suppurativa, and in July 2016, adalimumab became the first immunosuppressive drug FDA-approved for adult noninfectious intermediate uveitis, posterior uveitis, and panuveitis and was approved in September 2018 additionally for the treatment of pediatric patients 2 years old or older with noninfectious intermediate uveitis, posterior uveitis, and panuveitis. It is administered via subcutaneous injection. For the treatment of adults with noninfectious uveitis, a loading dose of 80 mg is utilized, followed by 40 mg 1 week later, and a subsequent maintenance dose of 40 mg every 2 weeks. For the treatment of adult patients with rheumatoid arthritis, psoriatic arthritis, and ankylosing spondylitis, the recommended dose is 40 mg every 2 weeks. For pediatric patients 2 years and older with JIA, the recommended dosing is based on weight: 10 mg every other week for those weighing 10 to <15 kg, 20 mg every other week for those weighing 15 to <30 kg, and 40 mg every 2 weeks for those weighing 30 kg or more. A loading regimen of 80 mg followed by 40 mg 1 week later has also been studied and approved in plaque psoriasis, and a loading dose of 160 mg followed by 80 mg 2 weeks later has been approved for adult Crohn's disease, ulcerative colitis, and hidradenitis suppurativa, with maintenance dosing then of 40 mg every other week. The majority of published literature and FDA approval supports maintenance dosing every 2 weeks in children and adults, but there is published experience in children and substantial experiential data in adults that suggest weekly dosing may benefit some patients with incomplete response to dosing every 2 weeks [38].

Several case reports, case series, and a few prospective non-comparative trials have been published since 2006 demonstrating the efficacy of adalimumab in the treatment of a number of entities of refractory uveitis including JIA-associated uveitis [39–43], Behçet's disease [40, 44], VKH disease [40], uveitis associated with ankylosing spondylitis [40], sarcoid uveitis [40, 45] (Fig. 7.2), birdshot chorioretinitis [40], pars planitis [40], or idiopathic uveitis [39, 40]. In a prospective case series of 26 patients with posterior segment involving sarcoidosis followed for 12 months, adalimumab was shown to achieve an improvement in intraocular inflammation in 22 (85%) of the patients [45]. In that study, adalimumab was shown to induce the resolution of vasculitis and CME. Another prospective trial of adalimumab in refractory uveitis in adults demonstrated initial efficacy in 68% of patients with a sustained response in 39% of the cohort at 50 weeks [46]. A prospective non-comparative trial of 131 patients with refractory uveitis found that 84.7% of subjects were able to reduce their baseline immunosuppression by at least 50% 6 months after starting adalimumab [40]. Several patients unresponsive to infliximab or who lost responsiveness to infliximab had improved control of uveitis after switching to adalimumab [41, 43, 47]. There is some evidence that use of adalimumab as a first-line agent in refractory childhood uveitis is more effective than when used as a second-line therapy [42]. In one study, intravitreal injection of adalimumab was not effective in decreasing CME refractory to steroid therapy [48].

More recently, the results of two industry-supported randomized controlled trials of adalimumab for the treatment of noninfectious intermediate uveitis, posterior uveitis, and pan-

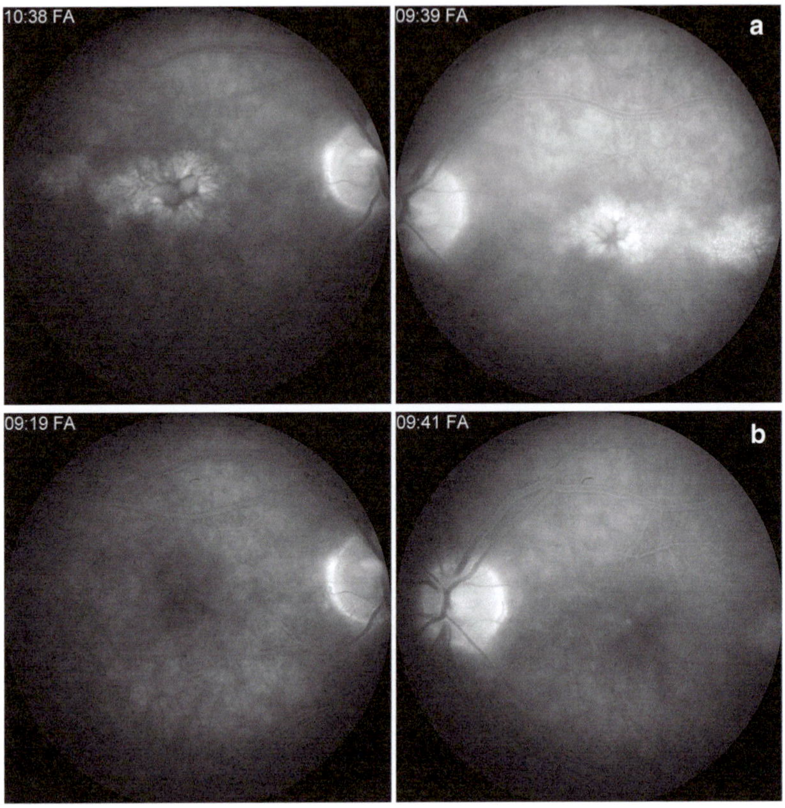

Fig. 7.2 Resolution of cystoid macular edema after treatment with adalimumab. Fluorescein angiography of a 58-year-old female with sarcoidosis panuveitis demonstrating cystoid macular edema (**a**) that resolved after the initiation of adalimumab (**b**)

uveitis were published [49, 50]. The VISUAL 1 study [49] enrolled 217 patients with active noninfectious uveitis, while the VISUAL 2 study [50] enrolled 226 corticosteroid-dependent patients with inactive noninfectious uveitis. Both studies randomized the patients to receive adalimumab or placebo subcutaneous injections, with a loading dose of 80 mg adalimumab (or placebo), 40 mg 1 week later, and then 40 mg every 2 weeks. A third study, VISUAL 3, was an open-label extension of the two randomized trials for patients who either experienced a study endpoint or completed 18 months in the study without a flare. VISUAL 1 required patients to undergo a 2-week prednisone burst to 60 mg with a forced taper off all corticosteroids by study week 15; VISUAL 2 did not require a steroid burst but required a corticosteroid taper over 19 weeks. Both studies used a primary endpoint of time to treatment failure (TTF), defined by a composite endpoint which included two-step worsening of anterior chamber cell or vitreous haze, the occurrence of new inflammatory retinal or retinovascular lesions, or a 15 letter worsening in vision on the Early Treatment Diabetic Retinopathy Study (ETDRS) chart. The primary outcome assessment for both studies was at 6 months, but patients were followed for a total of 18 months.

For the VISUAL 1 study, the median TTF was 24 weeks in the adalimumab group and 13 weeks in the placebo group. There was a 28% absolute reduction in risk of treatment failure (TF) in the adalimumab group relative to placebo at the 6-month time point. Hazard ratio for TF during 18 months of follow-up was 0.50, suggesting that risk of TF in the adalimumab group was reduced 50% relative to the placebo group over the duration of the study. For the VISUAL 2 study, the TTF was more than 18 months in the adalimumab group versus 8.3 months in the placebo group. The 40th percentile for TTF was found to be 10.2 and 4.8 months for adalimumab and placebo, respectively. Hazard ratio for TF during 18 months of follow-up was 0.57, suggesting 43% reduction of TF risk in the adalimumab group relative to placebo over the duration of the study.

VISUAL 3 reported on the additional long-term follow-up data generated on patients who had completed the two referent trials above [51]. In this open-label study, 242 of 371 (65%) patients had active uveitis; of these, 60% (145/242) achieved quiescence at week 78, and 66% of those were corticosteroid-free. Of the 129 patients entering with inactive uveitis, 74% (96/129, nonresponder imputation) achieved quiescence at week 78, and 93% of those were corticosteroid-free. Inflammatory lesions, anterior chamber inflammation grade, and vitreous haze grade, best corrected visual acuity, and mean dose of corticosteroids all showed improvement in patients with active uveitis and remained stable in patients with inactive uveitis.

The Sycamore study was an investigator-initiated randomized clinical trial conducted at tertiary hospitals in Great Britain, enrolling children with JIA with chronic uveitis despite the use of methotrexate. The study was terminated early after 90 patients were enrolled due to a high efficacy signal in favor of treatment with adalimumab over placebo, with an identified risk reduction of 75% (hazard ratio = 0.25) in the 60 adalimumab-treated patients relative to 30 patients who were treated with placebo [52]. This study was the primary underpinning of the subsequent decision of the FDA and the European Medicines Agency to approve adalimumab for its pediatric uveitis indication.

Golimumab

Golimumab (Simponi, Janssen Biotech, Horsham, PA) is an IgG1κ human monoclonal antibody against TNF that binds both the soluble and membrane forms of TNF. The FDA first approved golimumab in 2009 for the treatment of rheumatoid arthritis, psoriatic arthritis, and ankylosing spondylitis. Later on, it was also approved for the treatment of ulcerative colitis. It is administered as a subcutaneous injection at a dose of 50 mg every month for rheumatoid arthritis, psoriatic arthritis, and ankylosing spondylitis. For ulcerative colitis, it is given at loading doses of 200 mg at week 0 and 100 mg at week 2 followed by maintenance doses of 100 mg every 4 weeks.

An initial report on the use of golimumab in the treatment of uveitis appeared in 2011 [53]. That report described a patient with JIA-associated uveitis who had a relapse while on adalimumab and whose inflammation remained controlled on golimumab after a follow-up for 7 months. That report also described another patient with idiopathic retinal vasculitis who was switched from adalimumab to golimumab because of relapse of retinal vasculitis accompanied by macular edema. By 3 months after the initiation of treatment, the vitreous haze decreased, the retinal hemorrhages resolved, and the cystoid macular edema subsided (Fig. 7.3) with the inflammation remaining controlled after a follow-up for 6 months.

One retrospective case series of 13 patients with refractory uveitis due to psoriatic arthritis, sarcoidosis, axial spondyloarthritis, JIA, VKH disease, or Behçet's disease showed that golimumab controlled inflammation at 6 months in 12 of 13 patients, the majority of whom had previously failed treatment with infliximab or adalimumab [54]. Another retrospective case series of 17 patients with JIA- or HLA-B27-associated uveitis demonstrated response to golimumab therapy in 14 patients, in 12 of whom the uveitis was inactive after a mean follow-up for 21.9 months [55].

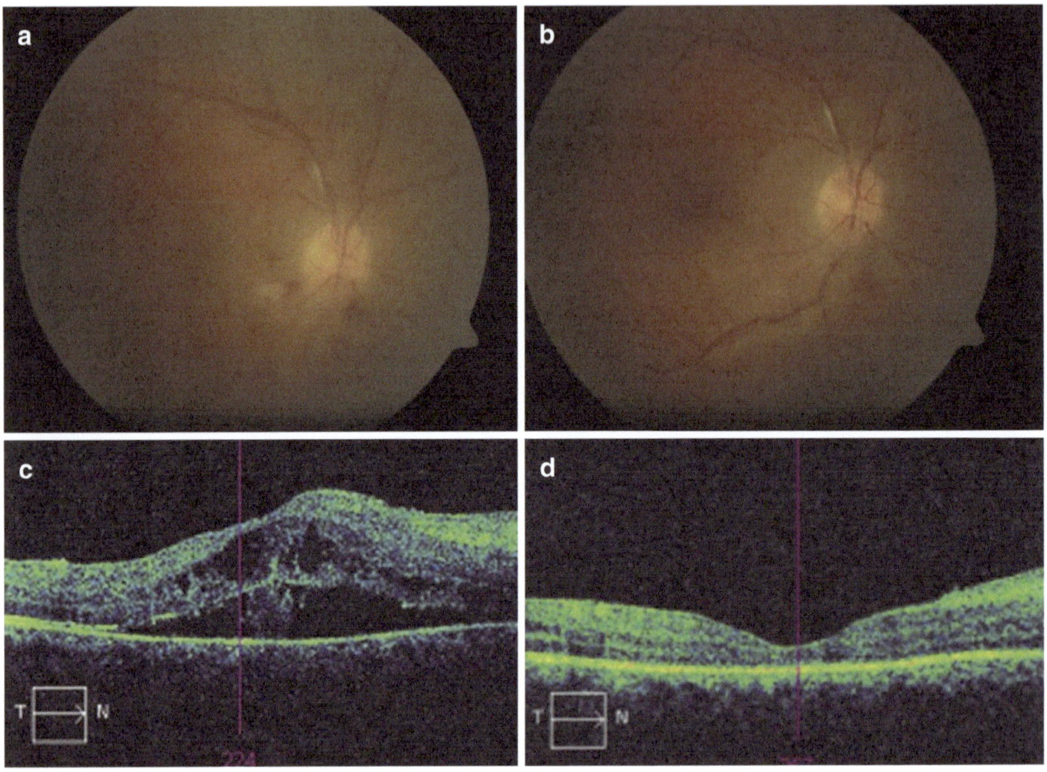

Fig. 7.3 Resolution of inflammation from idiopathic retinal vasculitis with golimumab. Color fundus photography showing vitreous haze, retinal hemorrhage, and a cotton-wool spot in the right eye of a 28-year-old male (**a**) that markedly resolved 3 months after the initiation of golimumab (**b**). Optical coherence tomography showing cystoid macular edema in the right eye (**c**) that resolved 3 months after treatment with golimumab (**d**). (Adapted with permission from reference [53])

In addition, case reports or additional small case series on the success of golimumab in treating uveitis associated with JIA [56, 57], Behçet's disease [58], and ankylosing spondylitis or psoriatic arthritis [59] have also been reported.

Certolizumab

Certolizumab pegol (pegylated certolizumab) (Cimzia, UCB Inc., Smyrna, GA) is a recombinant, humanized Fab' fragment of anti-TNF antibody conjugated to polyethylene glycol. It binds and neutralizes both the soluble and membrane forms of TNF. It was first approved by the FDA in 2008 for the treatment of Crohn's disease. Subsequently, it was also approved for the treatment of rheumatoid arthritis, psoriatic arthritis, ankylosing spondylitis, non-radiographic axial spondyloarthritis and plaque psoriasis. It is administered as a subcutaneous injection, with loading doses of 400 mg given at 0, 2, and 4 weeks and with maintenance doses of 200 mg other week or 400 mg every 4 weeks thereafter. The recommended dose for plaque psoriasis is 400 mg every other week.

There is very limited data on the use of certolizumab in uveitis. In 2014, one retrospective case series reported that five of seven patients showed quiescence of uveitis after a mean follow-up of 10.4 months while on treatment on certolizumab after having been previously being refractory to at least one of the other TNF inhibitors, namely, infliximab, adalimumab, or golimumab [60]. The patients who responded to certolizumab had uveitis or scleritis associated with Behçet's disease, psoriatic arthritis, inflammatory bowel disease, idiopathic retinal vasculitis, ankylosing spondylitis, or relapsing polychondritis. The two patients who failed to achieve remission had uveitis associated with ankylosing spondylitis or psoriatic arthritis.

A double-masked randomized clinical trial looking at the effect of certolizumab for treatment of axial spondyloarthropathy performed an analysis on rates of uveitis in patients with history of spondyloarthropathy-associated uveitis and randomized to either certolizumab or placebo and found a significant reduction in risk of uveitis flare over 96 weeks of study in certolizumab-treated patients [61]. Also, a case report in 2012 showed that certolizumab was effective in controlling refractory scleritis in a patient with rheumatoid arthritis [62]. In contrast, another report described a patient with rheumatoid arthritis well-controlled on certolizumab who developed bilateral uveitis which was thought to be secondary to the certolizumab [63].

Etanercept

Etanercept (Enbrel, Immunex Corporation, Thousand Oaks, CA) is a recombinant dimeric fusion protein that consists of the extracellular ligand-binding portion of TNFR2 linked to the Fc portion of human IgG1. It binds both the soluble and membrane forms of TNF. It is administered by a subcutaneous injection with the usual dose being 50 mg once weekly. The FDA first approved etanercept in 1998 for the treatment of rheumatoid arthritis. Subsequently, it was also approved for the treatment of polyarticular JIA, psoriatic arthritis, ankylosing spondylitis, and plaque psoriasis.

A number of reports have appeared since 2001 on the use of etanercept in the treatment of uveitis. Even though a few reports described the beneficial effects of etanercept in refractory childhood uveitis [64], JIA-associated uveitis [65], uveitis associated with ankylosing spondylitis [66], and intermediate uveitis [67], the results from other studies have been non-promising [68–70]. A randomized placebo-controlled clinical trial in pediatric JIA patients with uveitis did not identify a difference in anterior segment inflammation in subjects taking etanercept compared with placebo [70]. Even in those studies that have demonstrated an efficacy of etanercept in controlling uveitis, the etanercept was found to be less effective than infliximab in controlling inflammation [65, 66]. Also, new uveitis events have been reported in patients on etanercept compared to those patients on infliximab or adalimumab, suggesting that etanercept might induce uveitis in some patients [71]. However, it is possible that, rather than causing uveitis, etanercept is simply less effective than the other TNF inhibitors in preventing the development of uveitis in susceptible patients. Given the above observations, etanercept is not currently recommended for the use in the treatment of uveitis.

Indications for Biologics Targeting TNF in the Treatment of Uveitis

At the present time, only two biologics that target TNF, namely, infliximab and adalimumab, have significant supporting evidence for their use in the treatment of noninfectious uveitis. The evidence for their efficacy comes from case reports, case series, a few prospective non-comparative clinical trials, and, in the case of adalimumab, also randomized clinical trials (Table 7.2). Two large phase 3 clinical trials evaluating the efficacy of adalimumab in adult patients with active or inactive noninfectious uveitis (intermediate uveitis, posterior uveitis, and panuveitis) have shown beneficial effect of adalimumab in these populations, and a third large randomized trial using adalimumab for pediatric uveitis in Europe also revealed benefit leading to its approval for this indication [4, 49, 50, 52, 72].

Adalimumab has been approved by the FDA for use in adult patients and in pediatric patients 2 years or older with noninfectious intermediate uveitis, posterior uveitis, and panuveitis. Infliximab has not yet been approved by the FDA for use in the treatment of uveitis, and its use in uveitis is off-label. Both drugs are very expensive. Adalimumab has the advantage of being given via subcutaneous injection which the patient can self-administer, whereas infliximab is administered via intravenous infusion. Recently, an expert panel has recommended considering the use of infliximab or adalimumab as a first-line immunomodulating agent in treating the ocular manifestations of Behçet's disease and as a potential second-line immunomodulating therapy in the treatment of JIA-associated uveitis [73].

Table 7.2 Ophthalmic indications of anti-TNF biologic drugs

Drug	Specific conditions[a]
Infliximab	Behçet's disease JIA-associated anterior uveitis HLA-B27-associated anterior uveitis Sarcoid uveitis Birdshot chorioretinitis Uveitis secondary to Crohn's disease Vogt-Koyanagi-Harada disease Scleritis Idiopathic posterior uveitis
Adalimumab	Noninfectious intermediate uveitis, posterior uveitis, and panuveitis (FDA-approved)[b] Behçet's disease JIA-associated uveitis Uveitis associated with ankylosing spondylitis Sarcoid uveitis Birdshot chorioretinitis Pars planitis Idiopathic uveitis

[a]Based on the findings of case reports, case series, and prospective non-comparative clinical trials
[b]Evidence from three randomized controlled trials

Not all patients with uveitis respond to infliximab or adalimumab therapy. One possible explanation is that the inflammatory process in those patients may be primarily mediated by other inflammatory cytokines, such as IL-1 or IL-6 instead of TNF. Alternatively, some patients can develop antibodies against infliximab or adalimumab and such antibodies have been detected in the sera of patients [74, 75]. Such antibodies could bind the respective drug and prevent it from binding to TNF. This mechanism could result in loss of responsiveness to infliximab or adalimumab in some patients after an initial response. Switching from one of the two drugs to the other could be beneficial in those cases. Sometimes treatment with biologic agents directed at inflammatory molecules other than TNF might also be beneficial.

Safety of Biologics Targeting TNF in the Treatment of Uveitis

Malignancy and Infection Risks

In general, the biologics targeting TNF have a good safety profile. All of the biologic anti-TNF agents carry boxed warnings about increased risk of malignancy or serious infection (Table 7.3). A large retrospective study of uveitis patients (the Systemic Immunosuppressive Therapy for Eye Diseases, or SITE Research Study) treated with immunosuppression identified an increased risk of overall mortality [adjusted hazard ratio 1.99] and cancer-specific mortality [adjusted hazard ratio 3.83] in patients treated with TNF inhibitors [76], although this finding notably was not replicated in the same study cohort with expanded patient numbers and longer patient follow-up [77]. Data from the rheumatologic literature is mixed. A meta-analysis of randomized, placebo-controlled trials of infliximab and adalimumab in rheumatoid arthritis patients identified a pooled odds ratio for malignancy of 3.3, with a dose-dependent effect [78]. However, a systematic literature review of observational studies and registries did not identify any increased risk of cancer in rheumatoid arthritis patients treated with TNF inhibitors compared to those treated with other immunosuppressive agents, although the risk of melanoma may be slightly increased with anti-TNF therapy [79]. The 2015 American College of Rheumatology guidelines for treating rheumatoid arthritis recommend using other immunosuppressant agents over TNF inhibitors in patients with previously treated or untreated skin cancer (including melanoma) and previously treated lymphoproliferative disorders,

Table 7.3 Contraindications for the use of TNF inhibitors

Drug	Manufacturer-specified contraindications
Infliximab	Moderate or severe heart failure (infliximab >5 mg/kg) History of severe hypersensitivity reaction to infliximab Known hypersensitivity to inactive components of the pharmaceutical product Known hypersensitivity to any murine protein
Adalimumab	None
Golimumab	None
Certolizumab	History of hypersensitivity to certolizumab pegol or to any of the excipients
Etanercept	Sepsis
Relative contraindications for TNF inhibitors	
Active infection	
Latent tuberculosis	
Chronic hepatitis B	
Known demyelinating disease	
Moderate to severe heart failure	
Solid malignancy or nonmelanoma skin cancer within the last 5 years	
History of skin melanoma	
History of lymphoproliferative malignancy	

but do not recommend alternative therapy considerations in the setting of previously treated solid organ malignancy [80]. The use of TNF inhibitors in conjunction with azathioprine or 6-mercaptopurine has been reported to increase the risk of T cell non-Hodgkin lymphoma, most commonly the hepatosplenic T cell lymphoma subtype, in patients with inflammatory bowel disease [81]. This is a rare malignancy, but can be fatal and is included in the black box warnings for TNF inhibitors.

As a class, the TNF inhibitors increase the risk of developing severe infections including invasive fungal infections, particularly if being used in the setting of a concomitant immunosuppressive drug. Latent tuberculosis may undergo reactivation with the use of anti-TNF agents, making it necessary to screen patients for tuberculosis prior to starting treatment. Patients with a positive tuberculosis test should be treated for active or latent tuberculosis as appropriate; after adequate tuberculosis treatment, the patient can begin anti-TNF therapy. In patients at risk for ongoing tuberculosis exposure, yearly screening for tuberculosis is recommended. Similarly, chronic hepatitis B carriers can develop reactivation of the hepatitis B virus with TNF suppression, and hence, hepatitis screening is necessary prior to treatment.

Other Adverse Effects

Hypersensitivity and injection site reactions are among the most common adverse effects of anti-TNF treatment. Hypersensitivity reactions may be mitigated with premedication with antihistamines, acetaminophen, and even corticosteroids. Similarly, injection site reactions can also be reduced with antihistamines, icing the injection site and rotating injection locations. The TNF inhibitors as a class may worsen congestive heart failure and are not recommended for use in patients with New York Heart Association class III or IV disease. Case reports of drug-induced lupus-like syndrome [34], granulomatous sarcoidosis-like disease [82], and psoriasis [83] have been reported in association with TNF inhibition. Demyelinating diseases, including multiple sclerosis and optic neuritis, have also been reported in patients receiving anti-TNF therapy [84, 85]. Given the known association between multiple sclerosis and intermediate uveitis, it is incumbent upon treating physicians to rule out demyelinating disease prior to starting a TNF blocker. As TNF inhibition may exacerbate preexisting demyelinating disease, use of these agents is not recommended in patients with a known history of demyelinating disease.

Vaccination and Anti-TNF Agents

The American College of Rheumatology makes several recommendations about vaccination of patients undergoing treatment with TNF inhibitors for rheumatoid arthritis that are applicable to uveitis patients [86]. Vaccination against pneumococcal pneumonia, influenza, hepatitis B (in high-risk populations), human papillomavirus, and herpes zoster should be completed prior to starting treatment with a TNF inhibitor. If a patient is already on anti-TNF therapy, vaccinations with killed vaccines (pneumococcal, hepatitis B, and injectable influenza) and recombinant vaccines (human papillomavirus) are safe; however, live vaccines such as for herpes zoster and the nasal influenza vaccine are not recommended. In the pediatric population, the vaccination schedule should be discussed with the patient's pediatrician with the goal of completing vaccinations as able.

Use in Special Populations

All of the TNF inhibitors are pregnancy category B, as there are no adequate and well-controlled studies in pregnant women to assess for fetal risk. Animal reproduction studies have not identified fetal harm due to these drugs. There is evidence that all of the TNF inhibitors cross the placenta; however, observational surveillance of women who continued on TNF inhibitors during their pregnancies has not identified increased risks to the fetus. These pregnancy surveillance programs are ongoing. At present, it is reasonable to continue anti-TNF therapy during pregnancy after careful discussion with the patient if the benefits of treatment are thought to outweigh any theoretical risks. There are no clear recommendations for nursing mothers treated with TNF inhibitors.

Several of the anti-TNF agents have been specifically studied in children for treatment of childhood inflammatory disease. Infliximab is approved for the treatment of pediatric Crohn's disease and ulcerative colitis in patients 6–17 years of age. Adalimumab has similarly been approved for treatment of pediatric Crohn's disease in patients 6 years of age or older. Adalimumab was found safe and effective in the treatment of JIA and noninfectious intermediate uveitis, posterior uveitis and panuveitis in children aged 2 and older and has been approved for these indications; it has not been studied in children less than 2 or weighing less than 10 kg. Infliximab has been used off-label to treat childhood uveitis. Etanercept is also approved for treating children 2 years or older with polyarticular JIA, although use in treatment of uveitis is not recommended as previously discussed. Certolizumab and golimumab do not have any approved indications for use in children, although there are case reports of using golimumab to treat refractory JIA-associated uveitis without an adverse event in children [56, 59]. There are no specific recommendations to alter treatment in the elderly; however, given the increased risk for infection and malignancy in this patient population, appropriate counseling and close monitoring are advised.

Laboratory Monitoring

In addition to screening for infections, baseline laboratory evaluation including a complete blood count, liver function tests, and serum creatinine should be obtained before starting a TNF inhibitor. Similar laboratory evaluation should be completed several weeks after starting therapy and following any significant dose modifications as elevation of liver function tests and rarely cytopenia have been observed with TNF inhibitor therapy. Interval monitoring should be conducted every 3–6 months in patients without additional risk factors for hepatic or renal disease, although concurrent therapy with other immunosuppressive agents may require more frequent laboratory monitoring.

Acknowledgments LJK has served as a coinvestigator in clinical trials sponsored by AbbVie, Bristol-Myers-Squibb, Genentech, pSivida, and the National Eye Institute and was also supported by institutional grants to the Casey Eye Institute from the National Eye Institute and Research to Prevent Blindness. AS is supported by a Mallinckrodt Foundation Research Fellowship Award. In addition, AS has participated as a coinvestigator in clinical trials sponsored by AbbVie, Bristol-Myers-Squibb, pSivida, and Genentech, the National Eye Institute, University of Pennsylvania, Research to Prevent Blindness, and Allergan.

References

1. De Vos AF, Van Haren MA, Verhagen C, Hoekzema R, Kijlstra A. Kinetics of intraocular tumor necrosis factor and interleukin-6 in endotoxin-induced uveitis in the rat. Invest Ophthalmol Vis Sci. 1994;35(3):1100–6.
2. Santos LM, Marcos MC, Gallardo Galera JM, Gomez Vidal MA, Collantes EE, Ramirez CR, et al. Aqueous humor and serum tumor necrosis factor-alpha in clinical uveitis. Ophthalmic Res. 2001;33(5):251–5.
3. Ozdamar Y, Berker N, Bahar G, Soykan E, Bicer T, Ozkan SS, et al. Inflammatory mediators and posterior segment involvement in ocular Behcet disease. Eur J Ophthalmol. 2009;19(6):998–1003.
4. Kopplin LJ, Shifera AS, Suhler EB, Lin P. Biological response modifiers in the treatment of noninfectious uveitis. Int Ophthalmol Clin. 2015;55(2):19–36.
5. Wajant H, Pfizenmaier K, Scheurich P. Tumor necrosis factor signaling. Cell Death Differ. 2003;10(1):45–65.
6. Tracey KJ, Cerami A. Tumor necrosis factor: a pleiotropic cytokine and therapeutic target. Annu Rev Med. 1994;45:491–503.
7. Chu WM. Tumor necrosis factor. Cancer Lett. 2013;328(2):222–5.
8. Willermain F, Rosenbaum JT, Bodaghi B, Rosenzweig HL, Childers S, Behrend T, et al. Interplay between innate and adaptive immunity in the development of non-infectious uveitis. Prog Retin Eye Res. 2012;31(2):182–94.
9. Dick AD, Forrester JV, Liversidge J, Cope AP. The role of tumour necrosis factor (TNF-alpha) in experimental autoimmune uveoretinitis (EAU). Prog Retin Eye Res. 2004;23(6):617–37.
10. De Vos AF, Van Haren MA, Verhagen C, Hoekzema R, Kijlstra A. Tumour necrosis factor-induced uveitis in the Lewis rat is associated with intraocular interleukin 6 production. Exp Eye Res. 1995;60(2):199–207.
11. Rosenbaum JT, Howes EL Jr, Rubin RM, Samples JR. Ocular inflammatory effects of intravitreally-injected tumor necrosis factor. Am J Pathol. 1988;133(1):47–53.
12. Smith JR, Levinson RD, Holland GN, Jabs DA, Robinson MR, Whitcup SM, et al. Differential efficacy of tumor necrosis factor inhibition in the management of inflammatory eye disease and associated rheumatic disease. Arthritis Rheum. 2001;45(3):252–7.
13. Sfikakis PP, Theodossiadis PG, Katsiari CG, Kaklamanis P, Markomichelakis NN. Effect of infliximab on sight-threatening panuveitis in Behcet's disease. Lancet. 2001;358(9278):295–6.
14. Arayssi T, Hamra R, Homeidan F, Uthman I, Awwad ST, Mroue K, et al. The efficacy of a single dose of infliximab in the treatment of Behcet's disease uveitis. Clin Exp Rheumatol. 2005;23(3):427.
15. Mansour AM. Infliximab treatment of posterior uveitis. Ophthalmology. 2004;111(1):197–8.
16. itez-Del-Castillo JM, Martinez-de-la-Casa JM, Pato-Cour E, Mendez-Fernandez R, Lopez-Abad C, Matilla M, et al. Long-term treatment of refractory posterior uveitis with anti-TNFalpha (infliximab). Eye (Lond). 2005;19(8):841–5.
17. Joseph A, Raj D, Dua HS, Powell PT, Lanyon PC, Powell RJ. Infliximab in the treatment of refractory posterior uveitis. Ophthalmology. 2003;110(7):1449–53.
18. Tugal-Tutkun I, Mudun A, Urgancioglu M, Kamali S, Kasapoglu E, Inanc M, et al. Efficacy of infliximab in the treatment of uveitis that is resistant to treatment with the combination of azathioprine, cyclosporine, and corticosteroids in Behcet's disease: an open-label trial. Arthritis Rheum. 2005;52(8):2478–84.
19. Wechsler B, Sable-Fourtassou R, Bodaghi B, Huong DL, Cassoux N, Badelon I, et al. Infliximab in refractory uveitis due to Behcet's disease. Clin Exp Rheumatol. 2004;22(4 Suppl 34):S14–6.
20. Kruithof E, Kestelyn P, Elewaut C, Elewaut D, Van Den BF, Mielants H, et al. Successful use of infliximab in a patient with treatment resistant spondyloarthropathy related uveitis. Ann Rheum Dis. 2002;61(5):470.
21. El-Shabrawi Y, Hermann J. Anti-tumor necrosis factor-alpha therapy with infliximab as an alternative to corticosteroids in the treatment of human leukocyte antigen B27-associated acute anterior uveitis. Ophthalmology. 2002;109(12):2342–6.
22. El-Shabrawi Y, Hermann J. Case series of selective anti-tumor necrosis factor alpha therapy using infliximab in patients with nonresponsive chronic HLA-B27-associated anterior uveitis: comment on the articles by Brandt et al. Arthritis Rheum. 2002;46(10):2821–2.
23. Kahn P, Weiss M, Imundo LF, Levy DM. Favorable response to high-dose infliximab for refractory childhood uveitis. Ophthalmology. 2006;113(5):860–4.
24. Rajaraman RT, Kimura Y, Li S, Haines K, Chu DS. Retrospective case review of pediatric patients with uveitis treated with infliximab. Ophthalmology. 2006;113(2):308–14.
25. Murphy CC, Ayliffe WH, Booth A, Makanjuola D, Andrews PA, Jayne D. Tumor necrosis factor alpha blockade with infliximab for refractory uveitis and scleritis. Ophthalmology. 2004;111(2):352–6.
26. Mangge H, Heinzl B, Grubbauer HM, El-Shabrawi Y, Schauenstein K. Therapeutic experience with infliximab in a patient with polyarticular juve-

nile idiopathic arthritis and uveitis. Rheumatol Int. 2003;23(5):258–61.
27. Baughman RP, Bradley DA, Lower EE. Infliximab in chronic ocular inflammation. Int J Clin Pharmacol Ther. 2005;43(1):7–11.
28. Doty JD, Mazur JE, Judson MA. Treatment of sarcoidosis with infliximab. Chest. 2005;127(3):1064–71.
29. Pritchard C, Nadarajah K. Tumour necrosis factor alpha inhibitor treatment for sarcoidosis refractory to conventional treatments: a report of five patients. Ann Rheum Dis. 2004;63(3):318–20.
30. Fries W, Giofre MR, Catanoso M, Lo GR. Treatment of acute uveitis associated with Crohn's disease and sacroileitis with infliximab. Am J Gastroenterol. 2002;97(2):499–500.
31. Ally MR, Veerappan GR, Koff JM. Treatment of recurrent Crohn's uveitis with infliximab. Am J Gastroenterol. 2008;103(8):2150–1.
32. Rispo A, Scarpa R, Di GE, Cozzolino A, Lembo G, Atteno M, et al. Infliximab in the treatment of extra-intestinal manifestations of Crohn's disease. Scand J Rheumatol. 2005;34(5):387–91.
33. Niccoli L, Nannini C, Benucci M, Chindamo D, Cassara E, Salvarani C, et al. Long-term efficacy of infliximab in refractory posterior uveitis of Behcet's disease: a 24-month follow-up study. Rheumatology (Oxford). 2007;46(7):1161–4.
34. Suhler EB, Smith JR, Giles TR, Lauer AK, Wertheim MS, Kurz DE, et al. Infliximab therapy for refractory uveitis: 2-year results of a prospective trial. Arch Ophthalmol. 2009;127(6):819–22.
35. Markomichelakis N, Delicha E, Masselos S, Sfikakis PP. Intravitreal infliximab for sight-threatening relapsing uveitis in Behcet disease: a pilot study in 15 patients. Am J Ophthalmol. 2012;154(3):534–41.
36. Giganti M, Beer PM, Lemanski N, Hartman C, Schartman J, Falk N. Adverse events after intravitreal infliximab (Remicade). Retina. 2010;30(1):71–80.
37. Wu L, Hernandez-Bogantes E, Roca JA, Arevalo JF, Barraza K, Lasave AF. Intravitreal tumor necrosis factor inhibitors in the treatment of refractory diabetic macular edema: a pilot study from the Pan-American Collaborative Retina Study Group. Retina. 2011;31(2):298–303.
38. Correll CK, Bullock DR, Cafferty RM, Vehe RK. Safety of weekly adalimumab in the treatment of juvenile idiopathic arthritis and pediatric chronic uveitis. Clin Rheumatol. 2018;37(2):549–53.
39. Vazquez-Cobian LB, Flynn T, Lehman TJ. Adalimumab therapy for childhood uveitis. J Pediatr. 2006;149(4):572–5.
40. Diaz-Llopis M, Salom D, Garcia-De-Vicuna C, Cordero-Coma M, Ortega G, Ortego N, et al. Treatment of refractory uveitis with adalimumab: a prospective multicenter study of 131 patients. Ophthalmology. 2012;119(8):1575–81.
41. Biester S, Deuter C, Michels H, Haefner R, Kuemmerle-Deschner J, Doycheva D, et al. Adalimumab in the therapy of uveitis in childhood. Br J Ophthalmol. 2007;91(3):319–24.
42. Simonini G, Taddio A, Cattalini M, Caputo R, de LC, Parentin F, et al. Superior efficacy of adalimumab in treating childhood refractory chronic uveitis when used as first biologic modifier drug: adalimumab as starting anti-TNF-alpha therapy in childhood chronic uveitis. Pediatr Rheumatol Online J. 2013;11:16.
43. Tynjala P, Kotaniemi K, Lindahl P, Latva K, Aalto K, Honkanen V, et al. Adalimumab in juvenile idiopathic arthritis-associated chronic anterior uveitis. Rheumatology (Oxford). 2008;47(3):339–44.
44. Mushtaq B, Saeed T, Situnayake RD, Murray PI. Adalimumab for sight-threatening uveitis in Behcet's disease. Eye (Lond). 2007;21(6):824–5.
45. Erckens RJ, Mostard RL, Wijnen PA, Schouten JS, Drent M. Adalimumab successful in sarcoidosis patients with refractory chronic non-infectious uveitis. Graefes Arch Clin Exp Ophthalmol. 2012;250(5):713–20.
46. Suhler EB, Lowder CY, Goldstein DA, Giles T, Lauer AK, Kurz PA, et al. Adalimumab therapy for refractory uveitis: results of a multicentre, open-label, prospective trial. Br J Ophthalmol. 2013;97(4):481–6.
47. Bawazeer A, Raffa LH, Nizamuddin SH. Clinical experience with adalimumab in the treatment of ocular Behcet disease. Ocul Immunol Inflamm. 2010;18(3):226–32.
48. Androudi S, Tsironi E, Kalogeropoulos C, Theodoridou A, Brazitikos P. Intravitreal adalimumab for refractory uveitis-related macular edema. Ophthalmology. 2010;117(8):1612–6.
49. Jaffe GJ, Dick AD, Brezin AP, Nguyen QD, Thorne JE, Kestelyn P, et al. Adalimumab in patients with active noninfectious uveitis. N Engl J Med. 2016;375(10):932–43.
50. Nguyen QD, Merrill PT, Jaffe GJ, Dick AD, Kurup SK, Sheppard J, et al. Adalimumab for prevention of uveitic flare in patients with inactive non-infectious uveitis controlled by corticosteroids (VISUAL II): a multicentre, double-masked, randomised, placebo-controlled phase 3 trial. Lancet. 2016;388(10050):1183–92.
51. Suhler EB, Adán A, Brézin AP, Fortin E, Goto H, Jaffe GJ, Kaburaki T, Kramer M, Lim LL, Muccioli C, Nguyen QD, Van Calster J, Cimino L, Kron M, Song AP, Liu J, Pathai S, Camez A, Schlaen A, van Velthoven MEJ, Vitale AT, Zierhut M, Tari S, Dick AD. Safety and efficacy of adalimumab in patients with noninfectious uveitis in an ongoing open-label study: VISUAL III. Ophthalmology. 2018;125(7):1075–87.
52. Ramanan AV, Dick AD, Jones AP, McKay A, Williamson PR, Compeyrot-Lacassagne S, Hardwick B, Hickey H, Hughes D, Woo P, Benton D, Edelsten C, Beresford MW, SYCAMORE Study Group. Adalimumab plus methotrexate for uveitis in juvenile idiopathic arthritis. N Engl J Med. 2017;376(17):1637–46.

53. Cordero-Coma M, Salom D, Diaz-Llopis M, Lopez-Prats MJ, Calleja S. Golimumab for uveitis. Ophthalmology. 2011;118(9):1892–4.
54. Cordero-Coma M, Calvo-Rio V, Adan A, Blanco R, Alvarez-Castro C, Mesquida M, et al. Golimumab as rescue therapy for refractory immune-mediated uveitis: a three-center experience. Mediat Inflamm. 2014;2014:717598.
55. Miserocchi E, Modorati G, Pontikaki I, Meroni PL, Gerloni V. Long-term treatment with golimumab for severe uveitis. Ocul Immunol Inflamm. 2014;22(2):90–5.
56. William M, Faez S, Papaliodis GN, Lobo AM. Golimumab for the treatment of refractory juvenile idiopathic arthritis-associated uveitis. J Ophthalmic Inflamm Infect. 2012;2(4):231–3.
57. Miserocchi E, Modorati G, Pontikaki I, Meroni P, Gerloni V. Golimumab treatment for complicated uveitis. Clin Exp Rheumatol. 2013;31(2):320–1.
58. Mesquida M, Victoria HM, Llorenc V, Pelegrin L, Espinosa G, Dick AD, et al. Behcet disease-associated uveitis successfully treated with golimumab. Ocul Immunol Inflamm. 2013;21(2):160–2.
59. Faez S, Lobo AM, Sobrin L, Papaliodis GN. Treatment of seronegative spondyloarthropathy-associated uveitis with golimumab: retrospective case series. Clin Exp Ophthalmol. 2014;42(4):392–5.
60. Llorenc V, Mesquida M, Sainz de la MM, Blanco R, Calvo V, Maiz O, et al. Certolizumab Pegol, a new anti-TNF-alpha in the armamentarium against ocular inflammation. Ocul Immunol Inflamm. 2016;24(2):167–72.
61. Rudwaleit M, Rosenbaum JT, Landewe R, Marzo-Ortega H, Sieper J, van der HD, et al. Observed incidence of uveitis following Certolizumab Pegol treatment in patients with axial Spondyloarthritis. Arthritis Care Res (Hoboken). 2016;68(6):838–44.
62. Tlucek PS, Stone DU. Certolizumab pegol therapy for rheumatoid arthritis-associated scleritis. Cornea. 2012;31(1):90–1.
63. Moisseiev E, Shulman S. Certolizumab-induced uveitis: a case report and review of the literature. Case Rep Ophthalmol. 2014;5(1):54–9.
64. Reiff A, Takei S, Sadeghi S, Stout A, Shaham B, Bernstein B, et al. Etanercept therapy in children with treatment-resistant uveitis. Arthritis Rheum. 2001;44(6):1411–5.
65. Tynjala P, Lindahl P, Honkanen V, Lahdenne P, Kotaniemi K. Infliximab and etanercept in the treatment of chronic uveitis associated with refractory juvenile idiopathic arthritis. Ann Rheum Dis. 2007;66(4):548–50.
66. Braun J, Baraliakos X, Listing J, Sieper J. Decreased incidence of anterior uveitis in patients with ankylosing spondylitis treated with the anti-tumor necrosis factor agents infliximab and etanercept. Arthritis Rheum. 2005;52(8):2447–51.
67. Manzano RP, Carvounis PE, Albini TA, Holz ER. Etanercept monotherapy induces complete resolution of cystoid macular edema in a patient with intermediate uveitis. Retin Cases Brief Rep. 2007;1(4):261–3.
68. Foster CS, Tufail F, Waheed NK, Chu D, Miserocchi E, Baltatzis S, et al. Efficacy of etanercept in preventing relapse of uveitis controlled by methotrexate. Arch Ophthalmol. 2003;121(4):437–40.
69. Schmeling H, Horneff G. Etanercept and uveitis in patients with juvenile idiopathic arthritis. Rheumatology (Oxford). 2005;44(8):1008–11.
70. Smith JA, Thompson DJ, Whitcup SM, Suhler E, Clarke G, Smith S, et al. A randomized, placebo-controlled, double-masked clinical trial of etanercept for the treatment of uveitis associated with juvenile idiopathic arthritis. Arthritis Rheum. 2005;53(1):18–23.
71. Shifera AS, Kopplin L, Lin P, Suhler EB. Drug-induced uveitis. Int Ophthalmol Clin. 2015;55(2):47–65.
72. Hawkins MJ, Dick AD, Lee RJ, Ramanan AV, Carreno E, Guly CM, et al. Managing juvenile idiopathic arthritis-associated uveitis. Surv Ophthalmol. 2016;61(2):197–210.
73. Levy-Clarke G, Jabs DA, Read RW, Rosenbaum JT, Vitale A, Van Gelder RN. Expert panel recommendations for the use of anti-tumor necrosis factor biologic agents in patients with ocular inflammatory disorders. Ophthalmology. 2014;121(3):785–96.
74. Measurement of infliximab and anti-infliximab antibody levels can help distinguish maintenance versus loss of response. Gastroenterol Hepatol (NY). 2012;8(2):131–4.
75. Vogelzang EH, Kneepkens EL, Nurmohamed MT, van Kuijk AW, Rispens T, Wolbink G, et al. Anti-adalimumab antibodies and adalimumab concentrations in psoriatic arthritis; an association with disease activity at 28 and 52 weeks of follow-up. Ann Rheum Dis. 2014;73(12):2178–82.
76. Kempen JH, Daniel E, Dunn JP, Foster CS, Gangaputra S, Hanish A, et al. Overall and cancer related mortality among patients with ocular inflammation treated with immunosuppressive drugs: retrospective cohort study. BMJ. 2009;339:b2480.
77. Kempen JH, Newcomb CW, Foster CS, Jabs DA, Levy-Clarke G, Rosenbaum JT, Nida Sen H, Suhler EB, Thorne JE, Bhatt NP, Buchanich JM. Risk of overall and cancer mortality after immunosuppression of patients with non-infectious ocular inflammatory diseases. Invest Ophthalmol Vis Sci. 2019;60:ARVO E-Abstract 3854.
78. Bongartz T, Sutton AJ, Sweeting MJ, Buchan I, Matteson EL, Montori V. Anti-TNF antibody therapy in rheumatoid arthritis and the risk of serious infections and malignancies: systematic review and meta-analysis of rare harmful effects in randomized controlled trials. JAMA. 2006;295(19):2275–85.
79. Ramiro S, Gaujoux-Viala C, Nam JL, Smolen JS, Buch M, Gossec L, et al. Safety of synthetic and biological DMARDs: a systematic literature review informing the 2013 update of the EULAR recommen-

dations for management of rheumatoid arthritis. Ann Rheum Dis. 2014;73(3):529–35.
80. Singh JA, Saag KG, Bridges SL Jr, Akl EA, Bannuru RR, Sullivan MC, et al. 2015 American College of Rheumatology guideline for the treatment of rheumatoid arthritis. Arthritis Care Res (Hoboken). 2016;68(1):1–25.
81. Deepak P, Sifuentes H, Sherid M, Stobaugh D, Sadozai Y, Ehrenpreis ED. T-cell non-Hodgkin's lymphomas reported to the FDA AERS with tumor necrosis factor-alpha (TNF-alpha) inhibitors: results of the REFURBISH study. Am J Gastroenterol. 2013;108(1):99–105.
82. Tong D, Manolios N, Howe G, Spencer D. New onset sarcoid-like granulomatosis developing during anti-TNF therapy: an under-recognised complication. Intern Med J. 2012;42(1):89–94.
83. Famenini S, Wu JJ. Infliximab-induced psoriasis in treatment of Crohn's disease-associated ankylosing spondylitis: case report and review of 142 cases. J Drugs Dermatol. 2013;12(8):939–43.
84. Mohan N, Edwards ET, Cupps TR, Oliverio PJ, Sandberg G, Crayton H, et al. Demyelination occurring during anti-tumor necrosis factor alpha therapy for inflammatory arthritides. Arthritis Rheum. 2001;44(12):2862–9.
85. Foroozan R, Buono LM, Sergott RC, Savino PJ. Retrobulbar optic neuritis associated with infliximab. Arch Ophthalmol. 2002;120(7):985–7.
86. Singh JA, Furst DE, Bharat A, Curtis JR, Kavanaugh AF, Kremer JM, et al. 2012 update of the 2008 American College of Rheumatology recommendations for the use of disease-modifying antirheumatic drugs and biologic agents in the treatment of rheumatoid arthritis. Arthritis Care Res (Hoboken). 2012;64(5):625–39.

Biologics Targeting B- and T-Cell Activation

8

George R. Mount

Abbreviations

APC	Antigen-presenting cell
COPD	Chronic obstructive pulmonary disease
CTLA4	Cytotoxic T-lymphocyte-associated antigen 4
FDA	Food and Drug Administration
GPA	Granulomatosis with polyangiitis
JIA	Juvenile idiopathic arthritis
MPA	Microscopic polyangiitis
PML	Progressive multifocal leukoencephalopathy

Pearls

- Rituximab is a monoclonal antibody which blocks CD-20, a cell surface marker found on B-lymphocytes but not on plasma cells.
- Rituximab is commonly administered as paired 1000 mg intravenous doses given 2 weeks apart, and repeated every 6 months if benefit is realized.
- Peri-infusional corticosteroids may be useful with initial infusions to prevent a transient worsening due to a tumor lysis-like response.
- Abatacept is a fusion protein combining the Fc portion of human IgG1 with soluble CTLA4 immunoglobulin, which reduces T-cell activation by blocking T-cell co-stimulation, and may be given either intravenously or subcutaneously.

Disclosure The views expressed are those of the author and do not reflect the official policy of the Department of the Army, the Department of Defense, or the U.S. Government.

G. R. Mount (✉)
Casey Eye Institute, Oregon Health and Science University, Portland, OR, USA

Madigan Army Medical Center, Tacoma, WA, USA
e-mail: george.r.mount.mil@mail.mil

Introduction

Biologics are medications manufactured by recombinant DNA technology to target specific pathways that contribute to the inflammatory response. These pathways include cytokine-directed therapies, interference of T- and B-cell interactions, B-cell depletion, induction of tolerance, interference with immune complex formation, and chemokine modulation. Biologics are approved and employed in the treatment of a variety of systemic inflammatory diseases, to include entities such as rheumatoid arthritis, psoriatic arthritis, spondyloarthritis, and inflammatory bowel disease. The off-label use of biologic agents offers an alternative therapeutic approach

P. Lin, E. Suhler (eds.), *Treatment of Non-infectious Uveitis*,
https://doi.org/10.1007/978-3-030-22827-9_8

for the patient with ocular inflammation who has failed or poorly tolerated traditional immunosuppressive agents.

Many of the more commonly used biologics target specific cytokines that play a key role in the inflammatory process. An alternative approach focuses on preventing B- or T-cell activation. Rituximab is a chimeric mouse–human IgG1κ monoclonal antibody directed against the extracellular domain of CD20 antigen on B cells, targeting of which allows for selective elimination of B cells. Abatacept, a fully human fusion protein comprising the extracellular portion of CTLA4 and the Fc fragment of IgG1, binds to a receptor target on the antigen-presenting cell preventing proper interaction with the T cell, and therefore, proper T-cell activation.

Targeting B-Cell Activation

Anti-CD20 Therapy (Rituximab)

B cells are antigen-specific, antibody-secreting lymphocytes produced in the bone marrow and released into the circulation. Upon encountering the antigenic peptide for which its immunoglobulin receptor is specific, a B cell is activated to participate in several important immune response mechanisms. These include interactions with T cells resulting in the production of inflammatory cytokines, generation of memory B cells, and development of long- and short-lived plasma cells [1]. CD20 is a 33- to 37-kDa, non-glycosylated phosphoprotein expressed on the surface of mature B cells that have exited the bone marrow to enter the blood. CD20 is expressed on the surface of all B cells except stem cells and plasma cells that have returned to the bone marrow (Fig. 8.1). As such, targeting CD20 allows for selective elimination of B cells with subsequent B-cell regeneration from unaffected stem cells, effectively rebooting the B-cell-driven immune response [2]. Likewise, the selective sparing of plasma cells allows for the preservation of immunoglobulin levels.

Rituximab (Rituxan®, Genentech, Inc.) is a chimeric mouse/human monoclonal antibody directed against the B lymphocyte surface antigen CD20 (Fig. 8.2) [3]. Rituximab was initially

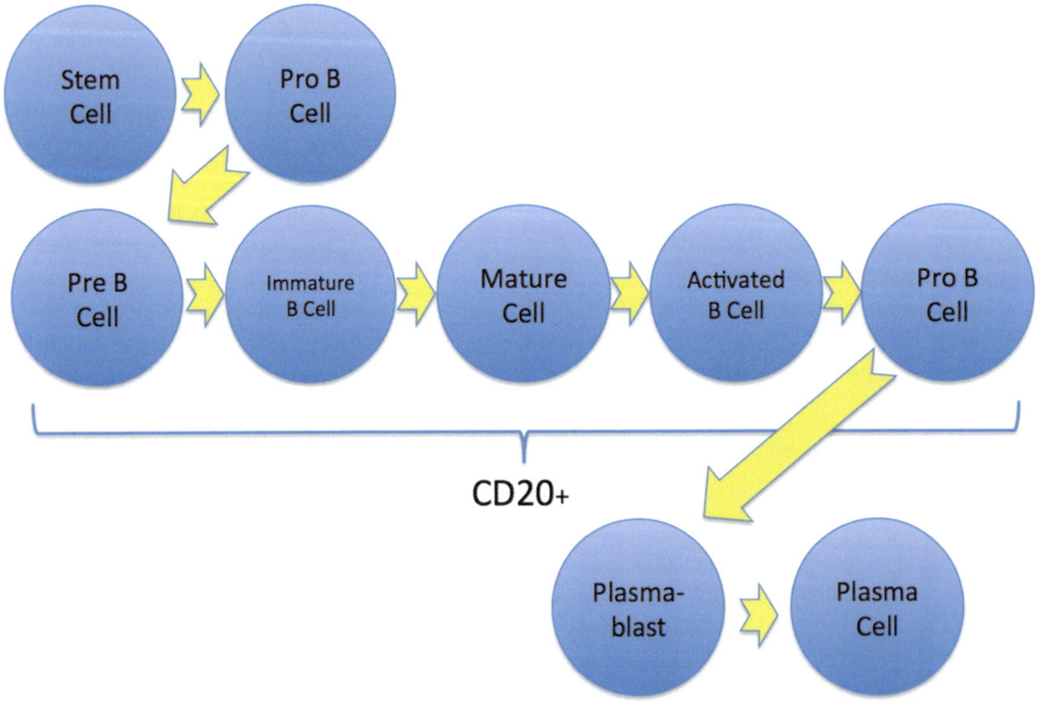

Fig. 8.1 B-Cell CD20 Distribution

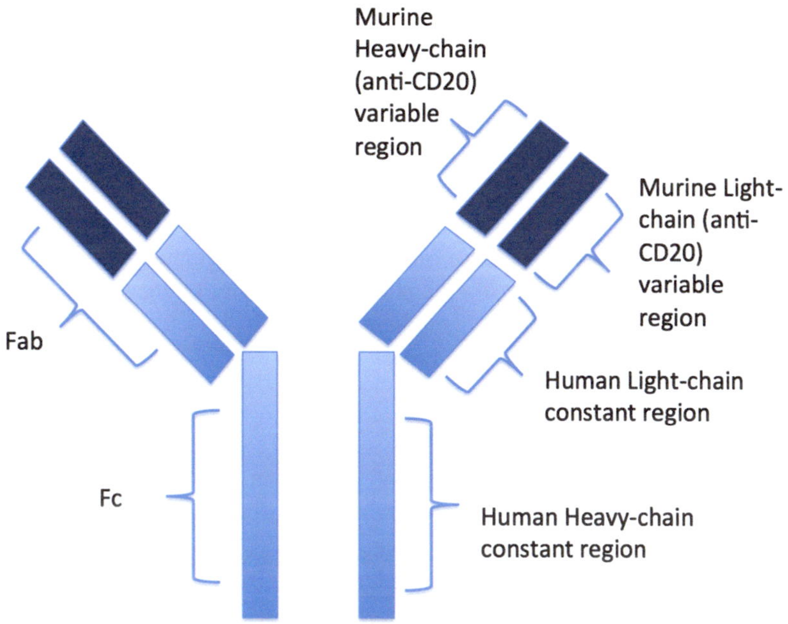

Fig. 8.2 Rituximab Structure

developed and trialed for the treatment of B-cell lymphomas, and in 1997, it became the first therapeutic monoclonal antibody approved by the Food and Drug Administration (FDA) for the treatment of non-Hodgkin's lymphoma [4]. Given the important role B cells play in the pathogenesis of autoimmune disease, anti-CD20 therapy has been extended to the treatment of autoimmune disease. Additional FDA indications for rituximab now include rheumatoid arthritis and ANCA-associated vasculitis (including granulomatosis with polyangiitis (GPA) and microscopic polyangiitis (MPA)). Similarly, B-cell directed therapy, employed in an off-label fashion, has shown promising results in the treatment of uveitis, scleritis, and orbital inflammatory disease.

Data to support the use of rituximab in treating uveitis are limited to case reports and case series. In these reports, uveitis was primarily associated with an underlying autoimmune disorder such as rheumatoid arthritis or juvenile idiopathic arthritis. An early case report detailed the successful use of rituximab in a 49-year-old woman with chronic, bilateral anterior uveitis refractory to corticosteroids and typical immunotherapeutics [5]. The same group later described their experience using rituximab in severe uveitis associated with juvenile idiopathic arthritis (JIA), demonstrating control of active disease in 7 of 10 patients who were refractory to other typical immunosuppressive therapies [6].

The data supporting the use of rituximab in patients with scleritis and orbital inflammatory disease are perhaps stronger. Again, the effective use of rituximab was initially described in several case reports and case series [7, 8]. More recently, two-phase 1/2 clinical trials evaluated the effectiveness of rituximab treatment for orbital inflammation and refractory scleritis [9, 10]. In patients with noninfectious orbital disease, rituximab was safe and effective in 7 of 10 patients. Similarly, rituximab was effective for 9 of 12 patients with refractory, noninfectious scleritis. Treatment with rituximab in these patient groups was well tolerated, although some patients had peri-infusional worsening with initial infusions which did not affect the eventual outcome. The authors ascribed this phenomenon to a tumor lysis-like response due to widespread B-cell lysis and noted that adjunctive corticosteroids were useful in blunting this response. There is also literature suggesting benefit of rituximab therapy in the treatment of ocular cicatricial pemphigoid with the adjunctive use of intravenous immunoglobulin [11].

Rituximab is administered by intravenous infusion, with patients typically receiving a

1000 mg dose followed by a repeat 1000 mg dose two weeks later [12]. Repeat dosing usually occurs at 6-month intervals, although this is often dependent on the initial response to therapy and recurrence of disease activity. Data suggest a role for the use of a reduced dose single infusion (500 mg) in maintenance dosing schemes [13]. Concomitant use of non-biologic immunotherapy is frequently employed, with methotrexate often used in combination with rituximab. In an effort to reduce the risk for infusion reaction, pretreatment with acetaminophen, diphenhydramine, and intravenous methylprednisolone is typical.

Data regarding the safety of rituximab is primarily derived from its use in patients with rheumatoid arthritis [14]. With premedication and careful administration of a patient's infusion, the risk for serious infusion reaction is minimal (<1%). As with all immunosuppressive agents, the use of rituximab engenders an increased risk for infection. Serious infection rates are low, estimated at 2–3%. The risk for infection potentially increases with the development of hypogammaglobulinemia, which is more commonly seen in patients receiving multiple courses of therapy [14]. As such, monitoring IgG levels in patients receiving multiple rounds of rituximab is a common practice [15].

Given the important role B cells play in control of viral-mediated infections, concern for reactivation of viral infection in patients receiving rituximab is high. Screening for hepatitis B exposure is recommended prior to initiation of rituximab therapy, with avoidance of use in those patients demonstrating evidence of prior exposure (positivity for hepatitis B surface antibody (HBsAb) or hepatitis B core antibody (anti-HBc)) [16]. Rare, yet devastating, reactivation of JC virus leading to progressive multifocal leukoencephalopathy (PML) has been reported [17]. The risk of reactivation is variable, and often reflects the underlying autoimmune condition. Given the widespread exposure to the JC virus and low risk of reactivation, serologic screening for JC virus exposure is not recommended. The use of live vaccines is not recommended during treatment with rituximab [18].

Other B-cell inhibitors in development or use for the treatment of inflammatory disease include the B-cell activating factor (BAFF) inhibitors belimumab (Benlysta, GlaxoSmithKline) as well as the fully humanized anti-CD20 blocker ocrelizumab (Genentech) [19]. There is no published evidence for the use of these newer agents in the treatment of ocular inflammation as of the time of this publication.

Targeting T-Cell Activation

Blocking Co-stimulation (Abatacept)

T cells play a vital role in the development and propagation of the normal immune response, and the aberrant immune response leading to autoimmunity in a variety of clinical conditions. The activation of T cells requires not only the recognition of antigen, but also an important step of co-stimulation. With appropriate co-stimulation, T-cell activation leads to differentiation, migration, and penetration of T cells into inflamed tissue. With additional T-cell proliferation, inflammatory cytokines are released, further regulating downstream immune responses. The initial signal in co-stimulation involves the presentation of antigen to a corresponding T-cell receptor. The second, obligatory signal, involves the interaction of an antigen-presenting cell surface ligand with a corresponding T-cell surface receptor (Fig. 8.3) [20]. Absence of this second signal results in T-cell anergy. One important co-stimulatory pathway involves the interaction of the antigen-presenting cell (APC) CD80/86 molecular complex with the T-cell receptor CD28, which, when expressed, serves as a positive co-stimulatory signal [21]. Cytotoxic T-lymphocyte-associated antigen (CTLA4), serves as an important downregulator of this positive co-stimulatory pathway [22]. When expressed, CTLA4 binds to CD80/86 with a significantly higher affinity than CD28, resulting in blockade of the obligatory co-stimulatory signal (Fig. 8.4). T-cell activation results in increased expression of CTLA4 providing the mechanism for a negative, downregulatory process in the immune response [23].

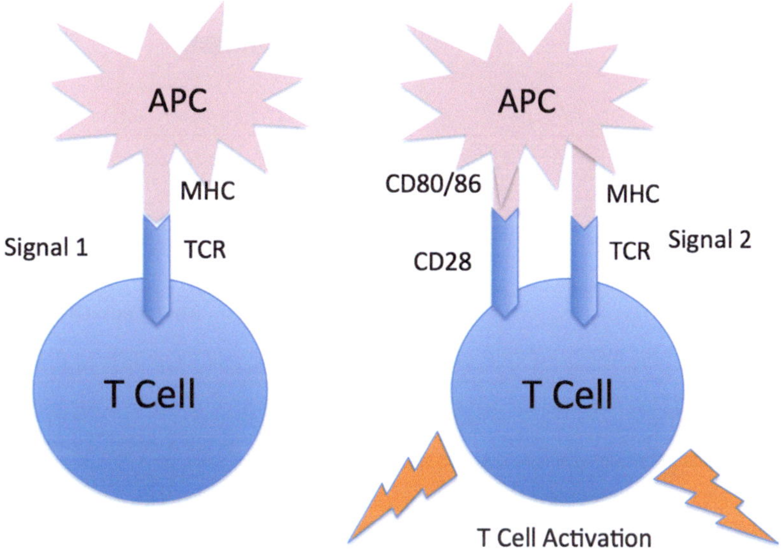

Fig. 8.3 T-Cell Activation Requires Co-stimulation. APC Antigen-Presenting Cell, MHC Major Histocompatibility Complex, TCR T-Cell Receptor

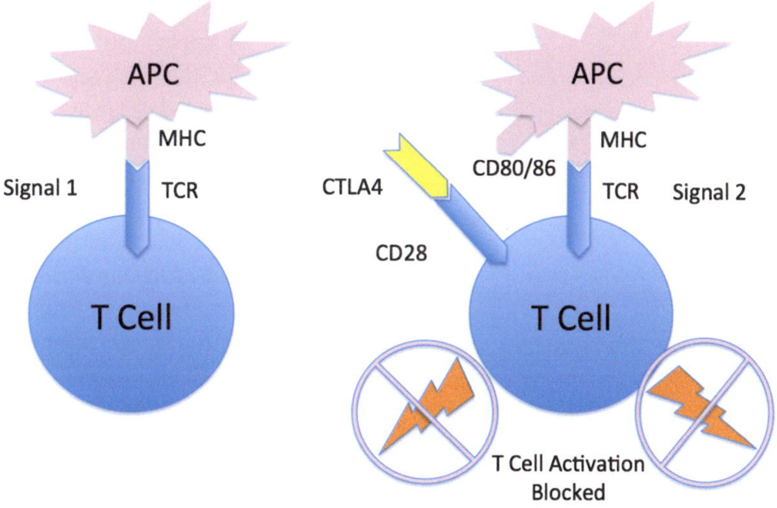

Fig. 8.4 CTLA4 Blocks T-Cell Co-stimulation. APC Antigen-Presenting Cell, MHC Major Histocompatibility Complex, TCR T-Cell Receptor

Abatacept (Orencia®, Bristol-Meyers Squibb Company), is a fully human fusion protein comprising the extracellular portion of cytotoxic T-lymphocyte-associated antigen-4 (CTLA4) and the Fc fragment of IgG1 (Fig. 8.5). As such, abatacept exploits the T-cell co-stimulation pathway through its ability to bind to CD80/86 on the APC, preventing proper interaction of co-stimulatory molecules with the T cell, and therefore, downregulating T-cell activation (Fig. 8.6). Abatacept is FDA-approved for use in patients with rheumatoid arthritis, psoriatic arthritis, and JIA who do not respond adequately to methotrexate.

Several case reports and case series document the use of abatacept in JIA-associated uveitis [24, 25]. One case series describes its use in 7 patients with JIA-associated uveitis refractory to typical immunosuppressive and anti-TNF therapies. The use of abatacept resulted in sustained improvement in all but one patient, and treatment was well tolerated [26]. A subsequent update on the progress of these patients, with a median follow-up of

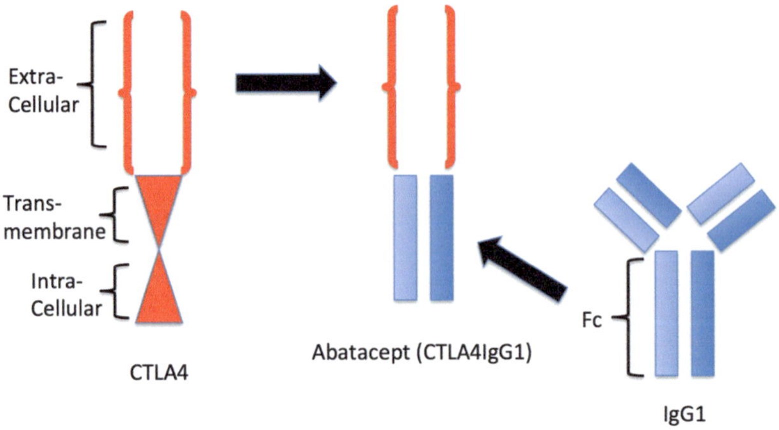

Fig. 8.5 Abatacept (CTLA4IgG1)

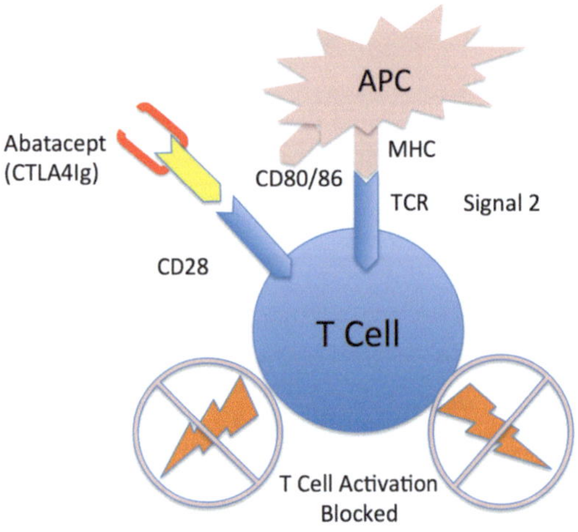

Fig. 8.6 Abatacept (CTLA4Ig) Blocks T-Cell Co-stimulation. APC Antigen-Presenting Cell, MHC Major Histocompatibility Complex, TCR T-Cell Receptor

21 months, revealed that 5 of these 6 patients demonstrated a sustained response. One patient relapsed as manifest by increased arthritis and uveitic activity [27]. A subsequent report of 2 patients with refractory JIA-associated uveitis supported these findings, and suggested a more sustained response, with remission extending to 16 months in one patient [28]. A more recent study published by the European Multinational Interdisciplinary Working Group for Uveitis in Childhood published a retrospective study of 21 children with active uveitis, 18 of whom also had active arthritis [29]. Arthritis inactivity was achieved in 7 of 18 patients, while uveitis inactivity was achieved in 11 of 21, but recurred later in 8 patients, while remaining active in 10. Systemic corticosteroids or immunosuppression were tapered in 3 patients, but uveitis recurred in all of them during further follow-up.

Abatacept is available in both subcutaneous and intravenous formulations. Intravenous dosing is weight-based and generally occurs at 4-week intervals after an initial loading schedule (0, 2, and 4 weeks) [30]. Interestingly, the use of abatacept for the treatment of JIA-associated uveitis at a reduced frequency (infusions every 6–7 weeks) demonstrated sustained efficacy [26]. Infusions are quickly administered, typically taking 30–45 minutes. Infusion reactions are uncommon, and therefore, premedication is generally not required. Subcutaneous dosing may be administered as initial therapy or after a loading IV infusion, and injections are given weekly at a dose of 125 mg.

Rates of serious infection are similar to other biologic agents, with perhaps a lower risk for reactivation of tuberculosis [31]. An exception may exist in patients with chronic obstructive pulmonary disease (COPD), where pneumonia was noted to develop at an increased rate compared to patients without COPD [32]. In patients with rheumatoid arthritis, the use of abatacept was not associated with an increased risk for malignancy [33]. As with all biologic immunotherapies, administration of live vaccines while a patient is receiving abatacept is not recommended. As with rituximab, the use of abatacept in patients with rheumatoid arthritis was associated with a reduced response to inactivated vaccines (e.g., conjugated pneumococcal vaccine) [34]. (Table 8.1). Both in the case of rituximab

Table 8.1 Characteristics, route of administration, dosage, use in ocular inflammation, and potential side effects for rituximab and abatacept

Generic Name	Trade Name	Mechanism of Action	Route	FDA Indications	Dosage	Use in Ocular Inflammation	Special Considerations	Potential Adverse Effects
Rituximab	Rituxan®	B-cell inhibition (anti-CD20)	IV	Moderate to severe rheumatoid arthritis in adult patients with inadequate response to anti-TNF therapy ANCA-associated vasculitis	500 or 1000 mg IV at week 0 and 2, may repeat every 6–12 months (RA dosing); 375 mg/m^2 weekly × 4 (vasculitis dosing)	Case reports, series in uveitis Phase 1/2 trial in refractory scleritis Phase 1/2 trial is refractory orbital inflammation	Latent tuberculosis and viral hepatitis (especially HBV status) screening prior to initiation Monitor CBC and metabolic panel prior to subsequent infusions Live vaccines should not be given concurrently or within 3 months of discontinuation Rare cases of progressive multifocal leukoencephalopathy (PML) reported with use	Increased susceptibility to infection Infusion reactions Cardiovascular events Headache
Abatacept	Orencia®	T-cell inhibition (co-stimulation)	IV, SQ	Rheumatoid arthritis Juvenile idiopathic arthritis Psoriatic arthritis	500, 750 or 1000 mg IV every 4 weeks after loading, 125 mg SQ weekly; JIA 10 mg/kg, max 1000 mg IV at weeks 0, 2, 4, and then every 4 weeks	Case reports, series in JIA-associated uveitis	Latent tuberculosis and viral hepatitis screening prior to initiation Live vaccines should not be given concurrently or within 3 months of discontinuation	Increased susceptibility to infection Allergic reaction Headache Nausea

and abatacept, co-administration with other biologics has not been demonstrated as safe or effective, and consecutive use should be undertaken with caution, with washout periods on the order of five half-lives of the respective drugs a reasonable consideration.

References

1. Hoyer BF, Manz RA, Radbruch A, Hiepe F. Long-lived plasma cells and their contribution to autoimmunity. Ann N Y Acad Sci. 2005;1050:124–33.
2. Cragg MS, Walshe CA, Ivanov AO, Glennie MJ. The biology of CD20 and its potential as a target for mAb therapy. Curr Dir Autoimmun. 2005;8:140–74.
3. Reff ME, Carner K, Chambers KS, Chinn PC, Leonard JE, Raab R, et al. Depletion of B cells in vivo by a chimeric mouse human monoclonal antibody to CD20. Blood. 1994;83:435–45.
4. Grillo-Lopez AJ. Rituximab: an insider's historical perspective. Semin Oncol. 2000;27(Suppl 12):9–16.
5. Tappeiner C, Heinz C, Specker C, Heiligenhaus A. Rituximab as a treatment option for refractory endogenous anterior uveitis. Ophthalmic Res. 2007;39:184–6.
6. Heiligenhaus A, Miserocchi E, Heinz C, Gerloni V, Kotaniemi K. Treatment of severe uveitis associated with juvenile idiopathic arthritis with anti-CD20 monoclonal antibody (rituximab). Rheumatology (Oxford). 2011;50:1390–4.
7. Kurz PA, Suhler EB, Choi D, Rosenbaum JT. Rituximab for treatment of ocular inflammatory disease: a series of four cases. Br J Ophthalmol. 2009;93(4):546–8.
8. Pelegrin L, Jakob E, Schmidt-Bacher A, Schwenger V, Becker M, Max R, et al. Experiences with rituximab for the treatment of autoimmune diseases with ocular involvement. J Rheumatol. 2014;41:84–90.
9. Suhler EB, Lim LL, Beardsley RM, Giles TR, Pasadhika S, Lee ST, et al. Rituximab therapy for refractory orbital inflammation: results of a phase 1/2, dose-ranging, randomized clinical trial. JAMA Ophthalmol. 2014;132:572–8.
10. Suhler EB, Lim LL, Beardsley RM, Giles TR, Pasadhika S, Lee ST, et al. Rituximab therapy for refractory scleritis: results of a phase I/II dose-ranging, randomized, clinical trial. Ophthalmology. 2014;121:1885–91.
11. Foster CS, Chang PY. A combination of rituximab and intravenous immunoglobulin for recalcitrant ocular cicatricial pemphigoid: a preliminary report. Ophthalmology. 2010;117(5):861–9.
12. Genentech Inc., and Biogen Idec Inc. [Internet] Rituximab Prescribing Information [Updated August 2014]. Available from: http://www.gene.com/download/pdf/rituxan_prescribing.pdf.
13. Guillevin L, Pagnoux C, Karras A, Khouatra C, Aumaître O, Cohen P, et al. Rituximab versus azathioprine for maintenance in ANCA-associated vasculitis. N Engl J Med. 2014;371(19):1771–80.
14. van Vollenhoven RF, Emery P, Bingham CO 3rd, Keystone EC, Fleischmann R, Furst DE, et al. Longterm safety of patients receiving rituximab in rheumatoid arthritis clinical trials. J Rheumatol. 2010;37(3):558–67.
15. Buch MH, Smolen JS, Betteridge N, Breedveld FC, Burmester G, Dörmer T, et al. Updated consensus statement on the use of rituximab in patients with rheumatoid arthritis. Ann Rheum Dis. 2011;70(6):909–20.
16. Pyrpasopoulou A, Douma S, Vassiliadis T, Chatzimichailidou S, Triantafyllou A, Aslanidis S. Reactivation of chronic hepatitis B virus infection following rituximab administration for rheumatoid arthritis. Rheumatol Int. 2011;31:403–4.
17. Carson KR, Evens AM, Richey EA, Habermann TM, Focosi D, Seymour JF, et al. Progressive multifocal leukoencephalopathy after rituximab therapy in HIV-negative patients: a report of 57 cases from the Research on Adverse Drug Events and Reports project. Blood. 2009;113:4834–40.
18. van Assen S, Agmon-Levin N, Elkayam O, Cervera R, Doran MF, Dougados M, et al. EULAR recommendations for vaccination in adult patients with autoimmune inflammatory rheumatic diseases. Ann Rheum Dis. 2011;70:414–22.
19. Lin P, Suhler EB, Rosenbaum JT. The future of uveitis therapy. Ophthalmology. 2014;121:365–76.
20. Carreno BM, Collins M. The B7 family of ligands and its receptors: new pathways for costimulation and inhibition of immune responses. Annu Rev Immunol. 2002;20:29–53.
21. Lindsley PS, Ledbatter JA. The role of CD28 receptor during T cell responses to antigen. Ann Rev Immunol. 1993;11:191–212.
22. Brunner MC, Chambers CA, Chan FK, Hanke J, Winoto A, Allison JP. CLTA-4 mediated inhibition of early events of T cell proliferation. J Immunol. 1999;162(10):5813–20.
23. Alegre ML, Shiels H, Thompson CB, Gajewski TF. Expression and function of CTLA-4 in Th1 and Th2 cells. J Immunol. 1998;161:3347–56.
24. Angeles-Han S, Flynn T, Lehman T. Abatacept for refractory juvenile idiopathic arthritis-associated uveitis – a case report. J Rheumatol. 2008;35:1897–8.
25. Kenawy N, Cleary G, Mewar D, Beare N, Chandna A, Pearce I. Abatacept: a potential therapy in refractory cases of juvenile idiopathic arthritis-associated uveitis. Graefes Arch Clin Exp Ophthalmol. 2011;249(2):297–300.
26. Zulian F, Balzarin M, Falcini F, Martini G, Alessio M, Cimaz R, et al. Abatacept for severe anti-tumor necrosis factor alpha refractory juvenile idiopathic arthritis-related uveitis. Arthritis Care Res. 2010;62(6):821–5.
27. Zulian F, Zannin ME. Reply to: Abatacept for refractory juvenile idiopathic arthritis-associated uveitis: two new cases. Arthritis Care Res. 2011;63(2):308.

28. Elhai M, Deslandre CJ, Kahan A. Abatacept for refractory juvenile idiopathic arthritis-associated uveitis: two new cases. Arthritis Care Res. 2011;63(2):307–8.
29. Tappeiner C, Misericchi E, Bodaghi B, Kotaniemi K, Mackensen F, Gerloni V, et al. Abatacept in the treatment of severe, longstanding, and refractory uveitis associated with juvenile idiopathic arthritis. J Rheumatol. 2015 Apr;42:706–11.
30. Bristol-Myers Squibb Co. [Internet] Abatacept Prescribing Information [Updated June 2015]. Available from: http://packageinserts.bms.com/pi/pi_orencia.pdf.
31. Souto A, Maneiro JR, Salgado E, Carmona L, Gomez-Reino JJ. Risk of tuberculosis in patients with chronic immune-mediated inflammatory diseases treated with biologics and tofacitinib: a systematic review and meta-analysis of randomized controlled trials and long-term extension studies. Rheumatology (Oxford). 2014;53(10):1872–85.
32. Rozelle AL, Genovese MC. Efficacy results from pivotal clinical trials with abatacept. Clin Exp Rheumatol. 2007;25(5 Suppl 46):S30–4.
33. Weinblatt M, Combe B, Covucci A, Aranda R, Becker JC, Keystone E. Safety of the selective costimulation modulator abacept in rheumatoid arthritis patients receiving background biologic and non biologic disease modifying antirheumatic drugs. Arthritis Rheum. 2006;54:2807–16.
34. Crnkic Kapetanovic M, Saxne T, Jönsson G, Truedsson L, Geborek P. Rituximab and abatacept but not tocilizumab impair antibody response to pneumococcal conjugate vaccine in patients with rheumatoid arthritis. Arthritis Res Ther. 2013;15(5):R171.

9 Targeting Interleukin-6 in Ocular Inflammatory Diseases

Marina Mesquida, Victor Llorenç, and Alfredo Adán

Pearls

- Serum and intraocular levels of IL-6 are significantly elevated in patients with active noninfectious uveitis and decrease during remission, thus implying that IL-6 has an active role in chronic disease.
- Studies about the role of IL-6 in the development of macular edema have shown that elevated intraocular levels of both VEGF and IL-6 were correlated with the presence and severity of macular edema in different conditions (uveitis, diabetic retinopathy, retinal vein occlusion).
- Tocilizumab is a fully humanized antibody that binds both to soluble and membrane-bound IL-6R. It has been approved for the treatment of RA and JIA, and is currently under investigation on several clinical trials for a wide variety of autoimmune conditions, including uveitis and thyroid eye disease.
- The clinical success of tocilizumab as the first biologic to target IL-6 has triggered the development of new therapies blocking IL-6, and presently a number of novel IL-6/IL-6R inhibitors are being tested in clinical trials and preclinical studies.

None of the authors has any proprietary/financial interest to disclose.
This study received no financial support.

M. Mesquida (✉)
Institut Clinic d'Oftalmologia, Hospital Clinic de Barcelona, Universitat de Barcelona, Barcelona, Spain

Ophthalmology Clinical Research Unit, Fundació Clínic per a la Recerca Biomèdica, IDIBAPS, Barcelona, Spain
e-mail: mesquida@clinic.ub.es

V. Llorenç · A. Adán
Institut Clinic d'Oftalmologia, Hospital Clinic de Barcelona, Universitat de Barcelona, Barcelona, Spain

Introduction

Interleukin-6 (IL-6) was identified three decades ago by Kishimoto and colleagues as a T-cell-derived factor inducing activated B cells to differentiate into antibody-producing cells [1]. IL-6 is a soluble mediator formerly known as B-cell stimulatory factor (BSF-2), interferon (IFN)-beta 2, and hepatocyte stimulating factor, based on the above-stated function, antiviral activity, and acute phase protein synthesis, respectively [2]. When the BSF-2 complementary DNA was successfully cloned in 1986 [3], it turned out that

P. Lin, E. Suhler (eds.), *Treatment of Non-infectious Uveitis*,
https://doi.org/10.1007/978-3-030-22827-9_9

these molecules with different names studied by various groups were in fact identical, resulting in the single name IL-6 [2]. Since its molecular discovery, major advances have taken place in understanding the biology of IL-6 and its fundamental role in inflammation, immune regulation, hematopoiesis, host defense, homeostasis, and tissue regeneration. IL-6 is often referred to as a pleiotropic cytokine being produced by a wide range of hematopoietic and somatic cells that influences numerous cell types with multiple biological functions. However, abnormal IL-6 production has been associated with the development of a wide variety of systemic immune-mediated, chronic diseases, and even neoplasms [1]. From the ocular perspective, significant elevation of IL-6 has been found in aqueous (AqH) or vitreous humor derived from diabetic macular edema (DME), retinal vein occlusion (RVO), and refractory/chronic uveitis patients [4–6]. Over the last decade, tocilizumab, a humanized monoclonal antibody (mAb) that binds the IL-6 receptor (IL-6R), has gained approval for the treatment of rheumatoid arthritis (RA) in more than 100 countries worldwide [7]. It is also approved for the treatment of systemic and polyarticular juvenile idiopathic arthritis (sJIA and pJIA, respectively), and for Castleman's disease in Japan. Furthermore, it has been reported to be effective in various immune-mediated disorders including noninfectious uveitis and its associated macular edema [4]. Due to the clinical success of IL-6-blockade, a number of new biologics targeting IL-6 signaling are currently being tested in clinical trials or in preclinical studies. It is expected that this strategy will have wider applicability in numerous immune-mediated diseases [7–9].

IL-6 Biology

IL-6 Signaling Pathways

Human IL-6 is a 26 kDa protein made up of 212 amino acids codified by a gene located in chromosome 7p21 [7]. The biology and signaling of IL-6 are now better comprehended principally due to the outstanding work of Dr. Tadamitsu Kishimoto from Osaka University and Dr. Stefan Rose-John from the University of Kiehl. IL-6 triggers signal transduction after binding the IL-6 receptor (IL-6R). There are two forms of the IL-6R, the 80 kDa transmembrane receptor protein and the 55 kDa soluble form (sIL6-R). During the so-called classic signaling, IL-6 binds its cognate transmembrane IL-6R forming the IL-6/IL-6R complex [7–9]. Signaling is only initiated when the IL-6/IL-6R complex associates with a second protein, the 130 kDa transmembrane glycoprotein named gp130 [10]. The association of gp130 with IL-6/IL-6R leads to the formation of the high affinity activated IL-6/IL-6R/gp130 complex, adopting a hexameric structure consisting of two molecules each of IL-6, IL-6R, and gp130, thereby triggering the initiation of the intracellular signal transduction pathway via activation of Janus kinase (JAK) and signal transducer and activator of transcription 3 (STAT3) as well as the JAK-SHP2-Ras-mitogen-activated protein kinase (MAPK) pathways, eliciting the downstream signal cascade leading to specific changes of intra-nuclear gene expression of various sets of IL-6-responsive genes [10]. The activation of STAT3 in turn induces the suppressor of cytokine signaling 1 (SOCS1) and SOCS3, which bind tyrosine-phosphorylated JAK and gp130 respectively, to stop IL-6 signaling by means of a negative feedback loop, as a mechanism of counter-regulation [11, 12].

In the last years, a new paradigm in IL-6 signaling has been elucidated [12, 13]. In addition to the signaling through the membrane-bound IL-6R (classic signaling), IL-6 can provide signal transduction in cells lacking the cognate transmembrane IL-6R through binding the sIL-6R in association with gp130, in the so-called trans-signaling pathway [13]. Whilst it is known that almost all cells of the body express gp130, only few cells possess the transmembrane IL-6R, mainly hepatocytes and some leukocyte subpopulations (monocytes, neutrophils, T cells, and B cells). In trans-signaling, IL-6 binds the sIL-6R, and the IL-6/sIL-6 complex subsequently binds gp130 on cells that do not express the transmembrane IL-6R (and are therefore unable to respond to IL-6 in the absence of sIL-6R) [12]. In other words, this pathway allows cells that do not express surface IL-6R to respond to the presence of IL-6 [13].

To ensure that IL-6/sIL-6R trans-signaling is tightly regulated, there is counter-regulation by a soluble form of gp130 (sgp130), present at high concentrations in serum of healthy individuals (range, 250–400 ng/ml), as part of the physiological IL-6 buffer in the blood [13, 14]. This natural inhibitor forms a complex with IL-6/sIL-6R, preventing the binding of IL-6/sIL-6R to membrane-bound gp130 [12–14].

It is believed that the pleiotropic effect of IL-6 derives from the broad range of cells expressing gp130, which highlights the importance of trans-signaling [13]. The signal-transducing protein gp130 is shared by all members of the IL-6 cytokine family (including IL-35, IL-27, IL-11, leukemia inhibitory factor, oncostatin M, ciliary neurotrophic factor, among others). The fact that all the IL-6 family members use gp130 as a common signal transducer suggests why the aforementioned cytokines display pleiotropy and redundancy [14]. In summary, IL-6 binding to its transmembrane receptor leads to the activation of the so-called classic signaling pathway, whereas the IL-6/sIL-6R complex triggers the so-called trans-signaling pathway. Various studies have shown that classic signaling via the membrane-bound receptor is regenerative and protects from bacterial infections, whereas trans-signaling via the soluble receptor is inflammatory [15]. Therefore, it has been hypothesized that the sole blockade of IL-6 trans-signaling may be more beneficial than global IL-6 inhibition, maintaining the regenerative functions of IL-6 and specifically suppressing only pathophysiologic inflammatory activity [13, 15].

IL-6 Biological Functions

IL-6 is an essential mediator in host defense against environmental stress, alerting about the occurrence of an emergent event and sending out a warning sign to the entire body [9]. Under physiological conditions IL-6 is barely detectable in serum (1–5 pg/ml), although its levels can increase more than 100,000-fold during early phases of inflammation [8, 9]. A myriad of cell types in the body can synthesize IL-6, including cells of the innate immune system such as neutrophils and monocytes/macrophages. As mentioned, IL-6 is important in the integrated host defense against numerous pathogens including bacteria, fungi, viruses, and mycobacteria [16]. During infectious inflammation, IL-6 is promptly produced by monocytes and macrophages after the stimulation of Toll-like receptors (TLRs) with distinct pathogen-associated molecular patterns (PAMPs) [17]. In noninfectious inflammation such as burn or traumatic injury, damage-associated molecular patterns (DAMPs) from injured or dying cells stimulate TLRs to produce IL-6 [17]. PAMPs and DAMPs stimulate a number of signaling pathways including NF-κB, and upregulate the transcription of the mRNA of inflammatory cytokines such as IL-6, tumor necrosis factor alpha (TNF-α), and IL-1β. TNF-α and IL-1β in turn can activate transcription factors to synthesize IL-6 [13]. The local encounter of these innate immune cells with danger signals in early stages of the immune response is thereby translated into systemic dissemination of IL-6 through the bloodstream and the rapid elevation of serum IL-6 levels [8]. Liver hepatocytes respond to the IL-6 stimulus inducing the synthesis of acute-phase proteins such as C-reactive protein (CRP), serum amyloid A, fibrinogen, haptoglobin, and alpha-1-antichymotrypsin [18]. CRP is a well-known biomarker of inflammation and is used as such in clinical laboratory tests. Importantly, its expression principally depends on IL-6 [19]. Alpha-1-antichymotrypsin and serum amyloid A persistent elevation may lead to the generation of amyloid A amyloidosis and amyloid fibril deposition, which have been related to the deterioration of various organs and pathogenesis of Alzheimer's disease [20, 21]. IL-6 also stimulates hepcidin production, which antagonizes the action of the iron transporter ferroportin 1 on the gut, therefore reducing serum iron levels, suggesting that the IL-6-hepcidin axis is responsible for the hypoferremia and anemia associated with chronic inflammation [22]. In addition, IL-6 upregulates the expression of zinc importer ZIP14, favoring the hypozincemia seen in chronic inflammation [23]. Conversely, IL-6 downregulates the expression of fibronectin, albumin, and transferrin [24]. These changes in acute phase response protein levels are used for the evaluation of inflammation severity in routine clinical laboratory tests. Apart from its role in host defense, IL-6 has many other relevant biological functions. In hematopoiesis, IL-6 induces maturation of megakaryocytes into platelets and activation of stem cells [25]. IL-6 generated in the bone marrow stromal cells upregulates the receptor activator of nuclear factor kappa-B ligand (RANKL), which activates osteoclasts leading to bone resorption and osteoporosis [26]. In addition to immune cells, many other cell types are involved in the production of IL-6 in response to various stimuli, including mesenchymal cells, endothelial cells, adipocytes, and fibroblasts. Importantly, the production of IL-6 in inflamed tissues induces an excess of vascular endothelial growth factor (VEGF), which results in increased angiogenesis and vascular permeability [27]. Upon IL-6 stimulation, endothelial cells release chemokines to induce recruitment of more immune cells. In dermal keratinocytes, IL-6 promotes their proliferation and fibroblast collagen production, which may contribute to the pathogenesis of autoimmune diseases such as psoriasis, systemic sclerosis, and thyroid eye disease [28, 29]. Table 9.1 summarizes the IL-6 principal biological functions.

IL-6 in Immunity and Inflammation

B cells are stimulated under the influence of IL-6. Indeed, plasmocytoid dendritic cells can produce IL-6, thereby promoting the differentiation of B cells into antibody-producing plasma cells [1, 2]. On the other hand, IL-6 may indirectly induce antibody production by triggering the synthesis of IL-21 by $CD4^+$ T cells to drive STAT3-dependent plasma cell differentiation in B cells [30]. Moreover, IL-6 constitutes a key regulator of $CD4^+$ T-cell differentiation. It maintains the balance between Th1 and Th2 effector functions, inhibiting Th1 differentiation through interfering with IFN-γ production by upregulation of SOCS1 or SOCS3 in $CD4^+$ T cells [30, 31], and promot-

Table 9.1 IL-6 biological functions

IL-6 production site	Action	Target	Biological effect	Possible clinical implication	References
Liver hepatocytes	Stimulation	C-reactive protein	Endothelial dysfunction	Atherothrombosis	[18, 19]
		Serum amyloid A	Amyloid-fibril deposition	Amyloid A amyloidosis	[20]
		alpha1-antichymotrypsin	Amyloid-fibril formation	Alzheimer's disease	[21]
		Fibrinogen	Hypercoagulation	Cardiovascular disease	
		Haptoglobin	Reduced serum iron levels	Iron deficiency anemia associated with chronic inflammation	[22]
		ZIP14	Enhances zinc importer	Hypozincemia associated with chronic inflammation	[23]
	Inhibition	Fibronectin	Cell adhesion and migration	Abnormal would healing, tumorigenicity	
		Albumin	Hypoalbuminemia	Edema	
		Transferrin	Reduced iron transport	Iron deficiency anemia associated with chronic inflammation	[24]
Bone marrow	Stimulation	Megacaryocyte maturation	Increased platelet count	Thrombocytosis associated with inflammation	[25]

Table 9.1 (continued)

IL-6 production site	Action	Target	Biological effect	Possible clinical implication	References
Immune system	Stimulation	CD4 T-cell differentiation into Th17	IL-17 production	Autoimmune diseases (including noninfectious uveitis)	
		CD4 T follicular cell differentiation	IL-21 production	IgG4-related disease (including orbital inflammatory disease)	
		CD8 T-cell differentiation into cytotoxic T-cell			[37]
		B-cell differentiation into plasma B cell	Antibody production	Hypergammaglobulinemia and autoantibody production, multiple myeloma	
	Inhibition	CD4 T-cell differentiation into Th1	Balance toward Th2 differentiation		
		TGF-beta-induced Treg differentiation	Decreased Treg count	Autoimmune diseases (including noninfectious uveitis)	[34]
Synovial fibroblast	Stimulation	RANKL	Activation of osteoclasts	Bone resorption and osteoporosis	[26]
		VEGF	Increased angiogenesis and vascular permeability	Edema, neovascularization	[27]
Skin	Stimulation	Keratinocyte proliferation	Increased keratosis	Psoriasis	[28]
		Dermal fibroblasts	Increased collagen production	Systemic sclerosis	
Eye	Stimulation	VEGF	Increased vascular permeability	Blood-retinal barrier breakdown and macular edema pathogenesis	
		CD4 T-cell differentiation into Th17	IL-17 production	Autoimmune uveitis	[68]

Abbreviations: *CD* cluster of differentiation, *IL-17* interleukin-17, *IL-21* interleukin-21, *RANKL* receptor activator of nuclear factor kappa-B ligand, *TGF-beta* transforming growth factor beta, *Th1* T helper 1 cells, *Th2* T helper 2 cells, *Th17* T helper 17 cells, *VEGF* vascular endothelial growth factor

ing Th2 differentiation by the synthesis of two Th2-type cytokines, IL-4 and IL-13 [32].

Importantly, in combination with transforming growth factor-beta (TGF-β), IL-6 promotes the differentiation of Th17 cells, which play a crucial role in the induction of autoimmune tissue injury by activating transcription factors such as retinoic acid-related orphan receptor (ROR)γt and ROR-α [33]. IL-6 is also considered a regulator of the balance between Th17 and T regulatory cells (Treg), inhibiting Treg differentiation induced by TGF-β [34]. The resultant Th17/Treg imbalance leads to the breakdown of immunological tolerance and is of pathological relevance for the development of various autoimmune and chronic inflammatory diseases [35].

In addition, IL-6 is implicated in the early differentiation process of T follicular helper cells (Tfh), which is considered to be the principal Th cell subset that supports the germinal center for the induction, affinity maturation, and generation of memory B cells as well as long-lived plasma cells [36]. IL-6 can also induce naïve/rested $CD8^+$ T cells to be activated and acquire cytotoxic function [37].

IL-6 in Disease Pathogenesis

As it has been previously discussed, IL-6 is a pleiotropic cytokine performing a broad range of biological activities in inflammation, immune regulation, hematopoiesis, and oncogenesis [1, 8, 9]. Cytokines such as IL-6 are essential for life, and under physiological conditions its production has tight negative regulatory mechanisms. However, abnormal overproduction of IL-6 has been found responsible for the pathogenesis of various autoimmune, chronic inflammatory diseases, and even cancers [38]. In the late 1980s, Kishimoto's group from Osaka University reported the excessive production of IL-6 in the synovial tissues of patients with RA [39], and in the hyperplastic lymph nodes of patients with Castleman's disease [40]. Individuals suffering from this condition can display severe inflammatory symptoms including fever, anemia, increased levels of acute-phase proteins, and hypergammaglobulinemia, suggesting that the generation of IL-6 by cells in germinal centers of hyperplastic lymph nodes may be the key element responsible for the variety of clinical symptoms in this disease [40]. In 1990 it was found that cardiac myxoma, a benign heart tumor, can produce large amounts of IL-6, which could explain the systemic inflammatory symptoms that patients with this condition may suffer [41]. The reason(s) why such dysregulated, continuous IL-6 production is induced remains to be clarified. Elucidation of mechanisms underlying this abnormal, persistent IL-6 synthesis in such disparate diseases is of particular importance to tailor treatment and such investigations are in progress. Table 9.2 summarizes clinical diseases in which IL-6 plays a role in pathogenesis.

Table 9.2 IL-6 role in disease pathogenesis

Autoimmune/immune-mediated inflammatory diseases	Rheumatoid arthritis
	Juvenile idiopathic arthritis and Still's disease
	Castleman's disease
	Systemic sclerosis
	Inflammatory myopathies
	Large vessel vasculitis
	Systemic lupus erythematosus
	Relapsing polychondritis
	Cogan's syndrome
	Polymyalgia rheumatica
	Ankylosing spondylitis
	Behçet's disease
	Inflammatory bowel disease
	Graft-versus-host disease
	Autoimmune hemolytic anemia
	Acquired hemophilia A
	IgG4-related disease
	Atherosclerosis
	Diabetes mellitus
	Amyloid A amyloidosis
Autoinflammatory diseases	TNF-receptor-associated periodic syndrome
	Chronic inflammatory neurological cutaneous articular syndrome (CINCA)
Neoplastic diseases	Cardiac myxoma
	Multiple myeloma
	Colorectal cancer
	Prostate cancer
Neurological diseases	Alzheimer's disease
	Multiple sclerosis
	Neuromyelitis optica
Ocular diseases	Uveitis
	Diabetic retinopathy
	Retinal vein occlusion
	Macular edema
	Thyroid eye disease
	Cogan's syndrome

Targeting the IL-6 Response: From Bench to Bedside

In the past decades, the blockade of TNF-α with different biologics has revolutionized the treatment of autoimmune diseases such as RA and inflammatory bowel disease, leading to the concept of TNF-α as a master cytokine in these conditions. However, in spite of their remarkable clinical success, a number of patients remain unresponsive/intolerant to the TNF-α blockers, and therefore other treatment strategies are needed. Because of the biological activities of IL-6 and its prominent pathogenic role in various diseases, it was anticipated that IL-6 inhibition would constitute a promising novel treatment strategy for immune-mediated conditions [42]. Tocilizumab (Actemra outside the EU, and RoActemra inside the EU) is the first biologic designed to target IL-6 signaling. It is a humanized mAb developed by grafting the complimentary-determining regions of mouse anti-human IL-6R antibody onto human IgG1 [42]. Tocilizumab blocks IL-6-mediated signaling by binding to both soluble and transmembrane IL-6 receptors. It reduces IL-6 pleiotropic actions such as T-cell activation, Th17 differentiation (and resultant Th17/Treg misbalance), antibody secretion, and hepatic acute phase protein production such as CRP [35, 42]. Indeed, CRP level is a hallmark for checking whether IL-6 activity is completely blocked in vivo [8]. Tocilizumab was originated by the Japanese company Chugai Pharmaceutical in the 1990s by Tadamitsu Kishimoto and collaborators. In 1997 the first clinical trial in RA was conducted in Japan, and soon afterwards trials in Castleman's disease and sJIA commenced [42]. In 2002, a majority share in Chugai Pharmaceutical was acquired by Roche. It gained its first approval in 2005 to treat Castleman's disease in Japan, which was followed by subsequent approvals for RA, sJIA, and poliarticular JIA (pJIA) in the forthcoming years. Tocilizumab has been authorized by the food and drug administration (FDA) and the European medicines agency (EMA) for the treatment of patients with RA who have active disease despite having been treated with one or more disease modifying anti-rheumatic drugs (DMARDs), including other biologic response modifiers such as TNF inhibitors or methotrexate. It has also gained indication for use in children 2 years or older with sJIA. At present, tocilizumab is approved in more than 100 countries worldwide [42]. Table 9.3 depicts a brief history of IL-6, from bench to bedside.

Table 9.3 Brief history of IL-6: from bench to bedside

Milestone	Year	Authors (if applicable)
First report of the existence of soluble factors for the enhancement of IgG and IgE antibody responses	1973	Kishimoto and Ishizaka
Cloning of the IL-6 gene	1986	Hirano et al.
IL-6 found in cardiac myxoma tissue	1987	Hirano et al.
IL-6 found in synovial fluid in RA	1988	Houssiau et al.
Cloning of the IL-6 receptor	1988	Hirano et al.
IL-6 involved in lymph nodes in Castleman's disease	1989	Yoshizaki et al.
Cloning of gp130	1990	Hirano et al.
gp130 found to be a common signal transducer for IL-6 cytokine family	1991	Murakami et al.
Cloning of STAT3	1994	Akira et al.; Zhong et al.
Chugai Pharmaceutical begins the clinical development of TCZ	1997	
TCZ first clinical trial for RA in Japan	1997	
TCZ first clinical trial for Castleman's disease in Japan	2001	
TCZ first clinical trial for sJIA in Japan	2002	
Hoffmann–La Roche reaches agreement with Chugai Pharmaceutical	2003	
TCZ (iv) approved for Castleman's disease in Japan	2005	
TZC (iv) approved for RA, pJIA, and sJIA in Japan	2008	
TCZ (iv) approved for RA in EU	2009	
TCZ (iv) approved for RA in USA	2010	
TCZ (iv) approved for sJIA and pJIA in EU and USA	2011	
TCZ (sc) approved for RA, sJIA, pJIA, and Castleman's disease in Japan	2013	
TCZ (sc) approved for RA, sJIA, and pJIA in EU and USA	2014	
TCZ approved in >100 countries worldwide	2015	

Abbreviations: *IL*-6 interleukin-6, *STAT3* signal transducer and activator of transcription 3, *pJIA* polyarticular juvenile idiopathic arthritis, *RA* rheumatoid arthritis, *sJIA* systemic juvenile idiopathic arthritis, *TCZ* tocilizumab, *EU* European Union, *USA* United States of America

Apart from RA, sJIA, and Castleman's disease, published studies have suggested that tocilizumab may have broader application for other chronic, immune-mediated diseases. Indeed, off-label use of tocilizumab has been reported in lupus erythematosus, systemic sclerosis, inflammatory myopathies, systemic vasculitis, Behcet's disease, relapsing polychondritis, polymyalgia rheumatica, acquired hemophilia A, autoimmune hemolytic anemia, amyloid A amyloidosis, graft-versus-host disease, IgG4-related disease, as well as other non-organ-specific immune-related conditions such as atherosclerosis and diabetes mellitus [7–9, 42]. In addition, IL-6 blockade may be useful for neoplastic disorders such as cardiac myxoma, multiple myeloma, colorectal cancer, and prostate cancer [38]. All the aforementioned studies are not licensed and therefore must await formal clinical trials.

Dosing and Administration

Tocilizumab may be given through two different routes of administration: intravenous (iv) infusions or subcutaneous (sc) injections. Intravenous tocilizumab is registered for use in RA (alone or in combination therapy with other DMARDs), sJIA, pJIA, and Castleman's disease, and its dose is adjusted according to the patient's weight. The starting dose in adults is 4 milligrams (mg) of tocilizumab per kilogram (kg) of body weight (4 mg/kg), but the dose can be increased to 8 mg/kg if needed. In children, the recommended dose is 8 mg/kg in those weighing over 30 kg (66 pounds) and 12 mg/kg in those under 30 kg. Tocilizumab iv infusions are usually given every 4 weeks (q4w), although for children with JIA dosing can be as frequent as every 2 weeks (q2w) [7]. Subcutaneous tocilizumab constitutes a desirable alternative due to its ambulatory administration [43]. Its efficacy has been evaluated in three randomized controlled trials (RCT): BREVACTA, MUSASHI, and SUMMACTA, which demonstrated noninferiority compared to the iv route utilizing the following dosing: sc tocilizumab 162 mg injections q2w is equivalent to iv tocilizumab 4 mg/kg q4w; and sc tocilizumab 162 mg weekly injections is equivalent to iv 8 mg/kg q4w) [43, 44]. Subcutaneous tocilizumab is approved by the FDA and the EMA for use in RA but not for sJIA or pJIA yet.

Safety Profile of IL-6 Inhibition

The safety of IL-6 blockade both in clinical trials and in the "real-world" setting has been extensively reviewed [43–45]. The most frequently reported adverse events associated with tocilizumab are infections, infusion reactions, and gastrointestinal perforations [45–47]. Perhaps the most concerning potential side effect with tocilizumab therapy is the risk of infection, as it is with most biologic drugs. IL-6 is important in the host defense against numerous pathogens including bacteria (and mycobacteria), fungi, and viruses [2]. On the basis of this knowledge, it is not surprising that IL-6 blockade with tocilizumab has been associated with an increase in serious and opportunistic infections. Of note, these infection rates are similar to those seen with TNF inhibitors and other biologic agents in the treatment of RA and do not increase over time [45–48]. The most frequently reported infections are pneumonia, herpes zoster, acute bronchitis, and pyelonephritis. In a meta-analysis of six randomized, controlled trials of tocilizumab 4 and 8 mg/kg, Campbell et al. found that the risk of infection was significantly higher than in the placebo or control group (odds ratio 1.30, 95% CI 1.07–1.58) [47]. In patients treated with tocilizumab, active infections should be ruled out before treatment is commenced. Reactivation of tuberculosis (TB) during tocilizumab therapy occurs at 0.23 cases per 100 patient-years, and is low compared to anti-TNF therapy [45]. Nonetheless, it still remains a concern and screening for prior exposure to TB is recommended before starting tocilizumab therapy as well as hepatitis B serology. Patients diagnosed with latent TB should undergo prophylaxis treatment before starting tocilizumab infusions. In case of developing a severe active infection once treatment with tocilizumab has been initiated, therapy should be interrupted. Screening and monitoring for TB and any other infection should be performed during treatment with tocilizumab [45–48].

Blockade of IL-6 with tocilizumab has also been associated with an increased risk of gastrointestinal perforations, which may occur predominantly in the large bowel [49]. The reported rate of serious gastrointestinal perforation in the global post-marketing safety database population was estimated to be at least 0.15 (95% confidence interval: 0.12, 0.18) events per 100 patient-years (PY) [48]. Therefore, tocilizumab should be used with caution in patients with a history of intestinal ulceration or diverticulitis. In case of signs or symptoms of abdominal pain, gastrointestinal hemorrhage, fever or changes in bowel movement habits, prompt evaluation should be performed in order to discard gastrointestinal disease and a risk of concomitant perforation [48, 49].

With regards to laboratory abnormalities, tocilizumab, especially when used with methotrexate, may cause an increase in hepatic transaminase levels [48]. Although no increased risk of clinical hepatitis was noted, the initiation of treatment with tocilizumab should be evaluated carefully in patients with hepatic transaminases 1.5 fold higher than normal serum values and it is not recommended at all when the serum levels are fivefold higher than normal [48]. In addition, treatment with tocilizumab is known to be associated with a reduction in peripheral blood neutrophil counts and a higher incidence of neutropenia [50, 51]. Mechanistic hypotheses include inhibition of IL-6-induced neutrophil survival, downregulation of other inflammatory cytokines, and facilitation of neutrophil migration from the circulation into tissues [50]. Paradoxically, the effects of tocilizumab on neutrophils may represent a therapeutic effect (as found in inflamed RA joints) rather than an adverse event [51].

Tocilizumab Safety in Pediatric Patients

A recent study from Yokota et al. reported the results of the safety and effectiveness of iv tocilizumab in sJIA from 1 year of post-marketing surveillance follow-up of 417 patients in a real-world setting [46]. The median age was 11.2 years. The overall incidence rate per 100 PYs for all serious adverse events (SAE) was 62.3. The most common SAEs were infections, with a rate of 18.2/100 patient-years, mostly bacterial pneumonia. The second most common SAEs were blood and lymphatic disorders, with a rate of 9.8/100 PYs. Of note, eight patients experienced serious infusion reactions, which occurred between the second and the fourth tocilizumab infusions. Six out of eight patients were tested for anti-drug antibodies, and five were positive. In conclusion, the results of this study demonstrated that tocilizumab was well tolerated and its safety profile was within an acceptable range for pediatric patients with sJIA [46].

Safety of Subcutaneous Versus Intravenous Tocilizumab

Recently, Burmester et al. have reported the safety of sc versus iv tocilizumab in combination with traditional DMARDs in patients with RA, showing that sc safety is similar to iv, albeit with a high frequency of injection site reactions. With careful patient selection, the benefit:risk ratio is apparently favorable, offering patients a convenient ambulatory administration route [44].

The New IL-6 Inhibitors

The launch of tocilizumab in 2010 as the first biological drug to target IL-6 constituted a key alternative to TNF-α blockers and its clinical success aroused the interest of the pharmaceutical industry for the investigation of other IL-6-blocking strategies. Indeed, at present a number of novel IL-6/IL-6R inhibitors are being tested in clinical trials and preclinical studies. These strategies include (1) targeting IL-6 itself with sirukumab, siltuximab, olokizumab, clazakinumab, and EBI-031; and (2) targeting the IL-6R with sarilumab and ALX-0061. Table 9.4 illustrates the ongoing clinical trials with tocilizumab and the latest IL-6 inhibitors.

Table 9.4 Currently ongoing clinical trials with IL-6 inhibitors

Drug	mAb structure	Target	Administration route	Studied indication	Clinicaltrials.gov identifier	Phase	Sponsor
Sirukumab	Fully human	IL-6	sc	Active RA despite DMARD therapy	NCT01604343	III	Janssen
			sc	Active RA despite anti-TNF therapy	NCT01606761	III	Janssen
			sc	Giant cell arteritis	NCT02531633	III	GlaxoSmithKline
			sc	Major depressive disorder	NCT02473289	II	Janssen
			iv	Active lupus nephritis	NCT01273389	II	Janssen
Siltuximab	Chimeric	IL-6	iv	Multicentric Castleman's disease	NCT01400503	II	Janssen
				Metastatic renal cell carcinoma	NCT00265135	I/II	Centocor, Inc.
				Solid tumors	NCT00841191	I/II	Centocor, Inc.
				High-risk smoldering multiple myeloma	NCT01484275	II	Janssen
				Type 1 diabetes	NCT02641522	0	Carla Greenbaum, Janssen
Olokizumab	Humanized	IL-6	sc	RA (Japanese patients)	NCT01533714	II	UCB pharma
				RA	NCT01533714	II	UCB pharma
Sarilumab	Fully human	IL-6Rα	sc	RA	NCT01146652	III	Sanofi
				RA unresponsive to anti-TNF	NCT01768572	III	Sanofi
				RA (Japanese patients)	NCT02293902	III	Sanofi
				Uveitis	NCT01900431	II	Sanofi
Clazakinumab	Humanized	IL-6	iv	RA	N/A	II	Alder BioPharmaceuticals
ALX-0061	Nanobody (heavy chain only)	IL-6R	iv	RA	NCT01284569	I/II	Ablynx
			sc	RA	NCT02287922	II	Ablynx
EBI-031	N/A	IL-6	intravitreal	DME, uveitis	N/A	0	Eleven biotherapeutics

Tocilizumab (non-RA trials)	Humanized	IL-6R	iv	Amyotrophic lateral sclerosis	NCT02469896	II	Barrow Neurological Institute
			iv	Hemophagocytic lymphohistiocytosis	NCT02007239	II	Children's Hospital of Philadelphia
			iv	B-cell chronic lymphocytic leukemia	NCT02336048	I	Hoffmann-La Roche
			iv	Treated HIV infection	NCT02049437	I	Case Western Reserve University
			iv	Non-ST elevation myocardial infarction	NCT01491074	II	Oslo University Hospital
			sc	Myocardial infarction	NCT02419937	N/A	Keesler Air Force Base Medical Center
			iv	Schizophrenia	NCT02034474	IV	New York State Psychiatric Institute
			iv	Schizophrenia	NCT01696929	I	Georgia Regents University
			iv	Steroid-refractory acute graft-versus-host disease	NCT01475162	I/II	Medical College of Wisconsin
			iv	Prevention of graft versus host disease	NCT02206035	II	William R. Drobyski, MD, Medical College of Wisconsin
			iv	Renal graft inflammation	NCT02108600	II	University of California, San Francisco
			iv	New-onset type 1 diabetes	NCT02293837	II	National Institute of Allergy and Infectious Diseases (NIAID)
			iv	KSHV-associated multicentric Castleman disease	NCT01441063	II	National Cancer Institute (NCI)
			iv	Fibrous dysplasia of bone	NCT01791842	II	Hospices Civils de Lyon
			iv	Hand osteoarthritis	NCT02477059	III	Assistance Publique – Hôpitaux de Paris
			sc	Systemic JIA	NCT01904292	I	Hoffmann-La Roche
			sc	Polyarticular-course JIA	NCT01904279	I	Hoffmann-La Roche
			sc	Polyarticular-course JIA	NCT02165345	I	Hoffmann-La Roche
			iv	Systemic JIA (patients less than 2 years old)	NCT01455701	I	Hoffmann-La Roche
			iv	Refractory polymyositis and dermatomyositis	NCT02043548	II	University of Pittsburgh
			iv	Polymyalgia rheumatica	NCT01396317	II	Hospital for Special Surgery, New York
			iv	Takayasu arteritis	NCT02101333	III	Assistance Publique – Hôpitaux de Paris
			iv	Giant cell arteritis	NCT01450137	II	University Hospital Inselspital, Berne
			sc	Systemic sclerosis	NCT02453256	III	Hoffmann-La Roche
			iv	Primary Sjögren's syndrome	NCT01782235	II	University Hospital, Strasbourg, France
			iv	Uveitis	NCT01717170	I/II	Johns Hopkins University
			iv	Uveitis associated with JIA	NCT01603355	I/II	Oregon Health & Science University
			iv	Thyroid eye disease	NCT01297699	III	Hospital Clinico Universitario de Santiago
			iv	DME	NCT02511067	II	University of Nebraska

Abbreviations: *DMARD* disease-modifying anti-rheumatic drugs, *DME* diabetic macular edema, *JIA* juvenile idiopathic arthritis, *IL-6* interleukin-6, *IL-6R* interleukin-6 receptor, *iv* intravenous, *N/A* not available, *sc* subcutaneous, *RA* rheumatoid arthritis

Agents Targeting IL-6

Sirukumab is a fully human mAb directed against IL-6. Results from a phase II (proof-of-concept and dose-finding) study in patients with active RA despite methotrexate therapy have been recently published [52]. Sirukumab given subcutaneously 100 mg q2w achieved the primary endpoint of ACR50 (which refers to a 50% improvement in RA activity as determined by the American College of Rheumatology score) at week 12 (26.7% versus 3.3% with placebo) [52]. Currently, sirukumab is being tested in phase III clinical trials in patients with RA and giant cell arteritis, and phase II trials for major depressive disorder and active lupus nephritis.

Siltuximab is a chimeric mAb that targets IL-6. It is approved for the treatment of patients with multicentric Castleman's disease by the FDA with the dose of 11 mg/kg intravenous infusion q3w. Siltuximab can neutralize the IL-6 effect in a number of human malignancies, reducing cancer-related anorexia and cachexia [53]. Phase I/II studies with siltuximab are ongoing in patients with multicentric Castleman's disease, metastatic renal cell carcinoma, solid tumors, and multiple myeloma.

Olokizumab is a humanized mAb that acts on site 3 of IL-6 and prevents IL-6 binding its signaling co-receptor gp130 [54], therefore blocking the assembly of the IL-6 signaling complex. A phase II clinical trial completed in 2012 showed clinical effectiveness of olokizumab for RA [55] and at present it is undergoing a phase II study for RA in Japanese patients.

Clazakinumab is also a humanized anti-IL-6 agent. It showed greater affinity and prolonged half-life in comparison with olokizumab [56]. Clazakinumab proved clinical efficacy in a phase II study in patients with RA compared to placebo [57]. However, there are no ongoing clinical trials with clazakinumab listed in clinicaltrials.gov at present.

Lastly, it is noteworthy to mention that an intravitreal anti-IL-6 mAb named EBI-031 is presently being tested in preclinical studies for its potential use in patients with DME with promising preliminary results [58]. Phase 1 clinical trials with EBI-031 are expected to begin in 2016.

Agents Targeting the IL-6R

Sarilumab (Sanofi, Regeneron Pharmaceuticals) is a fully human anti-IL-6Rα mAb that binds both the membrane-bound and the soluble forms of IL-6Rα with high affinity, thereby blocking classic and trans-signaling pathways. Preclinical studies showed a higher affinity to IL-6R compared to tocilizumab [59]. The results from the pivotal phase III study SARIL-RA-TARGET have just been published [60]. The study comprised 546 RA patients intolerant/unresponsive to anti-TNF who were treated with sarilumab (150 mg or 200 mg every 2 weeks) in combination with methotrexate. Results showed that both doses provided sustained clinical efficacy, as shown by significant improvements in symptomatic, functional, and radiographic outcomes. Sarilumab was generally well tolerated, and the adverse events observed in this study were consistent with the effects of IL-6 signaling blockade [60].

Apart from RA, sarilumab is also being investigated for the treatment of patients with noninfectious uveitis in the phase II SARIL-SATURN study.

The other agent targeting the IL-6R is ALX-001, a mAb composed of two nanobodies with a molecular weight of 13 kDa. ALX-0061 predominantly modulates IL-6 trans-signaling pathway and has a greater affinity for the soluble and transmembrane IL-6R in comparison to tocilizumab as well as an extended half-life [61]. Preclinical pharmacology studies support its clinical development and it is now being investigated in a phase I/II trial for RA.

With regards to safety, in the absence of published results about the occurrence of adverse events in long-term clinical trials with the newer IL-6 inhibitors, it remains to be determined whether similar profiles of adverse events (that is, a class effect) will be observed in the IL-6-blockade strategy and whether agents selectively targeting the trans-signaling (and therefore sparing classic IL-6 signaling) will offer any advantage from a safety profile perspective [59]. While these data are still pending, early reports from clinical trials show that totally human IL-6-specific and IL-6R mAbs behave similarly to tocilizumab in terms of their effects on standard laboratory tests (lipids levels, liver enzymes, effect on acute phase proteins, etc.).

IL-6 and IL-6 Blockade in Noninfectious Uveitis

Various studies have found significant elevation of IL-6 in ocular fluids derived from refractory/chronic uveitis patients and animal models [62–64]. Experimental autoimmune uveitis (EAU) is a rodent model of human uveoretinitis, and several publications have revealed that highly inflammatory IL-17-producing Th17 cells play a pivotal role in the development of EAU, human uveitis, and other experimental autoimmune diseases [64]. Evidence shows that autoreactive Th1 and Th17 cells mediate EAU, and IL-6 is was recognized as an essential factor in inducing early phase of Th17 differentiation from naïve T cells in combination with TGF-β [65, 66]. Th17 cells further produce IL-17, IL-6, and TNF-α, and these cytokines perpetuate inflammation by stimulating fibroblasts, endothelial cells, and macrophages to produce chemokines, with the subsequent recruitment of more neutrophils and macrophages to the retina, which results in tissue damage and chronic inflammation [65, 66]. Several studies have demonstrated that IL-6 gene deficiency or the blockage of the IL-6 molecule with an antibody inhibited the development of uveitis by suppression of the Th17 response [67, 68]. Yoshimura et al. studied the role of Th17 cells on EAU by using IL-6- and IL-23-deficient mice, and confirmed that EAU development was reduced in these animals [5]. They found that systemic administration of recombinant anti-IL-6R antibody ameliorates EAU interfering with antigen-specific Th17 differentiation/expansion, and concluded that IL-6 blockade can suppress acute Th17 responses and ameliorate chronic/refractory intraocular inflammation. On the other hand, TGF-β alone promotes naive T cells to differentiate into Treg, which are considered immunosuppressive helper T cells [5]. Th17 and Treg cells are distinct subsets of helper T cells, and IL-6 signaling together with TGF-β promotes Th17 cells and inhibits Treg cell differentiation. Haruta et al. found that the IL-6 signaling blockade not only inhibited Th17 cell differentiation but also promoted antigen-specific Treg cells, which, in turn, suppressed the inflammatory effects of antigen-specific Th1 cells [68]. Thus, the inhibitory effect of the IL-6 blockade in the development of EAU is associated with suppression of the induction of both Th1 and Th17 effects in this disease.

Currently there are two ongoing randomized clinical trials studying tocilizumab therapy for uveitis: the STOP-UVEITIS study (clinicaltrials.gov identifier, NCT01717170), which is a study of the safety, tolerability, and bioactivity of tocilizumab in adult patients with noninfectious uveitis, and an open-label trial of tocilizumab in the management of JIA-associated uveitis (clinicaltrials.gov identifier, NCT01603355). As these trials are yet to complete, the literature on tocilizumab efficacy in uveitis remain sparse and are limited to case reports or short series, as shown in Table 9.5. Many of these reports suggest that IL-6R blockade can be a useful therapy to treat uveitis patients with macular edema. In 2011, Muselier et al. firstly reported on tocilizumab's efficacy in two uveitis patients diagnosed with birdshot chorioretinopathy and idiopathic granulomatous panuveitis who were refractory to conventional immunosuppressive drugs [69]. Tocilizumab induced uveitis control in both patients and also macular edema resolution in one case. Shortly afterwards, Tappeiner et al. [70] reported that tocilizumab was effective for the treatment of intraocular inflammation in 2 out of 3 JIA patients with uveitis refractory to several classical DMARDs and anti-TNF agents. Similarly, the efficacy of tocilizumab in patients with uveitis associated with Behçet's, Castelman's disease and Cogan's syndrome has also been reported [70–73].

Table 9.5 Reported studies with tocilizumab therapy for uveitis

First author	Year of publication	Type of study	No. of patients included	Type of uveitis	Outcome measures		Rate of efficacy (primary)	Median follow-up (months)	Side effects
					Primary	Secondary			
Deuter	2016	CS	5	JIA ($n = 2$), AS ($n = 1$), RA ($n = 2$)	CFT	VA	75%	14	None
Suhler	2015 ARVO annual meeting abstract	RCT	2	JIA	IOI	CFT	50%	N/A	None
Mesquida	2014	CS	7	BCR ($n = 3$), JIA ($n = 3$), and idiopathic panuveitis ($n = 1$)	CFT	VA, IOI	100%	15	None
Papo	2014	CS	8	BCR ($n = 1$), BD ($n = 1$) and idiopathic panuveitis ($n = 6$)	IOI	VA	75%	8	Bronchitis ($n = 1$) and grade 1 leukopenia ($n = 1$) and thrombocytopenia ($n = 1$)
Calvo-Rio	2014	CS	3	RA ($n = 1$), BD ($n = 2$)	IOI	VA	100%	7	None
Tsang	2014	CR	1	JIA	IOI	VA	100%	6	None
Adán	2014	CR	1	JIA	Vasoproliferative retinal tumor size	CFT, IOI, VA	100%	6	None
Adán	2013	CS	5	BCR ($n = 3$), JIA ($n = 1$), idiopathic panuveitis ($n = 1$)	CFT	IOI, VA	100%	6	None
Adán	2013	CR	1	Idiopathic panuveitis	CFT	IOI, VA	100%	6	None
Shibuya	2013	CR	1	Cogan's syndrome	IOI	VA	100%	N/A	N/A
Oshitari	2012	CR	1	Castleman's disease	IOI	VA	100%	12	None
Hirano	2012	CR	1	BD	IOI	VA	100%	N/A	None
Tappeiner	2012	CS	3	JIA	IOI	VA, arthritis activity	75%	9	None
Muselier	2011	CS	2	BCR ($n = 1$), idiopathic panuveitis ($n = 1$)	IOI	CFT, VA	100%	N/A	None

Abbreviations: *BCR* birdshot chorioretinopathy, *BD* Behçet's disease, *CFT* central foveal thickness, *CR* case report, *CS* case series, *IOI* intraocular inflammation, *JIA* juvenile idiopathic arthritis, *IOI* intraocular inflammation, *RA* rheumatoid arthritis, *RCT* randomized clinical trial, *VA* visual acuity, *N/A* not available

Distinctively, our research has focused on tocilizumab's particular efficacy in uveitis-related macular edema [74–79]. In 2014, we reported the long-term efficacy and safety of tocilizumab for refractory uveitis-related macular edema in 11 eyes of 7 patients [77]. In all cases, macular edema was the principal cause of impaired visual acuity (VA). A complete or partial resolution of the macular edema was found in all eyes after 12 months of tocilizumab therapy, with a significant decrease in the mean central foveal thickness (CFT). A statistically significant reduction in CFT was seen beginning in month 1, and that improvement in macular edema continued being statistically significant at months 3, 6, and 12 of tocilizumab therapy. In addition, a statistically significant improvement in visual acuity was observed at months 3, 6, and 12. No patients experienced a worsening in vision during follow-up. Importantly, the improvement in VA was not as rapid as the CFT reduction, likely due to the long duration of macular edema, raising the possibility that early administration of tocilizumab in selected cases may lead to better functional results. We concluded that tocilizumab was effective for uveitic macular edema which has been previously refractory to local/systemic steroids, traditional immunosuppressive agents, and other biologic therapies including anti-TNF.

Analogously, in 2016, Deuter et al. evaluated the efficacy of tocilizumab in a cohort of 5 patients (8 eyes) suffering from noninfectious uveitis in whom chronic macular edema was the principal cause of visual loss [80]. These patients also showed refractoriness to systemic corticosteroids, conventional immunosuppressive medication/s, and to at least one biologic drug (mainly anti-TNF-α). The cohort included 2 uveitis associated with JIA, 2 with unrelated but co-existing RA, and 1 with ankylosing spondylitis (AS). At 3 months, a ≥ 25% reduction in CFT was observed in 6 eyes (75.0%) of 5 patients. During follow-up, complete resolution of macular edema was achieved in 5 eyes (62.5%) of 4 patients. Improvement of VA was observed in 3 eyes of 3 patients, and stabilization in 3 eyes of 3 patients. With regards to intraocular inflammatory signs, tocilizumab had to be discontinued in one patient with uveitis and RA due to persistent active anterior uveitis. Tocilizumab was well-tolerated, and no severe side effects occurred. Deuter et al. concluded that treatment with tocilizumab may be considered in chronic uveitic macular edema even if previous immunomodulatory therapy has failed [80].

Conclusions

Despite the benefits attributable to current biological targeted interventions, in most studies 50% or more of patients with noninfectious uveitis treated with anti-TNF are unresponsive/intolerant. This unmet need for effective interventions in noninfectious uveitis clearly mandates further research, especially when the objective, today, is clinical remission. Nonresponsiveness to TNF blockade and/or residual disease activity, as well as the continuing, albeit slower progression of structural damage in a proportion of patients treated with TNF inhibitors suggest that TNF is not the sole biological target in the disease process, and therefore further novel agents and novel strategies are needed.

Major discoveries have come out in IL-6-related research, which have favored the establishment of IL-6 targeted therapy for immune-mediated diseases. Basic research clarified the molecular basis and characteristics of the IL-6 cytokine redundancy and pleiotropy, whereas clinical research revealed its pathological significance in disease development. These findings led to the concept that IL-6 targeting would constitute a novel therapeutic strategy for immune-mediated diseases, and indeed tocilizumab, a humanized anti-IL-6R antibody, became an innovative biologic for the treatment of several intractable diseases. Given the prominent role of IL-6 in various pathological conditions, it is expected that this strategy would be widely applicable for other immune-mediated diseases including noninfectious uveitis and macular edema.

References

1. Kishimoto T, Hirano T, Kikutani H, Muraguchi A. Delineation of human B cell differentiation: immunological and molecular characterization of human B cell differentiation factor (BSF-2). Adv Exp Med Biol. 1987;213:177–88.
2. Wolvekamp MC, Marquet RL. Interleukin-6: historical background, genetics and biological significance. Immunol Lett. 1990;24:1–9.
3. Yamasaki K, Taga T, Hirata Y, Yawata H, Kawanishi Y, Seed B, Taniguchi T, Hirano T, Kishimoto T. Cloning and expression of the human interleukin-6 (BSF-2/IFN beta 2) receptor. Science. 1988;241:825–8.
4. Lin P. Targeting interleukin-6 for noninfectious uveitis. Clin Ophthalmol. 2015;9:1697–702.
5. Yoshimura T, Sonoda KH, Ohguro N, Ohsugi Y, Ishibashi T, Cua DJ, Kobayashi T, Yoshida H, Yoshimura A. Involvement of Th17 cells and the effect of anti-IL-6 therapy in autoimmune uveitis. Rheumatology (Oxford). 2009;48:347–54.
6. Perez VL, Papaliodis GN, Chu D, Anzaar F, Christen W, Foster CS. Elevated levels of interleukin 6 in the vitreous fluid of patients with pars planitis and posterior uveitis: the Massachusetts eye & ear experience and review of previous studies. Ocul Immunol Inflamm. 2004;12:193–201.
7. Kang S, Tanaka T, Kishimoto T. Therapeutic uses of anti-interleukin-6 receptor antibody. Int Immunol. 2015;27:21–9.
8. Tanaka T, Narazaki M, Kishimoto T. IL-6 in inflammation, immunity, and disease. Cold Spring Harb Perspect Biol. 2014;6:a016295.
9. Calabrese LH, Rose-John S. IL-6 biology: implications for clinical targeting in rheumatic disease. Nat Rev Rheumatol. 2014;10:720–7.
10. Boulanger MJ, Chow DC, Brevnova EE, Garcia KC. Hexameric structure and assembly of the interleukin-6/IL-6 alpha-receptor/gp130 complex. Science. 2003;300:2101–4.
11. Schmitz J, Weissenbach M, Haan S, Heinrich PC, Schaper F. SOCS3 exerts its inhibitory function on interleukin-6 signal transduction through the SHP2 recruitment sites of gp130. J Biol Chem. 2000;275:12848–56.
12. Narazaki M, Yasukawa K, Saito T, Ohsugi Y, Fukui H, Koishihara Y, Yancopoulos GD, Taga T, Kishimoto T. Soluble forms of the interleukin-6 signal-transducing receptor component gp130 in human serum possessing a potential to inhibit signals through membrane-anchored gp130. Blood. 1993;82:1120–6.
13. Rose-John S. IL-6 trans-signaling via the soluble IL-6 receptor: importance for the pro-inflammatory activities of IL-6. Int J Biol Sci. 2012;8:1237–47.
14. Kishimoto T, Akira S, Narazaki M, Taga T. Interleukin-6 family of cytokines and gp130. Blood. 1995;86:1243–54.
15. Scheller J, Chalaris A, Schmidt-Arras D, Rose-John S. The pro- and anti-inflammatory properties of the cytokine interleukin-6. Biochim Biophys Acta. 2011;181:878–88.
16. Hoge J, Yan I, Jänner N, et al. IL-6 controls the innate immune response against Listeria monocytogenes via classical IL-6 signaling. J Immunol. 2013;190:703–11.
17. Matzinger P. The danger model: a renewed sense of self. Science. 2002;296:301–4.
18. Heinrich PC, Castell JV, Andus T. Interleukin-6 and the acute phase response. Biochem J. 1990;265:621–36.
19. Devaraj S, Kumaresan PR, Jialal I. C-reactive protein induces release of both endothelial microparticles and circulating endothelial cells in vitro and in vivo: further evidence of endothelial dysfunction. Clin Chem. 2011;57:1757–61.
20. Jensen LE, Whitehead AS. Regulation of serum amyloid A protein expression during the acute-phase response. Biochem J. 1998;334:489–503.
21. Eriksson S, Janciauskiene S, Lannfelt L. Alpha 1-antichymotrypsin regulates Alzheimer beta-amyloid peptide fibril formation. Proc Natl Acad Sci U S A. 1995;92:2313–7.
22. Nemeth E, Tuttle MS, Powelson J, et al. Hepcidin regulates cellular iron efflux by binding to ferroportin and inducing its internalization. Science. 2004;306:2090–3.
23. Liuzzi JP, Lichten LA, Rivera S, et al. Interleukin-6 regulates the zinc transporter Zip14 in liver and contributes to the hypozincemia of the acute-phase response. Proc Natl Acad Sci U S A. 2005;102:6843–8.
24. Weiler HA, Jean-Philippe S, Cohen TR, Vanstone CA, Agellon S. Depleted iron stores and iron deficiency anemia associated with reduced ferritin and hepcidin and elevated soluble transferrin receptors in a multiethnic group of preschool-age children. Appl Physiol Nutr Metab. 2015;40:887–94.
25. Ishibashi T, Kimura H, Uchida T, Kariyone S, Friese P, Burstein SA. Human interleukin 6 is a direct promoter of maturation of megakaryocytes in vitro. Proc Natl Acad Sci U S A. 1989;86:5953–7.
26. Hashizume M, Hayakawa N, Mihara M. IL-6 trans-signaling directly induces RANKL on fibroblast-like synovial cells and is involved in RANKL induction by TNF-a and IL-17. Rheumatology (Oxford). 2008;47:1635–40.
27. Nakahara H, Song J, Sugimoto M, et al. Anti-interleukin-6 receptor antibody therapy reduces vascular endothelial growth factor production in rheumatoid arthritis. Arthritis Rheum. 2003;48:1521–9.
28. Grossman RM, Krueger J, Yourish D, et al. Interleukin 6 is expressed in high levels in psoriatic skin and stimulates proliferation of cultured human keratinocytes. Proc Natl Acad Sci U S A. 1989;86:6367–71.
29. Gillespie EF, Raychaudhuri N, Papageorgiou KI, et al. Interleukin-6 production in CD40-engaged fibrocytes in thyroid-associated ophthalmopathy: involvement of Akt and NF-κB. Invest Ophthalmol Vis Sci. 2012;53:7746–53.
30. Diehl SA, Schmidlin H, Nagasawa M, Blom B, Spits H. IL-6 triggers IL-21 production by human CD4+ T

cells to drive STAT3-dependent plasma cell differentiation in B cells. Immunol Cell Biol. 2012;90:802–11.
31. Diehl S, Anguita J, Hoffmeyer A, Zapton T, Ihle JN, Fikrig E, Rincón M. Inhibition of Th1 differentiation by IL-6 is mediated by SOCS1. Immunity. 2000;13:805–15.
32. Diehl S, Rincón M. The two faces of IL-6 on Th1/Th2 differentiation. Mol Immunol. 2002;39:531–6.
33. Miossec P, Korn T, Kuchroo VK. Interleukin-17 and type 17 helper T cells. N Engl J Med. 2009;361:888–98.
34. Kimura A, Kishimoto T. IL-6: regulator of Treg/Th17 balance. Eur J Immunol. 2010;40:1830–5.
35. Tanaka T. Can IL-6 blockade rectify imbalance between Tregs and Th17 cells? Immunotherapy. 2013;5:695–7.
36. Carbone A, Gloghini A. Emerging issues after the recognition of in situ follicular lymphoma. Leuk Lymphoma. 2014;55:482–90.
37. Okada M, Kitahara M, Kishimoto S, Matsuda T, Hirano T, Kishimoto T. IL-6/BSF-2 functions as a killer helper factor in the in vitro induction of cytotoxic T cells. J Immunol. 1988;141:1543–9.
38. Ho LJ, Luo SF, Lai JH. Biological effects of interleukin-6: clinical applications in autoimmune diseases and cancers. Biochem Pharmacol. 2015;97:16–26.
39. Hirano T, Matsuda T, Turner M, et al. Excessive production of interleukin 6/B cell stimulatory factor-2 in rheumatoid arthritis. Eur J Immunol. 1988;18:1797–801.
40. Yoshizaki K, Matsuda T, Nishimoto N, et al. Pathogenic significance of interleukin-6 (IL-6/BSF-2) in Castleman's disease. Blood. 1989;74:1360–7.
41. Zhang XG, Chaptal PA, Klein B. Constitutive production of interleukin-6 and immunologic features in cardiac myxomas. Arthritis Rheum. 1990;33:398–402.
42. Kishimoto T. Interleukin-6: from basic science to medicine – 40 years in immunology. Annu Rev Immunol. 2005;23:1–21.
43. Mitchel EL, Jones G. Subcutaneous tocilizumab for the treatment of rheumatoid arthritis. Expert Rev Clin Immunol. 2016;12:103–14.
44. Burmester GR, Rubbert-Roth A, Cantagrel A, et al. Efficacy and safety of subcutaneous tocilizumab versus intravenous tocilizumab in combination with traditional DMARDs in patients with RA at week 97 (SUMMACTA). Ann Rheum Dis. 2016;75:68–74.
45. Curtis JR, Perez-Gutthann S, Suissa S, Napalkov P, Singh N, Thompson L, Porter-Brown B, Actemra Pharmacoepidemiology Board. Tocilizumab in rheumatoid arthritis: a case study of safety evaluations of a large postmarketing data set from multiple data sources. Semin Arthritis Rheum. 2015;44:381–8.
46. Yokota S, Itoh Y, Morio T, et al. Tocilizumab in systemic juvenile idiopathic arthritis in a real-world clinical setting: results from 1 year of postmarketing surveillance follow-up of 417 patients in Japan. Ann Rheum Dis. 2016;75(9):1654–60.
47. Campbell L, Chen C, Bhagat SS, Parker RA, Östör AJ. Risk of adverse events including serious infections in rheumatoid arthritis patients treated with tocilizumab: a systematic literature review and meta-analysis of randomized controlled trials. Rheumatology (Oxford). 2011;50:552–62.
48. Nishimoto N, Miyasaka N, Yamamoto K, Kawai S, Takeuchi T, Azuma J. Long-term safety and efficacy of tocilizumab, an anti-IL-6 receptor monoclonal antibody, in monotherapy, in patients with rheumatoid arthritis (the STREAM study): evidence of safety and efficacy in a 5-year extension study. Ann Rheum Dis. 2009;68:1580–4.
49. Pfeil J, Grulich-Henn J, Wenning D, Breil T, Günther P, Lutz T. Multiple upper gastrointestinal perforations in a 15-year-old patient treated with tocilizumab. Rheumatology (Oxford). 2014;53:1713–4.
50. Nakamura I, Omata Y, Naito M, Ito K. Blockade of interleukin 6 signaling induces marked neutropenia in patients with rheumatoid arthritis. J Rheumatol. 2009;36:459–60.
51. Wright HL, Moots RJ, Edwards SW. The multifactorial role of neutrophils in rheumatoid arthritis. Nat Rev Rheumatol. 2014;10:593–601.
52. Smolen JS, Weinblatt ME, Sheng S, Zhuang Y, Hsu B. Sirukumab, a human anti-interleukin-6 monoclonal antibody: a randomised, 2-part (proof-of-concept and dose-finding), phase II study in patients with active rheumatoid arthritis despite methotrexate therapy. Ann Rheum Dis. 2014;73:1616–25.
53. Chen R, Chen B. Siltuximab (CNTO 328): a promising option for human malignancies. Drug Des Devel Ther. 2015;9:3455–8.
54. Shaw S, Bourne T, Meier C, et al. Discovery and characterization of olokizumab: a humanized antibody targeting interleukin-6 and neutralizing gp130-signaling. MAbs. 2014;6:774–82.
55. Genovese MC, Fleischmann D, Furst N, et al. Efficacy and safety of olokizumab in patients with rheumatoid arthritis with an inadequate response to TNF inhibitor therapy: outcomes of a randomised phase IIb study. Ann Rheum Dis. 2014;73:1607–15.
56. Shakib S, Francis B, Smith J. Safety, pharmacokinetics and pharmacodynamics of ALD518 (BMS-945429), a high-affinity monoclonal antibody directed against interleukin-6 administered by subcutaneous injection: a phase I trial. Arthritis Rheum. 2010;62(Suppl 10):1124.
57. Weinblatt ME, Mease P, Mysler E, et al. The efficacy and safety of subcutaneous clazakizumab in patients with moderate-to-severe rheumatoid arthritis and an inadequate response to methotrexate: results from a multinational, phase IIb, randomized, double-blind, placebo/active-controlled, dose-ranging study. Arthritis Rheumatol. 2015;67:2591–600.
58. Schmidt M, Matsumoto Y, Tisdale A, Lowden P, Kovalchin J, Wu P, Golden K, Dombrowski C, Lain B, Furfine ES. Optimised intravitreal IL-6 antagonist for the treatment of diabetic macular edema. The association for research in vision and ophthalmology (ARVO) annual meeting 2015 abstract.

59. Kim GW, Lee NR, Pi RH, Lim YS, Lee YM, Lee JM, Jeong HS, Chung SH. IL-6 inhibitors for treatment of rheumatoid arthritis: past, present, and future. Arch Pharm Res. 2015;38(5):575–84.
60. Genovese MC, Fleischmann R, Kivitz AJ, et al. Sarilumab plus methotrexate in patients with active rheumatoid arthritis and inadequate response to methotrexate: results of a phase III study. Arthritis Rheumatol. 2015;67:1424–37.
61. Van Roy M, Ververken C, Beirnaert E, et al. The preclinical pharmacology of the high affinity anti-IL-6R Nanobody® ALX-0061 supports its clinical development in rheumatoid arthritis. Arthritis Res Ther. 2015;17:135.
62. Curnow SJ, Falciani F, Durrani OM, Cheung CM, Ross EJ, Wloka K, Rauz S, Wallace GR, Salmon M, Murray PI. Multiplex bead immunoassay analysis of aqueous humor reveals distinct cytokine profiles in uveitis. Invest Ophthalmol Vis Sci. 2005;46:4251–9.
63. Horai R, Caspi RR. Cytokines in autoimmune uveitis. J Interferon Cytokine Res. 2011;31:733–44.
64. Caspi RR, Roberge FG, McAllister CG, el-Saied M, Kuwabara T, Gery I, Hanna E, Nussenblatt RB. T cell lines mediating experimental autoimmune uveoretinitis (EAU) in the rat. J Immunol. 1986;136:928–33.
65. Amadi-Obi A, Yu CR, Liu X, Mahdi RM, Clarke GL, Nussenblatt RB, Gery I, Lee YS, Egwuagu CE. TH17 cells contribute to uveitis and scleritis and are expanded by IL-2 and inhibited by IL-27/STAT1. Nat Med. 2007;13:711–8.
66. Bettelli E, Carrier Y, Gao W, Korn T, Strom TB, Oukka M, Weiner HL, Kuchroo VK. Reciprocal developmental pathways for the generation of pathogenic effector TH17 and regulatory T cells. Nature. 2006;441(7090):235–8.
67. Hohki S, Ohguro N, Haruta H, et al. Blockade of interleukin-6 signaling suppresses experimental autoimmune uveoretinitis by the inhibition of inflammatory Th17 responses. Exp Eye Res. 2010;91:162–70.
68. Haruta H, Ohguro N, Fujimoto M, et al. Blockade of interleukin-6 signaling suppresses not only th17 but also interphotoreceptor retinoid binding protein-specific Th1 by promoting regulatory T cells in experimental autoimmune uveoretinitis. Invest Ophthalmol Vis Sci. 2011;52:3264–71.
69. Muselier A, Bielefeld P, Bidot S, Vinit J, Besancenot JF, Bron A. Efficacy of tocilizumab in two patients with anti-TNF-alpha refractory uveitis. Ocul Immunol Inflamm. 2011;19:382–3.
70. Hirano T, Ohguro N, Hohki S, Hagihara K, Shima Y, Narazaki M, Ogata A, Yoshizaki K, Kumanogoh A, Kishimoto T, Tanaka T. A case of Behçet's disease treated with a humanized anti-interleukin-6 receptor antibody, tocilizumab. Mod Rheumatol. 2012;22:298–302.
71. Oshitari T, Kajita F, Tobe A, Itami M, Yotsukura J, Baba T, Yamamoto S. Refractory uveitis in patient with castleman disease successfully treated with tocilizumab. Case Rep Ophthalmol Med. 2012;2012:968180.
72. Shibuya M, Fujio K, Morita K, Harada H, Kanda H, Yamamoto K. Successful treatment with tocilizumab in a case of Cogan's syndrome complicated with aortitis. Mod Rheumatol. 2013;23:577–81.
73. Calvo-Río V, de la Hera D, Beltrán-Catalán E, Blanco R, Hernandez M, Martínez-Costa L, Loricera J, Cañal J, Ventosa J, Ortiz-Sanjuán F, Pina T, González-Vela MC, Rodríguez-Cundín P, González-Gay MA. Tocilizumab in uveitis refractory to other biologic drugs: a study of 3 cases and a literature review. Clin Exp Rheumatol. 2014;32:S54–7.
74. Adán A, Llorenç V, Mesquida M, Pelegrín L. Tocilizumab treatment for recalcitrant uveitic macular edema. Graefes Arch Clin Exp Ophthalmol. 2013;251:2249–50.
75. Adán A, Mesquida M, Llorenç V, Espinosa G, Molins B, Hernández MV, Pelegrín L. Tocilizumab treatment for refractory uveitis-related cystoid macular edema. Graefes Arch Clin Exp Ophthalmol. 2013;251:2627–32.
76. Adán A, Mesquida M, Llorenç V, Modesto C. Tocilizumab for retinal vasoproliferative tumor secondary to juvenile idiopathic arthritis-associated uveitis: a case report. Graefes Arch Clin Exp Ophthalmol. 2014;252:163–4.
77. Mesquida M, Molins B, Llorenç V, Sainz de la Maza M, Adán A. Long-term effects of tocilizumab therapy for refractory uveitis-related macular edema. Ophthalmology. 2014;121:2380–6.
78. Mesquida M, Leszczynska A, Llorenç V, Adán A. Interleukin-6 blockade in ocular inflammatory diseases. Clin Exp Immunol. 2014;176:301–9.
79. Mesquida M, Llorenç V, Adán A. In response to "Deuter CM, Zierhut M, Igney-Oertel A, Xenitidis T, Feidt A, Sobolewska B, Stuebiger N, Doycheva D. Tocilizumab in uveitic macular edema refractory to previous immunomodulatory treatment". Ocul Immunol Inflamm. 2017;25:215–20.
80. Deuter CM, Zierhut M, Igney-Oertel A, Xenitidis T, Feidt A, Sobolewska B, Stuebiger N, Doycheva D. Tocilizumab in uveitic macular edema refractory to previous immunomodulatory treatment. Ocul Immunol Inflamm. 2017;25:215–20.

Interferons and Intravenous Immunoglobulin

10

Durga S. Borkar and Nicholas J. Butler

Pearls

- Systemic interferon and intravenous immunoglobulin represent powerful, immunomodulatory treatment options in the armamentarium of the ocular inflammatory disease specialist, often employed in the setting of severe and refractory disease.
- The complex mechanisms of action for each of these agents are numerous and poorly understood.
- Due to high efficacy in certain patients, specific indications for their use are emerging, namely: Behçet disease, multiple sclerosis-associated uveitis, and uveitic cystoid macular edema for systemic interferon, and ocular mucous membrane pemphigoid and birdshot chorioretinitis for intravenous immunoglobulin.
- Side effects and adverse events are significant for interferon, though careful monitoring and patient-perceived benefit allow for low rates of discontinuation.
- Patients generally tolerate intravenous immunoglobulin very well; however, clinicians should be aware that serious complications may rarely occur.

Introduction

In the setting of seemingly intractable uveitis or other ocular inflammation, two relatively poorly understood immunomodulators, exogenous interferons and intravenous immunoglobulin (IVIg), may be considered in the treatment algorithm. More and more, though, as our understanding evolves with regard to their wholly disparate mechanisms of action, niche indications for these two agents have emerged. In the following, we discuss the current understanding of the mechanisms of action for systemically administered interferons and IVIg and how they may be applied discriminately to specific ocular inflammatory disease on a pathophysiological basis. Further, we review the available evidence for the efficacy of each of these treatments in specific uveitic, and other ocular immunological,

D. S. Borkar
Harvard Medical School, Massachusetts Eye and Ear Infirmary, Department of Ophthalmology, Boston, MA, USA

N. J. Butler (✉)
Harvard Medical School, Massachusetts Eye and Ear Infirmary, Department of Ophthalmology, Boston, MA, USA

Veterans Affairs Boston Healthcare System, Boston, MA, USA
e-mail: nicholas.butler4@va.gov

P. Lin, E. Suhler (eds.), *Treatment of Non-infectious Uveitis*,
https://doi.org/10.1007/978-3-030-22827-9_10

diseases, focusing on the most promising indications. Commonly utilized dosing regimens, side effect profiles, and other clinically relevant considerations are provided.

Interferon Therapy

Since the discovery of these endogenous cytokines in 1957, innumerable investigations of interferons have flooded the literature, vis-à-vis their role in the prevention of viral replication and as a potential biomarker in various diseases, their therapeutic utility in a vast array of neoplastic, infectious, and immunological disorders, and their de novo synthesis in sufficient quantity to treat disease in humans [1]. This immense body of study reflects the abstruse nature of interferons, in terms of their precise roles in immune responses and effects on the disease with exogenous administration; indeed, interferons have multifarious effects, including antiviral, antineoplastic, antiangiogenic, and immunomodulatory properties, among others.

The initial work from the dermatological literature that led to the use of exogenous interferon for ocular inflammatory disease involved three patients with poorly responsive Behçet disease. The investigators' rationale for attempting interferon treatment stemmed from the fact that in the earliest characterizations by Behçet himself in 1937, a viral etiology was suspected for this disorder [2]. In all three patients, a remarkable improvement in oral and genital ulcerations, thrombophlebitis, and arthritis was observed in as early as 2 days after initiating interferon alpha therapy; curiously, only one patient had eye manifestations and the uveitis failed to respond.

Mechanism of Action

Interferon alpha, a naturally occurring cytokine produced mainly by plasmacytoid dendritic cells (pDCs), has several therapeutic properties [3]. The other type I interferon, beta, is produced by fibroblasts. Production of both is upregulated in response to viral infection; they are the key component of the innate immune response to such pathogens. Recombinant interferon's exact mechanism of action in the treatment of uveitis is unknown; however, several hypotheses exist. Overall, it is thought to involve an intricate balance between excess tumor necrosis factor alpha (TNF alpha), promoting organ-specific autoimmunity, including uveitis, and excess interferon alpha, implicated in systemic autoimmunity, such as in autoimmune thyroiditis, diabetes, and systemic lupus erythematosus (SLE) [4].

One study of 11 patients with posterior uveitis and a complete response to interferon alpha-2b demonstrated that the pDCs of patients with uveitis secreted significantly less interferon alpha when stimulated in vitro, as compared to healthy controls [5]. This suggests that a functional impairment of pDCs in uveitis patients may be promoting their organ-specific autoimmunity, tipping the cross-regulatory balance between TNF alpha and interferon alpha in favor of TNF. In such a milieu, recombinant interferon alpha can be predicted to have success, as replacement therapy to address the endogenous deficiency. Further, they posit that functionally defective pDCs, with impaired interferon alpha production, may also be less effective at inducing regulatory T (Treg) cells in the setting of viral infection, which are the major regulators of autoreactive T cells. Exogenous interferon alpha may induce interleukin (IL)-10 producing Treg cells, mitigating the effects of autoreactive Th1 cells and encouraging immunotolerance over autoimmunity.

Invoking similar mechanisms, others have found that type I interferon treatment can suppress experimental autoimmune uveoretinitis (EAU) in Lewis rats [6]. In parallel experiments they detected decreased production of TNF alpha by stimulated splenocytes in interferon alpha/beta-treated rats, an explanation, at least in part, for the observed treatment effect.

Furthermore, experimental evidence indicates that interferon alpha increases the production of IL-1 receptor antagonist, thereby inhibiting the proinflammatory effects of IL-1 [7]. IL-1 plays a role in the pathophysiology of Behçet disease, which has shown a significant response to interferon therapy in clinical studies, as discussed below.

Beyond their therapeutic value in patients with uveitis, recombinant interferons have proven effectiveness for uveitic cystoid macular edema (CME); there is in vitro evidence that this may be mediated through enhanced barrier function at the level of the retinal vascular endothelium [8].

Indications for Therapy

Behçet Disease

The initial and most prevalent use of systemic interferon therapy for uveitis has been for the treatment of ocular Behçet disease, with particular utility in cases of persistent retinal vasculitis or macular involvement with significant vision loss [9]. In 1994, an initial case series detailed three patients with refractory intraocular inflammation secondary to Behçet disease who achieved rapid and complete suppression of their ocular inflammation with systemic interferon alpha-2b therapy [10]. In all three cases, after failing varying combinations of at least four immunosuppressive and cytotoxic agents, visual acuity improved significantly and remained stable with interferon. One patient improved from count fingers vision to 6/12 in his only seeing eye within 1 week of initiating therapy.

Similar case reports and small series supporting the high response rates of ocular Behçet disease to interferon alpha followed [11–14]. An open, prospective trial offered more definitive evidence, with interferon alpha inducing a complete remission of panuveitis in all seven enrolled patients [15]. In the same year, Zouboulis and Orfanos reviewed the available medical literature, conference proceedings, and abstracts for all Behçet disease patients treated with systemic interferon [16]. Of 144 patients treated, 39 had uveitis and 37 (95%) responded, either partially or completely, to interferon alpha.

Subsequently, investigators conducted a multicenter, non-randomized, prospective trial [17]. In 50 patients with Behçet disease and panuveitis or retinal vasculitis unresponsive to at least one immunosuppressive drug, systemic interferon alpha-2a induced high rates of clinical remission. More than 90% of patients responded to therapy and achieved quiescence within a median time period of 4 weeks; visual acuity improved significantly (0.56–0.84, $p < 0.0001$) by 24 weeks. Angiographic CME resolved in all patients in whom this complication preexisted ($n = 58$). In reviewing the literature 1 year later, these same investigators identified 182 Behçet disease patients with ocular disease and noted a partial or complete response to interferon alpha in 171 (94%) [18]. This comprised all known patients treated for this indication to date. They defined partial remission as ≥50% decrease in the number, severity, duration, and/or frequency of lesions or system-specific scores.

In 2006, Tugal-Tutken et al. retrospectively reviewed their experience with interferon alpha for the same indication and found a complete or partial response in 91% of 44 patients and sustained improvement in visual acuity in 95% [19]. Curiously, they found that only 36% remained recurrence-free during therapy and 20% had a sustained, drug-free remission. The authors suggest that a differential treatment effect may be observed between varying populations, as Kötter et al. had observed higher rates of treatment-induced (82%) and drug-free (40%) remissions [17].

From 2008 to 2011, two retrospective and two prospective studies definitively established the long-term safety and efficacy of exogenous interferon alpha, even in lower dose regimens in some cases, for refractory ocular Behçet disease [20–23]. Collectively, 175 patients were treated and followed for an extended period, ranging from 24 to 71 months. Of these, 160 (91%) responded favorably to interferon alpha. Rates of relapse of ocular inflammation decreased significantly, ranging from 5 to 15-fold. Drug-free remission was induced in all studies, from 28 to 89%, though the duration varied.

While a majority of studies describe interferon treatment in adults, children suffering from Behçet disease commonly develop ocular manifestations, which can often be more severe than in adults [24]. In 2007, Guillaume-Czitrom et al. described a case series of seven children with corticosteroid-dependent uveitis secondary to Behçet disease and their response to systemic interferon alpha [25]. Five out of seven children responded markedly and had remission maintenance with decreased corticosteroid dependency. However, it is notable that the remaining two children had significant adverse effects early in the initiation of interferon alpha therapy requiring treatment cessation.

Intermediate Uveitis

In addition to its use for the treatment of ocular Behçet disease, interferon therapy has increasing potential in the treatment of intermediate uveitis (IU) [26, 27]. Given the strong association with IU, many of the reported patients have a concurrent diagnosis of multiple sclerosis (MS), a disease for which exogenous interferon, primarily interferon beta, has long been employed [28]. More recently, investigators have found that, in addition to ameliorating the signs and symptoms of the underlying systemic disease, interferon beta effectively treats the associated ocular inflammation in patients with MS [26, 27, 29].

An initial study investigated 13 patients with multiple sclerosis and associated uveitis [27]. In this retrospective observational series, all patients except for one had bilateral IU. Thirteen eyes of seven patients additionally had CME. In all affected eyes, intraocular inflammation improved as measured by aqueous (average improvement 1.2 grades) and vitreous cell count (average improvement 1.7 grades). Additionally, vision improved in 17 eyes with visual acuity gains of three or more Snellen lines in 10 of these eyes. CME resolved completely in nine eyes (69%) with treatment. Although CME was still visible angiographically in two additional patients, it was reduced compared to before interferon therapy. These results unequivocally indicate that the ocular inflammation associated with MS rapidly responds to systemic interferon beta in a majority of patients, improving vision and lowering rates of uveitic complications such as CME.

While most studies assessing the use of interferon in the treatment of uveitis have been either retrospective chart reviews or prospective observational studies, a recent randomized controlled trial investigated the efficacy and safety of interferon beta in patients with IU and inflammatory CME compared to standard immunosuppressive therapy with subcutaneous (sc) methotrexate [26]. Although the sample size of the study was small with only 19 patients, the results after 3 months of treatment strongly favored interferon beta over methotrexate, both in terms of improvement in visual acuity and central macular thickness. The difference in visual acuity improvement was clinically significant with an approximately three-line improvement in the interferon arm compared to a one-line improvement in the methotrexate arm ($p = 0.04$). Change in macular thickness also supported the superiority of interferon, having decreased by a mean of 206 μm compared to an increase of 47 μm in those on methotrexate ($p < 0.0001$). In this study, a significant proportion of patients, approximately 26%, had multiple sclerosis.

Uveitic Cystoid Macular Edema

Observing Behçet disease patients treated with systemic interferons for refractory uveitis, investigators noticed incidental improvement in CME if present prior to initiating therapy [11, 17]. Others corroborated this finding, demonstrating a dramatic response of CME to interferon therapy in Behçet disease patients [15, 30]. More recently, mounting evidence supports the use of systemic interferon alpha for refractory, uveitic CME from a diverse array of noninfectious etiologies [31–35].

In 2006, Deuter et al. prospectively assessed the efficacy of interferon alpha-2a in the treatment of CME associated with endogenous uveitis in 15 eyes of eight non-Behçet disease patients [32]. In all cases, the uveitis was in complete remission but the CME had not responded to a combination of systemic corticosteroids and acetazolamide. In six patients, at least one additional immunosuppressant had also been tried. At initiation of interferon therapy, the doses of immunosuppressants were halved, acetazolamide was discontinued, and oral steroid was decreased to a maximum of 10 milligrams (mg) daily. Overall, CME resolved completely in 13 of 15 eyes, or seven out of eight patients, within 2–4 weeks of initiating treatment. Over long-term follow-up, four patients required reinstitution of therapy after completing the initial 6 month treatment phase, and the CME again responded and remained suppressed in all four patients with maintenance interferon dosing.

Subsequently, the same group retrospectively analyzed 24 consecutive, non-Behçet disease patients (40 eyes) treated with systemic interferon alpha-2a for uveitic CME [33]. The CME was long-standing, having been present for a mean duration of 36 months. Similar to their pilot study, the CME responded rapidly and completely in 25 of 40 eyes. Another 10 eyes were qualified as "partly effective" (incomplete resolution of CME or unable to taper interferon within 3 months), though central foveal thickness improved significantly, from 587 to 285 μm, in this group as well. Underscoring the strictness of their criteria for efficacy, approximately 50% of eyes in each group, "effective" and "partly effective", gained three or more lines during follow-up and the remainder demonstrated stable visual acuity.

Solely for reasons of availability, the first study to assess the efficacy of interferon alpha for uveitic CME in the United States used interferon alpha-2b, not alpha-2a [34]. Four patients with bilateral CME (eight eyes) were included; in all cases, they had recalcitrant CME, having failed numerous prior medical and surgical therapies and been present for an average duration of greater than 31 months. All eight eyes showed rapid improvement in mean central macular thickness from 563 to 267 μm ($p = 0.002$) followed by substantial gains in mean visual acuity from 20/129 at baseline to 20/56 at last visit ($p = 0.0004$). While the dosage was again tapered over the course of 6 months, all patients remained on a lower maintenance dose at the conclusion of the reported study period.

Although this was a smaller retrospective study, the results suggested similar efficacy between interferon alpha-2b and -2a in the treatment of refractory CME. The authors noted, however, that interferon alpha-2a may be more immunogenic than interferon alpha-2b, a claim suggested by others [34, 36–38]. As a result, neutralizing antibodies, with concomitant lack or loss of response to therapy, may be less commonly encountered with the interferon alpha-2b preparation. The results of the initial pilot study testing the efficacy of interferon alpha-2a for refractory CME support this [32]. One patient in this study showed no response to interferon therapy from the outset, and this patient was found to have preexisting neutralizing antibodies against interferon alpha. Another patient, after initially responding to therapy, eventually became nonresponsive to interferon alpha and similarly neutralizing antibodies were detected.

While this could be one explanation for the lack or loss of response seen in these patients, it is notable that the role of neutralizing antibodies is not completely clear. A recent study assessing the impact of neutralizing antibodies on the effectiveness of interferon alpha-2a for Behçet disease uveitis found no difference between those that developed anti-interferon alpha antibodies and those that did not [39]. Even more surprisingly, induction of commonly encountered autoantibodies, such as anti-nuclear antibody (ANA), anti-cardiolipin antibody, and anti-thyroid peroxidase antibody, a known complication of interferon therapy, lowered the attack rate of uveitis recurrences [39].

Etiologically Mixed Noninfectious Uveitis

Although predominantly used for uveitis associated with Behçet disease, interferon alpha has also been successful in treating uveitis associated with other etiologies [40, 41]. In 2007, Bodaghi et al. described the outcomes of 45 patients with a more heterogeneous range of uveitic entities treated with interferon alpha [40]. Approximately half of the patients had intraocular inflammation associated with Behçet disease and all cases were considered treatment resistant, with an average of more than three relapses despite steroid and additional immunosuppressive therapy. Etiological variability—including Vogt-Koyanagi-Harada (VKH) disease, birdshot chorioretinitis (BCR), IU, and idiopathic—comprised the other half of patients. Uveitis was controlled by interferon in more than 80% of patients with Behçet disease and close to 60% of patients with uveitis of other causes. In all cases, the daily prednisone requirement decreased significantly during the mean follow-up period of 30 months to a median dose of 10 mg per day.

A smaller study of 12 patients with uveitis of mixed causes, including Behçet disease ($n = 2$), sympathetic ophthalmia ($n = 1$), and idiopathic ($n = 9$), revealed a positive treatment response in terms of visual acuity and clinical activity of uveitis in 83% of patients within 1 month of commencing therapy with interferon alpha [41]. Additionally, CME, present in 14 eyes prior to interferon treatment, resolved in all cases.

Infectious Uveitis

While interferon alpha therapy is primarily used for noninfectious uveitis, there are limited case reports of interferon treatment for retinal vasculitis associated with both human T-cell lymphotropic virus type 1 (HTLV-1) and Kaposi sarcoma herpesvirus-associated uveitis [42, 43]. In all three of the patients included in these reports, there was a significant improvement within 1–2 months. In one case, maintenance interferon therapy was used for 34 months and in another, once interferon therapy was discontinued at 19 months, a relapse occurred which subsided with reinitiation of interferon [42]. These cases underscore the antiviral mechanism of action of interferons—inhibition of viral replication as opposed to virucidal activity.

Dosing

Standard dosing for interferon alpha for the treatment of uveitis is typically 3 million international units (IU) administered sc three times per week, although doses may range from 3 to 9 million IU and commence with daily dosing [17, 19, 20, 44, 45]. Concurrent taper of systemic corticosteroids to a dose of 10 mg prednisolone per day or less if possible is recommended, given the potential antagonistic effect of steroids [46]. Some clinicians recommend that other immunosuppressive agents be stopped prior to the initiation of interferon therapy, while others advocate combined treatment [47]. Although dosing is more standard for adults, the limited experience in children suggests weight-based dosing is appropriate. One case series of seven children with uveitis associated with Behçet disease described treatment with 1.5 or 3 million IU three times weekly in children 20–30 kg or 30–50 kg, respectively [25].

The introduction of pegylated interferon, which has a significantly longer half-life, allows for once weekly or once biweekly dosing with an improved side effect profile. This formulation is more commonly used in the treatment of hepatitis C, and the data for treatment of uveitis is limited. One initial case series described five patients with severe uveitis due to Behçet disease, all of whom achieved an extended, recurrence-free interval with weekly pegylated interferon, after controlling inflammation with standard interferon alpha [48]. Another recent study randomizing 72 patients with Behçet disease to either pegylated interferon or placebo suggested that pegylated interferon reduced corticosteroid need, improved quality of life, and induced increased levels of T regulatory lymphocytes [49]. Others have attempted to mitigate side effects and increase tolerability by employing lower initial doses of interferon with dose escalation as indicated, and results have been encouraging [20, 23, 50].

For the treatment of CME, most clinicians prescribe 3 to 6 million IU sc on a daily basis at the start of therapy [32–34]. Typically, the interferon is tapered on a monthly basis depending on the response. Dose reduction below 3 million IU daily often involves a lengthening of the interval (i.e., every other day, every third day, every fourth day, and so on). If the CME remains suppressed with once-weekly dosing, a reduction to 1.5 million IU sc weekly versus discontinuation may be attempted. One small uncontrolled study of patients with inflammatory CME found a 100% response rate to pegylated interferon [51]. A significant and rapid reduction of central retinal thickness, from 478 to 310 microns ($p < 0.05$), in ten eyes of seven patients was observed. Pegylated interferon doses typically start at 90–180 μg weekly, with subsequent schedule extension to every 2–4 weeks as able [49, 51].

Side Effects and Adverse Events

In general, numerous side effects and adverse events have been associated with systemic interferon treatment, which may negatively influence its use. It is important to note, however, that while adverse effects are commonly reported in interferon studies for uveitis, rarely do they lead to treatment cessation. More so, increasing adoption of pegylated formulations will decrease the incidence and severity of side effects and rates of discontinuation. Flu-like symptoms have been noted in 90% or more of patients and pretreatment with ibuprofen or acetaminophen may be beneficial [9]. This reaction is so common in fact that the absence of flu-like symptoms may indicate the presence of preexisting anti-interferon alpha neutralizing antibodies, potentially associated with decreased therapeutic response [18, 33, 40].

Additional adverse effects include mild erythema at the injection site, fatigue, cytopenias, alopecia, and depression. Depression may be exacerbated to the point of suicidal ideation; as such, careful mental health screening is mandatory for all patients commencing interferon therapy. Cytopenias (most commonly leukopenia and/or thrombocytopenia) may be rapid and severe, mandating close monitoring. Other relatively common side effects include transaminitis, gastrointestinal disturbance, and intermittent paresthesias [18, 33, 40]. Typically, these adverse effects are often manageable with either observation or dose reduction and lead to treatment cessation in only 4–7.5% of patients [17, 40]. While a majority of these estimates are based on adult cohorts, one case series of seven pediatric patients described two serious adverse events related to interferon alpha-2a therapy, retinal venous thrombosis and major depression [25].

Interferon therapy is not recommended in patients with sarcoidosis. This is based on reported cases of interferon-associated sarcoidosis, both with interferon alpha and beta treatment [52–55]. Similarly, interferon therapy may potentially exacerbate or trigger other autoimmune diseases, in genetically susceptible individuals [56–59]. Induction of numerous autoantibodies, such as ANA and anti-thyroid antibodies, has been well documented with recombinant interferon, especially with chronic therapy; this may be partly or wholly responsible for the increased autoimmunity seen in these patients.

Additionally, while the incidence of interferon alpha-related retinopathy in hepatitis C patients approaches 30%, it is not commonly described in uveitis patients [60]. In fact, among the entirety of the adult literature of interferon treatment for uveitis and/or CME, only one study, a prospective case series of 12 patients with noninfectious uveitis treated with interferon alpha-2b, commented on the development of retinopathy in a quarter of patients [41].

When considering the significant side effect profile of interferons, it is worth underscoring that this therapy does not predispose to infection. On the contrary, one may be able to leverage the antiviral properties of interferon when employing the treatment for a different primary indication (e.g., therapy of chronic CME in a patient with treated acute retinal necrosis, in whom local steroids may predispose to reactivation). Similarly, the lack of an association between interferon therapy and development of malignancy is noteworthy, especially in comparison to other treatments for sight-threatening uveitis.

Other Important Management Pearls

Careful laboratory monitoring in patients treated with systemic interferon is imperative. Baseline testing includes complete blood count (CBC) with differential and comprehensive metabolic panel (CMP). Rapid and life-threatening derangements in various hematological and chemical values may occur, including myelosuppression, especially neutropenia, thrombocytopenia, hypokalemia, and serum transaminase elevation, among others.

As such, frequent laboratory monitoring, on the order of once weekly or every other week, may be advisable for the initial month of therapy. Gradual lengthening of the monitoring interval can occur on an individualized basis. Most of these lab abnormalities will stabilize or normalize with dose reduction; in some cases, they may be closely monitored without a therapeutic change. Exceptionally, the uveitis specialist may enlist the assistance of a hematologist to reverse interferon-induced neutropenia with granulocyte colony-stimulating factor, if the benefits of continued therapy are deemed to outweigh the risks and costs.

As discussed above, chronic therapy with type I interferons may induce, exacerbate, or uncover silent autoimmunity in certain individuals. A careful screening for preexisting autoimmune disease is imperative prior to considering interferon therapy. Additionally, many clinicians will screen for the presence of ANA, and potentially other organ-specific autoantibodies based on history, at the start of therapy and every 3 months thereafter.

Lastly, the risk of aggravation of depressive symptoms with therapy cannot be overemphasized; suicidal ideation may rapidly ensue. A careful medical and neuropsychiatric history must be taken prior to prescribing interferon, and any patient with a history of depression should likely not be exposed to this agent.

Intravenous Immunoglobulin Therapy

For more than 60 years, IVIg has been given to immunodeficient patients with hypogammaglobulinemia for infection prophylaxis. In 1981, reports of dramatic improvement in platelet counts in children with idiopathic thrombocytopenic purpura (ITP) treated with IVIg infusions began to emerge [61], paving the way for its application in numerous other autoimmune diseases. Generally employed as a treatment of last resort, many of the described uveitis and ocular inflammatory patients were treated with IVIg after failing multiple other immunosuppressive agents. Given the presumed heterogeneity in the pathophysiology of immunological disorders of the eye, it is not surprising that the responses to IVIg for uveitis and other ocular inflammation have been variable, spanning the spectrum from lack of response to complete control of previously intractable disease. Overall though, the reported results have been favorable, especially in diseases such as ocular mucous membrane pemphigoid (MMP), where pathogenic autoantibodies are likely implicated. Below, we also review the present body of evidence in support of IVIg for sight-threatening, ocular inflammatory disease.

Mechanism of Action

Preparations of IVIg come from the pooled plasma of thousands (3000 to 10,000 or more) of healthy donors. As such, each infusion would be expected to contain a complete range of possible variable region binding sites (Fab) complementary to any given antigen encountered in normal sera. This property likely provides protection against infection in the setting of immunodeficiencies; however, the Fc (constant) region of antibodies in IVIg preparations—which enables directive interaction with B cells and phagocytes, among others, and the complement system—presumably plays a major role in the immunomodulatory properties of IVIg [62]. Blockade of Fcγ receptors on macrophages and other effector cells in the hematopoietic system by the Fc portion of exogenous IgG inhibits activation of these pathogenic cells, an important mechanism in the beneficial effect of IVIg in ITP and other autoantibody-mediated diseases [62]. The specific neonatal Fcγ receptor participates in the normal salvage and turnover of endogenous IgG; saturation of these receptors with IVIg may lead to rapid elimination of disease-associated autoantibodies [63]. Further, there is in vivo evidence that exogenous IgG may induce expression of the inhibitory Fcγ receptor IIB in macrophages, thereby tempering the inflammatory activity of autoantibody-associated disease [64]. A final Fc pathway through which IVIg may mediate an effect involves inhibition of antibody-dependent cell-mediated cytotoxicity, also via an Fcγ receptor blockade mechanism [62].

Unrelated to the Fc region, IVIg can also modulate B cells and their antibodies directly. Effects of IVIg on B cells include downregulation of antibody production; specific inhibition, via anti-CD5 IgG, of subsets of autoreactive B cells; and suppression of B cell migration from bone marrow to peripheral lymphoid organs [62, 63]. Beyond the direct effect on B cells, innumerable antiidiotypic antibodies present within a single IVIg preparation may bind the Fab region of pathogenic, circulating autoantibodies, thereby neutralizing them and attenuating their proinflammatory effects. Antiidiotypes against anti-neutrophil cytoplasmic antibody and other disease-associated autoantibodies, such as those to acetylcholine receptors, thyroglobulin, DNA, and factor VIII, have all been recovered from IVIg preparations [65].

Additionally, IVIg may mitigate the effects of autoreactive T cells by regulating differentiation of helper T (Th) cell populations and their associated cytokines, tipping the balance in favor of Th2 (anti-inflammatory) cytokine profiles over Th1 (proinflammatory) [62, 65]. Further, IVIg treatment, perhaps through induction of tolerogenic dendritic cells, encourages an expansion of Treg cells, which have immunosuppressive effects [65]. Beyond immunoglobulin, IVIg also contains numerous soluble factors such as T-cell receptors, CD4, CD8, and MHC, all of which may competitively interfere with normal binding and activation of autoreactive T cells by antigen-presenting cells; other soluble factors may be involved in directing apoptosis of autoreactive T cells [63]. Such T cell involving immunomodulatory pathways may be of particular relevance when considering the efficacy of IVIg in treating various uveitides, many of which are thought to be T-cell-mediated diseases.

The earliest evidence in support of IVIg in the treatment of uveitis comes from basic science. In 1993, investigators demonstrated that the development of EAU in rats immunized with S-antigen could be blocked by contemporaneous treatment with daily IVIg infusions [66]. They postulated that, via neutralizing antibody binding to rat T lymphocytes, infusions with IVIg may functionally deactivate these cells and induce a state of immunotolerance. Others subsequently determined that IVIg can similarly suppress the development of endotoxin-induced uveitis in rats, theorizing that the effects may be mediated through reduction of TNF alpha release [67].

In addition to its immunomodulatory effects, IVIg directly suppresses inflammation through several mechanisms. Exogenous immunoglobulin can bind C3b and C4b, complement proteins necessary for the initiation and propagation of the proteolytic cascade resulting in the membrane-attack complex, thereby scavenging these activated proteins from circulation and reducing complement-mediated tissue destruction [62, 65]. Moreover, IVIg can neutralize circulating immune complexes and microbial toxins, which may be responsible for potentiating inflammation [62]. The effects of other complement proteins, namely the anaphylatoxins C3a and C5a responsible for thromboxane and histamine release, may also be directly attenuated by exogenous immunoglobulin [65].

Indications for Therapy

The first reported use of IVIg for uveitis, in 1989, details a marked response in a single patient with steroid-resistant, severe posterior uveitis with phlebitis and retinal exudation [68]. Rosenbaum et al., in 1999, demonstrated the efficacy of IVIg in treating a heterogeneous group of ten patients with refractory, sight-threatening uveitis [69]. After seeing patent improvement in control of uveitis in one of two patients treated as part of a pilot study, four of eight patients were followed prospectively on a treatment protocol and derived substantial benefit from IVIg therapy. Benefit was determined based on visual acuity improvement and control of ocular inflammation. This was sustained over a median follow-up of 11 months, though disease worsened or recurred when therapy was interrupted.

In a retrospective, observational study of five consecutive patients with severe uveitis unresponsive to standard therapy, IVIg infusions controlled inflammation completely in 60% [70]. In two of the three responders, CME resolved as well. The third patient with a positive response to exogenous immunoglobulin had persistent CME; however, she also had poorly controlled diabetes which obfuscated the efficacy of IVIg in treating this complication. Importantly, none of the five patients experienced a complication or adverse reaction related to IVIg, and one patient had two successful pregnancies while under therapy.

More recently, Garcia-Geremias et al. retrospectively reviewed their experience over 10 years with IVIg for non-infectious uveitis [71]. The uveitis, though heterogeneous in disease association and phenotype (one case of BCR, one case of autoimmune retinopathy (AIR), and two patients with undifferentiated panuveitis), was severe and resistant to standard corticosteroid and immunomodulatory therapy in all cases. In three of the four patients, IVIg effected clinical improvement and/or stabilization of disease, based on exam parameters, visual field, and electrophysiological testing. In two patients, IVIg also permitted the reduction of systemic corticosteroid.

Disease-Specific Considerations

In the broader field of ocular immunology, the response of specific disease entities to IVIg has led to increasing awareness of niche indications for this therapy. The most important of these is ocular MMP, while the evidence in support of its use in other disease states continues to grow.

Ocular Mucous Membrane Pemphigoid

In patients with MMP, autoantibodies directed against the β4 integrin subunit, among others, in basal epithelial cells of skin and mucous membranes, leads to dysfunction of hemidesmosome adhesion and subsequent blistering of the epithelium [72]. Given the presumed pathophysiology of the disease, the rationale for the use of IVIg in this setting is well founded. Indeed, serum titers of anti-β4 integrin decrease in parallel with conjunctival inflammation on a monthly basis with IVIg therapy in these patients [73].

Published, expert consensus statements support the use of IVIg for patients with MMP and other mucocutaneous blistering diseases in whom there is insufficient response to or progression in spite of standard therapy (prednisone ≥60 mg/day for six or more weeks with concurrent immunosuppressive therapy for 10–12 weeks) [74]. Treatment-limiting adverse events associated with and/or contraindications to conventional therapy are additional indications to commence therapy with IVIg.

In 1999, Foster et al. published their initial experience with IVIg in ten patients with refractory ocular MMP [75]. The disease was severe and recalcitrant in all patients, having been present for a mean of 8.3 years (range, 3–14) and demonstrating refractoriness to numerous immunosuppressive agents, including tacrolimus, methotrexate, azathioprine, cytosine arabinoside, and cyclophosphamide. Within months of starting IVIg therapy, after a minimum of four and maximum of 12 cycles, the ocular disease was halted and chronic conjunctivitis resolved in all ten patients. Visual acuity improved or remained stable in all eyes.

This group later reported the long-term outcomes of these same ten patients [76]. The disease was severe (all ten patients had stage III disease or worse in at least one eye) and therapy with IVIg was protracted (total cycles: range, 20–42; mean, 32 and duration of therapy (months): range, 25–43; mean, 35). All patients were observed for 24–48 months after cessation of IVIg. Eight patients completed the IVIg treatment protocol [74]. Of these, all eight had no progression of the disease and seven of eight had stable or improved vision. Two of the ten patients, after initially responding to immunoglobulin, could not follow the protocol and the disease progressed, but only after treatment had been interrupted prematurely.

In a nonrandomized comparison, IVIg demonstrated superiority to conventional immunosuppressive therapy in the treatment of MMP with newly diagnosed ocular involvement [77]. There was a statistically significant benefit in favor of IVIg in controlling the disease activity more rapidly, preventing disease progression to a higher stage, reducing recurrences, and minimizing side effects. The single observer determining clinical activity and progression was not blinded to the treatment group, however, and it was unclear whether or not the data had been collected prospectively or retrospectively.

A minority of recalcitrant ocular MMP patients will still experience progression of the disease, ultimately to legal blindness (≤20/200), despite treatment with exogenous immunoglobulin. For these rare patients, Foster et al. have demonstrated that rituximab in conjunction with IVIg can be highly effective [78]. They note that, in addition to having a synergistic effect against disease-related autoantibodies, IVIg also provides significant protection against infection in these elderly patients whose peripheral B cells have been eliminated by rituximab.

Birdshot Chorioretinitis

In 2000, LeHoang et al. prospectively investigated 18 BCR patients with no prior history of immunosuppression, except for oral or injected corticosteroid in six patients [79]. All had been taken off steroid treatment for at least 2 months prior to initiation of monotherapy with IVIg. The response was significant with improved or stable vision in 33/36 eyes (92%), reduced vitritis in 34/36 eyes (94%), and reduced or resolved angiographic CME in 18/23 eyes (78%). In an additional study, this same group followed 37 patients, 19 retrospectively and 18 prospectively, with BCR and a documented drop in visual acuity prior to enrollment [80]. Over the course of extended follow-up (mean 2.7 ± 2.0 years), they observed an improvement in visual acuity in 53%, reduction in retinal vasculitis as confirmed by fluorescein angiography in 81%, and decrease in CME in 65% of patients.

Behçet Disease

In a series of six eyes of four patients with panuveitis associated with Behçet disease uncontrolled with topical and systemic corticosteroids with or without systemic cyclosporine, a complete response to IVIg was noted in all cases [81]. The effect was sustained with no recurrence of ocular inflammation up to a year after completing their IVIg treatment protocol.

A recent case report describes a 48-year-old female patient with Behçet disease with ocular involvement refractory to more than a dozen immunosuppressant agents, including infliximab and interferon alpha [82]. Given her poor response to therapy, an immunological investigation was undertaken and determined a secondary diagnosis of common variable immune deficiency. After initiating therapy with IVIg for the immune dysfunction, her Behçet disease and associated uveitis completely remitted and remained suppressed for more than 2 years.

There is little else in the literature regarding the use of IVIg for sight-threatening and/or treatment-resistant Behçet disease, likely owing to the profound response of this disease to interferon alpha or TNF alpha inhibition and their growing adoption as first-line agents. It is worth mentioning, though, that "the most dramatic improvement" (visual acuity OD: 4/200 to 20/40) among the eight uveitis patients treated with IVIg and followed prospectively by Rosenbaum et al. occurred in a male patient with Behçet disease [69].

Vogt-Koyanagi-Harada Disease

Two separate case reports suggest that IVIg may effectively treat VKH, though broader conclusions regarding its use in this condition require further study [83, 84]. One of these reports focused on the neurological involvement of VKH, and the eye findings and response to therapy were not well described [83].

Autoimmune Retinopathy

Circulating autoantibodies to retinal antigens, such as recoverin, α-enolase, and others, are demonstrable in all cases of AIR, whether associated with underlying malignancy (paraneoplastic AIR) or not (non-paraneoplastic AIR). It is not clearly understood whether or not these autoantibodies are causative of or resulting from the retinal destruction; nonetheless, their presence raises the possibility that IVIg therapy may be effective. Benefit, in some cases profound, has been demonstrated in cases of melanoma-associated retinopathy [85] and cancer-associated retinopathy [86]. Owing to the rarity of these diseases, the evidence in support of IVIg for AIR is limited to only a handful of reported patients and few conclusions regarding its efficacy can be drawn. However, the benefit of avoiding immunosuppression in the setting of a potentially undiscovered malignancy should be underscored, when considering IVIg for this indication.

Susac's Syndrome

Retinocochleocerebral vasculopathy, or Susac's syndrome, involves the clinical triad of sensorineural hearing loss, encephalopathy, and branch retinal artery occlusions, though patients commonly present with incomplete disease [87]. Evidence supports an immunological attack on endothelial cells in the target organs; patients with Susac's syndrome have high levels of anti-endothelial cell antibodies in their circulation [88]. Given this, therapy with IVIg is commonly employed with success, either alone or in conjunction with prednisone and/or other immunosuppressive agents [88–92].

Kawasaki Disease

In Kawasaki disease, an acute, systemic vasculitis associated with coronary artery disease in the pediatric and occasionally early adult populations, uveitis is the most commonly encountered ophthalmic manifestation [93]. The uveitis is generally mild and responsive to topical steroid drops, but IVIg is indicated for the management of the systemic disease [94]. Hence, ophthalmologists involved in the care of patients with Kawasaki disease should be aware of this point of intersection between IVIg and a specific disease entity.

Dosing

For the treatment of recalcitrant uveitis with IVIg, the majority of clinicians prescribe 1–2.5 g/kg per cycle, divided evenly in three consecutive, daily infusions [69–71]. Cycles are separated initially by 2–4 weeks and the interval is gradually extended based on treatment response, though some have spaced infusions further apart [71]. Reflecting a lack of consensus and the heterogeneity of indications, alternate protocols abound [79, 81, 86].

In the setting of ocular MMP, most employ an initial dose of 2–3 g/kg per cycle, also dividing the total cycle dose equally over three consecutive days [74]. Depending upon disease severity and clinical response, cycles are generally administered at 3–4 week intervals or as frequently as every 2 weeks in aggressive ocular MMP [74]. The interval can be gradually extended by 2 weeks, with complete control of the disease, until two infusion cycles have been administered 16 weeks apart. Many, at this point, consider this the end point of treatment [74].

Side Effects and Adverse Events

The vast majority of side effects and adverse events associated with IVIg are benign and self-limited, occurring in 1–5% and rarely necessitating discontinuation of therapy [62, 95]. Reactions occurring at the time of administration—headache, myalgias, nausea, dizziness, chills, fever, back pain, high blood pressure—resolve for the most part by decreasing the rate of or temporarily pausing the infusion [74]. Pretreatment with nonsteroidal anti-inflammatory agents, antihistamines, or even low-dose IV corticosteroid may obviate many of these side effects. Intravenous access site reactions, including phlebitis and dermatitis, occasionally occur [95].

IVIg may rarely be associated with serious complications, including aseptic meningitis, anaphylaxis, infection transmission from improperly screened donor serum, and thromboembolic events [96–98]. Anaphylactic reactions generally occur in IgA deficient patients and can be avoided by checking IgA levels prior to infusion. Preexisting hypertension and other risk factors for thromboembolism should be noted and optimized if possible. Fluid overload in patients with a history of cardiac impairment may lead to or exacerbate congestive heart failure [74].

Lastly, acute renal failure, especially in the elderly, patients with diabetes, and those with autoimmune disease involving the kidneys, such as granulomatous polyangiitis and SLE, may infrequently develop [62, 74]. The highest risk appears to be associated with IVIg preparations containing sucrose [74].

In terms of ocular adverse effects, extremely uncommon events have been reported as attributable to IVIg, including, paradoxically, two cases of uveitis with retinal vasculitis [99, 100] and a patient with bilateral central retinal vein occlusion [101]. Bilateral crystalline keratopathy also has been reported in patients exposed to exogenous immunoglobulin [102].

Other Important Management Pearls

Prior to commencing therapy with IVIg, baseline labs, including a CBC with differential and a CMP with liver and kidney function testing, as well as hepatitis B and C and human immunodeficiency virus screening, are recommended [74]. IgA levels and screening for cryoglobulin should also be performed, as patients with low or absent IgA may be at risk for anaphylaxis with IVIg infusions and cryoglobulin may predispose to acute renal failure [74].

Caution should be exercised in patients with a history of renal insufficiency or heart failure, as fluid overload may easily occur with IVIg infusions. To mitigate these adverse events, IVIg should be infused slowly over a period of 4–5 hours [74, 103].

Outside of these specific disease considerations, the relative safety of IVIg, especially in comparison to other agents often considered in the setting of intractable ocular inflammation, such as cyclophosphamide and chlorambucil, should be underscored. Importantly, IVIg is not contraindicated at extremes of age (children or elderly) or in pregnant women [74]. Also, similar to interferon therapy, patients are not at risk for opportunistic infection, as exogenous IVIg does not confer any systemic immunosuppression [104].

Given the present climate of healthcare economics, the exorbitant cost of IVIg therapy must be considered. Further, the therapy is quite time-consuming for the patients themselves, which may impart additional "cost" (e.g., time away from employment, reduced quality of life). Availability of supply may be an additional limitation to its use. Because of these potential considerations, many experts recommend that IVIg only be considered in truly refractory disease [96].

Only a small number of manufacturers supply IVIg in the United States [105]. Clinicians should recognize that the various preparations may differ in several ways, including composition of gammaglobulins and other immunologically active products, osmolarity and sodium concentration, sugar content, and others. These differences may affect patient outcomes, in terms of efficacy, adverse events, and side effects, though no head-to-head investigations have been undertaken. Standardization of preparation and comparison trials would be helpful in optimizing the product, one with physiologic osmolarity, low sodium, no sugar, minimized purification time, and high biological activity [74]. Also, in the recent past, critical shortages of IVIg have occurred. Premeditative and discriminate prescribing among clinicians will help to ensure that the patients likely to derive the greatest benefit, or already demonstrating a significant response, will have continued access to the drug.

Conclusion

In clinical practice, interferons and IVIg most commonly are employed in the setting of abject refractoriness, often after patients have failed to respond to numerous other immunosuppressive medications. This blanket application has pitfalls: diluting beneficial treatment effects and increasing cost and adverse events. Side effects and adverse events are far more common in patients treated with interferon, though importantly they are rarely treatment limiting; serious adverse reactions may rarely occur with exogenous immunoglobulin, despite its generally excellent tolerability.

As our understanding of the complex array of interactions and modulations these agents effect upon and within the human immune system evolves, more tailored patient selection can occur. By matching precise drug mechanisms of action to disease-specific, aberrant immune physiology of the eye, response rates will be optimized, while mitigating cost and side effects. This has already occurred, somewhat serendipitously for Behçet disease, MS-related IU, and uveitic CME with exogenous interferons and more thoughtfully for ocular MMP and BCR with IVIg. However, ongoing investigation of exact drug effects and further delineation of specific uveitic entities promise to enhance our application of these powerful immunomodulators in the future.

References

1. Isaacs A, Lindenmann J. Virus interference. I. The interferon. Proc R Soc Lond B Biol Sci. 1957;147(927):258–67.
2. Tsambaos D, Eichelberg D, Goos M. Behcet's syndrome: treatment with recombinant leukocyte alpha-interferon. Arch Dermatol Res. 1986;278(4):335–6.
3. Siegal FP, Fitzgerald-Bocarsly P, Holland BK, Shodell M. Interferon-alpha generation and immune reconstitution during antiretroviral therapy for human immunodeficiency virus infection. AIDS. 2001;15(13):1603–12.
4. Palucka AK, Blanck JP, Bennett L, Pascual V, Banchereau J. Cross-regulation of TNF and IFN-alpha in autoimmune diseases. Proc Natl Acad Sci U S A. 2005;102(9):3372–7.
5. Plskova J, Greiner K, Muckersie E, Duncan L, Forrester JV. Interferon-alpha: a key factor in autoimmune disease? Invest Ophthalmol Vis Sci. 2006;47(9):3946–50.
6. Okada AA, Keino H, Fukai T, Sakai J, Usui M, Mizuguchi J. Effect of type I interferon on experimental autoimmune uveoretinitis in rats. Ocul Immunol Inflamm. 1998;6(4):215–26.
7. Tilg H, Mier JW, Vogel W, Aulitzky WE, Wiedermann CJ, Vannier E, et al. Induction of circulating IL-1 receptor antagonist by IFN treatment. J Immunol. 1993;150(10):4687–92.
8. Gillies MC, Su T. Interferon-alpha 2b enhances barrier function of bovine retinal microvascular endothelium in vitro. Microvasc Res. 1995;49(3):277–88.
9. Zierhut M, Abu El-Asrar AM, Bodaghi B, Tugal-Tutkun I. Therapy of ocular Behcet disease. Ocul Immunol Inflamm. 2014;22(1):64–76.
10. Feron EJ, Rothova A, van Hagen PM, Baarsma GS, Suttorp-Schulten MS. Interferon-alpha 2b for refractory ocular Behcet's disease. Lancet. 1994;343(8910):1428.
11. Sanchez Roman J, Pulido Aguilera MC, Castillo Palma MJ, Ocana Medina C, Toral Pena A, Lopez-Checa F, et al. The use of interferon alfa-2r in the treatment of autoimmune uveitis (primary or associated with Behcet's disease). Rev Clin Esp. 1996;196(5):293–8.
12. Kotter I, Durk H, Eckstein A, Zierhut M, Fierlbeck G, Saal JG. Erosive arthritis and posterior uveitis in Behcet's disease: treatment with interferon alpha and interferon gamma. Clin Exp Rheumatol. 1996;14(3):313–5.
13. Pivetti-Pezzi P, Accorinti M, Pirraglia MP, Priori R, Valesini G. Interferon alpha for ocular Behcet's disease. Acta Ophthalmol Scand. 1997;75(6):720–2.
14. Wechsler B, Bodaghi B, Huong DL, Fardeau C, Amoura Z, Cassoux N, et al. Efficacy of interferon alfa-2a in severe and refractory uveitis associated with Behcet's disease. Ocul Immunol Inflamm. 2000;8(4):293–301.
15. Kotter I, Eckstein AK, Stubiger N, Zierhut M. Treatment of ocular symptoms of Behcet's disease with interferon alpha 2a: a pilot study. Br J Ophthalmol. 1998;82(5):488–94.
16. Zouboulis CC, Orfanos CE. Treatment of Adamantiades-Behcet disease with systemic interferon alfa. Arch Dermatol. 1998;134(8):1010–6.
17. Kotter I, Zierhut M, Eckstein AK, Vonthein R, Ness T, Gunaydin I, et al. Human recombinant interferon alfa-2a for the treatment of Behcet's disease with sight threatening posterior or panuveitis. Br J Ophthalmol. 2003;87(4):423–31.
18. Kotter I, Gunaydin I, Zierhut M, Stubiger N. The use of interferon alpha in Behcet disease: review of the literature. Semin Arthritis Rheum. 2004;33(5):320–35.
19. Tugal-Tutkun I, Guney-Tefekli E, Urgancioglu M. Results of interferon-alfa therapy in patients with Behcet uveitis. Graefes Arch Clin Exp Ophthalmol. 2006;244(12):1692–5.
20. Gueudry J, Wechsler B, Terrada C, Gendron G, Cassoux N, Fardeau C, et al. Long-term efficacy and safety of low-dose interferon alpha2a therapy in severe uveitis associated with Behcet disease. Am J Ophthalmol. 2008;146(6):837–44.e1.
21. Sobaci G, Erdem U, Durukan AH, Erdurman C, Bayer A, Koksal S, et al. Safety and effectiveness of interferon alpha-2a in treatment of patients with Behcet's uveitis refractory to conventional treatments. Ophthalmology. 2010;117(7):1430–5.

22. Deuter CM, Zierhut M, Mohle A, Vonthein R, Stobiger N, Kotter I. Long-term remission after cessation of interferon-alpha treatment in patients with severe uveitis due to Behcet's disease. Arthritis Rheum. 2010;62(9):2796–805.
23. Onal S, Kazokoglu H, Koc A, Akman M, Bavbek T, Direskeneli H, et al. Long-term efficacy and safety of low-dose and dose-escalating interferon alfa-2a therapy in refractory Behcet uveitis. Arch Ophthalmol. 2011;129(3):288–94.
24. Tugal-Tutkun I, Urgancioglu M. Childhood-onset uveitis in Behcet disease:a descriptive study of 36 cases. Am J Ophthalmol. 2003;136(6):1114–9.
25. Guillaume-Czitrom S, Berger C, Pajot C, Bodaghi B, Wechsler B, Kone-Paut I. Efficacy and safety of interferon-alpha in the treatment of corticodependent uveitis of paediatric Behcet's disease. Rheumatology (Oxford). 2007;46(10):1570–3.
26. Mackensen F, Jakob E, Springer C, Dobner BC, Wiehler U, Weimer P, et al. Interferon versus methotrexate in intermediate uveitis with macular edema: results of a randomized controlled clinical trial. Am J Ophthalmol. 2013;156(3):478–86 e1.
27. Becker MD, Heiligenhaus A, Hudde T, Storch-Hagenlocher B, Wildemann B, Barisani-Asenbauer T, et al. Interferon as a treatment for uveitis associated with multiple sclerosis. Br J Ophthalmol. 2005;89(10):1254–7.
28. Jacobs L, O'Malley J, Freeman A, Ekes R. Intrathecal interferon reduces exacerbations of multiple sclerosis. Science. 1981;214(4524):1026–8.
29. Interferon-alpha and transfer factor in the treatment of multiple sclerosis: a double-blind, placebo-controlled trial. AUSTIMS Research Group. J Neurol Neurosurg Psychiatry. 1989;52(5):566–74.
30. Deuter CM, Kotter I, Gunaydin I, Zierhut M, Stubiger N. Ocular involvement in Behcet's disease: first 5-year-results for visual development after treatment with interferon alfa-2a. Ophthalmologe. 2004;101(2):129–34.
31. Deuter C, Stubiger N, Zierhut M. Interferon-alpha therapy in noninfectious uveitis. Dev Ophthalmol. 2012;51:90–7.
32. Deuter CM, Koetter I, Guenaydin I, Stuebiger N, Zierhut M. Interferon alfa-2a: a new treatment option for long lasting refractory cystoid macular edema in uveitis? A pilot study. Retina. 2006;26(7):786–91.
33. Deuter CM, Kotter I, Gunaydin I, Stubiger N, Doycheva DG, Zierhut M. Efficacy and tolerability of interferon alpha treatment in patients with chronic cystoid macular oedema due to non-infectious uveitis. Br J Ophthalmol. 2009;93(7):906–13.
34. Butler NJ, Suhler EB, Rosenbaum JT. Interferon alpha 2b in the treatment of uveitic cystoid macular edema. Ocul Immunol Inflamm. 2012;20(2):86–90.
35. Paire V, Lebreton O, Weber M. Effectiveness of interferon alpha in the treatment of uveitis macular edema refractory to corticosteroid and/or immunosuppressive treatment. J Fr Ophtalmol. 2010;33(3):152–62.
36. Hanley JP, Haydon GH. The biology of interferon-alpha and the clinical significance of anti-interferon antibodies. Leuk Lymphoma. 1998;29(3–4):257–68.
37. Antonelli G, Currenti M, Turriziani O, Dianzani F. Neutralizing antibodies to interferon-alpha: relative frequency in patients treated with different interferon preparations. J Infect Dis. 1991;163(4):882–5.
38. Von Wussow P, Hehlmann R, Hochhaus T, Jakschies D, Nolte KU, Prummer O, et al. Roferon (rIFN-alpha 2a) is more immunogenic than intron A (rIFN-alpha 2b) in patients with chronic myelogenous leukemia. J Interferon Res. 1994;14(4):217–9.
39. Aydinoglu-Candan O, Araz-Ersan B, Gul A, Badur S, Tugal-Tutkun I. Anti-interferon alpha antibodies and autoantibodies in patients with Behcet's disease uveitis treated with recombinant human interferon alpha-2a. Graefes Arch Clin Exp Ophthalmol. 2015;253(3):457–65.
40. Bodaghi B, Gendron G, Wechsler B, Terrada C, Cassoux N, Huong du LT, et al. Efficacy of interferon alpha in the treatment of refractory and sight threatening uveitis: a retrospective monocentric study of 45 patients. Br J Ophthalmol. 2007;91(3):335–9.
41. Plskova J, Greiner K, Forrester JV. Interferon-alpha as an effective treatment for noninfectious posterior uveitis and panuveitis. Am J Ophthalmol. 2007;144(1):55–61.
42. Brasnu E, Wechsler B, Bron A, Charlotte F, Bliefeld P, Lehoang P, et al. Efficacy of interferon-alpha for the treatment of Kaposi's sarcoma herpesvirus-associated uveitis. Am J Ophthalmol. 2005;140(4):746–8.
43. Ishimoto S, Sakai Y, Ishibashi T, Khono T, Inomata H, Itoyama Y. Interferon-alpha for the treatment of retinal vasculitis associated with human T-lymphotropic virus type I myelopathy (HAM). Nippon Ganka Gakkai Zasshi. 1990;94(8):769–73.
44. Krause L, Altenburg A, Pleyer U, Kohler AK, Zouboulis CC, Foerster MH. Longterm visual prognosis of patients with ocular Adamantiades-Behcet's disease treated with interferon-alpha-2a. J Rheumatol. 2008;35(5):896–903.
45. Kotter I, Vonthein R, Zierhut M, Eckstein AK, Ness T, Gunaydin I, et al. Differential efficacy of human recombinant interferon-alpha2a on ocular and extra-ocular manifestations of Behcet disease: results of an open 4-center trial. Semin Arthritis Rheum. 2004;33(5):311–9.
46. Deuter CM, Kotter I, Wallace GR, Murray PI, Stubiger N, Zierhut M. Behcet's disease: ocular effects and treatment. Prog Retin Eye Res. 2008;27(1):111–36.
47. Hamuryudan V, Ozyazgan Y, Fresko Y, Mat C, Yurdakul S, Yazici H. Interferon alfa combined with azathioprine for the uveitis of Behcet's disease: an open study. Isr Med Assoc J. 2002;4(11 Suppl):928–30.
48. Bielefeld P, Devilliers H, Deschasse C, Saadoun D, Sève P, Muselier A, Creuzot-Garcher C, Besancenot

JF, Bron AM. Potential of Pegylated Interferon Alpha-2a in Behçet Uveitis: A Report of Five Cases. Ocul Immunol Inflamm. 2016 Oct;24(5):599-602.
49. Lightman S, Taylor SR, Bunce C, Longhurst H, Lynn W, Moots R, et al. Pegylated interferon-alpha-2b reduces corticosteroid requirement in patients with Behcet's disease with upregulation of circulating regulatory T cells and reduction of Th17. Ann Rheum Dis. 2015;74(6):1138–44.
50. Onal S, Kazokoglu H, Koc A, Akman M, Bavbek T, Direskeneli H, et al. Low dose and dose escalating therapy of interferon alfa-2a in the treatment of refractory and sight-threatening Behcet's uveitis. Clin Exp Rheumatol. 2009;27(2 Suppl 53): S113–4.
51. Stiefel HC, Kopplin LJ, Albini T, Chang M, Vegunta S, Suhler EB. Treatment of refractory cystoid macular edema with pegylated interferon alfa-2A: a retrospective chart review. Invest Ophthalmol Vis Sci. 2016;57, ARVO e-Abstract 1872.
52. Pietropaoli A, Modrak J, Utell M. Interferon-alpha therapy associated with the development of sarcoidosis. Chest. 1999;116(2):569–72.
53. Goldberg HJ, Fiedler D, Webb A, Jagirdar J, Hoyumpa AM, Peters J. Sarcoidosis after treatment with interferon-alpha: a case series and review of the literature. Respir Med. 2006;100(11):2063–8.
54. Doycheva D, Deuter C, Stuebiger N, Zierhut M. Interferon-alpha-associated presumed ocular sarcoidosis. Graefes Arch Clin Exp Ophthalmol. 2009;247(5):675–80.
55. Petousi N, Thomas EC. Interferon-beta-induced pulmonary sarcoidosis in a 30-year-old woman treated for multiple sclerosis: a case report. J Med Case Reports. 2012;6:344.
56. Kose S, Gozaydin A, Akkoclu G, Ece G. Chronic hepatitis B with type I diabetes mellitus and autoimmune thyroiditis development during interferon alpha therapy. J Infect Dev Ctries. 2012;6(4):364–8.
57. Dusheiko G. Side effects of alpha interferon in chronic hepatitis C. Hepatology. 1997;26(3 Suppl 1):112S–21S.
58. Dumoulin FL, Leifeld L, Sauerbruch T, Spengler U. Autoimmunity induced by interferon-alpha therapy for chronic viral hepatitis. Biomed Pharmacother. 1999;53(5–6):242–54.
59. Carella C, Mazziotti G, Amato G, Braverman LE, Roti E. Clinical review 169: Interferon-alpha-related thyroid disease: pathophysiological, epidemiological, and clinical aspects. J Clin Endocrinol Metab. 2004;89(8):3656–61.
60. Raza A, Mittal S, Sood GK. Interferon-associated retinopathy during the treatment of chronic hepatitis C: a systematic review. J Viral Hepat. 2013;20(9):593–9.
61. Imbach P, Barandun S, d'Apuzzo V, Baumgartner C, Hirt A, Morell A, et al. High-dose intravenous gammaglobulin for idiopathic thrombocytopenic purpura in childhood. Lancet. 1981;1(8232):1228–31.
62. Kazatchkine MD, Kaveri SV. Immunomodulation of autoimmune and inflammatory diseases with intravenous immune globulin. N Engl J Med. 2001;345(10):747–55.
63. Hartung HP. Advances in the understanding of the mechanism of action of IVIg. J Neurol. 2008;255 Suppl 3:3–6.
64. Samuelsson A, Towers TL, Ravetch JV. Anti-inflammatory activity of IVIG mediated through the inhibitory Fc receptor. Science. 2001;291(5503):484–6.
65. Kaveri SV, Lecerf M, Saha C, Kazatchkine MD, Lacroix-Desmazes S, Bayry J. Intravenous immunoglobulin and immune response. Clin Exp Immunol. 2014;178 Suppl 1:94–6.
66. Saoudi A, Hurez V, de Kozak Y, Kuhn J, Kaveri SV, Kazatchkine MD, et al. Human immunoglobulin preparations for intravenous use prevent experimental autoimmune uveoretinitis. Int Immunol. 1993;5(12):1559–67.
67. Obrador E, Peinado E, de Kozak Y, Ruiz-Moreno JM, Alio JL. Human immunoglobulin preparations for intravenous use prevent endotoxin-induced uveitis in rats. Ophthalmic Res. 1999;31(1):59–67.
68. Sunakawa M. High-dose intravenous gammaglobulin therapy for uveitis. Metab Pediatr Syst Ophthalmol. 1989;12(4):93–5.
69. Rosenbaum JT, George RK, Gordon C. The treatment of refractory uveitis with intravenous immunoglobulin. Am J Ophthalmol. 1999;127(5):545–9.
70. Onal S, Foster CS, Ahmed AR. Efficacy of intravenous immunoglobulin treatment in refractory uveitis. Ocul Immunol Inflamm. 2006;14(6):367–74.
71. Garcia-Geremias M, Carreno E, Epps SJ, Lee RW, Dick AD. Clinical outcomes of intravenous immunoglobulin therapy in refractory uveitis. Int Ophthalmol. 2015;35(2):281–5.
72. Chan RY, Bhol K, Tesavibul N, Letko E, Simmons RK, Foster CS, et al. The role of antibody to human beta4 integrin in conjunctival basement membrane separation: possible in vitro model for ocular cicatricial pemphigoid. Invest Ophthalmol Vis Sci. 1999;40(10):2283–90.
73. Letko E, Bhol K, Foster SC, Ahmed RA. Influence of intravenous immunoglobulin therapy on serum levels of anti-beta 4 antibodies in ocular cicatricial pemphigoid. A correlation with disease activity. A preliminary study. Curr Eye Res. 2000;21(2):646–54.
74. Ahmed AR, Dahl MV. Consensus statement on the use of intravenous immunoglobulin therapy in the treatment of autoimmune mucocutaneous blistering diseases. Arch Dermatol. 2003;139(8):1051–9.
75. Foster CS, Ahmed AR. Intravenous immunoglobulin therapy for ocular cicatricial pemphigoid: a preliminary study. Ophthalmology. 1999;106(11):2136–43.
76. Sami N, Letko E, Androudi S, Daoud Y, Foster CS, Ahmed AR. Intravenous immunoglobulin therapy in patients with ocular-cicatricial pemphigoid: a long-term follow-up. Ophthalmology. 2004;111(7):1380–2.

77. Letko E, Miserocchi E, Daoud YJ, Christen W, Foster CS, Ahmed AR. A nonrandomized comparison of the clinical outcome of ocular involvement in patients with mucous membrane (cicatricial) pemphigoid between conventional immunosuppressive and intravenous immunoglobulin therapies. Clin Immunol. 2004;111(3):303–10.
78. Foster CS, Chang PY, Ahmed AR. Combination of rituximab and intravenous immunoglobulin for recalcitrant ocular cicatricial pemphigoid: a preliminary report. Ophthalmology. 2010;117(5):861–9.
79. LeHoang P, Cassoux N, George F, Kullmann N, Kazatchkine MD. Intravenous immunoglobulin (IVIg) for the treatment of birdshot retinochoroidopathy. Ocul Immunol Inflamm. 2000;8(1):49–57.
80. Cassoux N, Goichot-Bonnat L, Karmochkine M, Georges F, Kullmann N, Lehoang P, et al. Efficacy of intravenous immunoglobulin in the treatment of Birdshot retinochoroiditis. J Fr Ophtalmol. 2002;25(1):23–30.
81. Seider N, Beiran I, Scharf J, Miller B. Intravenous immunoglobulin therapy for resistant ocular Behcet's disease. Br J Ophthalmol. 2001;85(11):1287–8.
82. Shutty B, Garg KJ, Swender D, Chernin L, Tcheurekdjian H, Hostoffer R. Optimal use of ivig in a patient with Behcet syndrome and common variable immunodeficiency. Ann Allergy Asthma Immunol. 2012;109(1):84.
83. Helveston WR, Gilmore R. Treatment of Vogt-Koyanagi-Harada syndrome with intravenous immunoglobulin. Neurology. 1996;46(2):584–5.
84. Gonzalez-Delgado M, Gonzalez C, Blazquez JI, Salas-Puig J, Castro J, Hernandez-Lahoz C. Intravenous immunoglobulin therapy in Vogt-Koyanagi-Harada syndrome. Neurologia. 2004;19(7):401–3.
85. Keltner JL, Thirkill CE, Yip PT. Clinical and immunologic characteristics of melanoma-associated retinopathy syndrome: eleven new cases and a review of 51 previously published cases. J Neuroophthalmol. 2001;21(3):173–87.
86. Guy J, Aptsiauri N. Treatment of paraneoplastic visual loss with intravenous immunoglobulin: report of 3 cases. Arch Ophthalmol. 1999;117(4):471–7.
87. Vodopivec I, Venna N, Rizzo JF 3rd, Prasad S. Clinical features, diagnostic findings, and treatment of Susac syndrome: a case series. J Neurol Sci. 2015;357(1–2):50–7.
88. Susac JO, Egan RA, Rennebohm RM, Lubow M. Susac's syndrome: 1975-2005 microangiopathy/autoimmune endotheliopathy. J Neurol Sci. 2007;257(1–2):270–2.
89. Mateen FJ, Zubkov AY, Muralidharan R, Fugate JE, Rodriguez FJ, Winters JL, et al. Susac syndrome: clinical characteristics and treatment in 29 new cases. Eur J Neurol. 2012;19(6):800–11.
90. Vodopivec I, Prasad S. Treatment of Susac Syndrome. Curr Treat Options Neurol. 2016;18(1):3.
91. Fox RJ, Costello F, Judkins AR, Galetta SL, Maguire AM, Leonard B, et al. Treatment of Susac syndrome with gamma globulin and corticosteroids. J Neurol Sci. 2006;251(1–2):17–22.
92. Petty GW, Engel AG, Younge BR, Duffy J, Yanagihara T, Lucchinetti CF, et al. Retinocochleocerebral vasculopathy. Medicine. 1998;77(1):12–40.
93. Bachmeyer C, Turc Y, Curan D, Duval-Arnould M. Anterior uveitis as the initial sign of adult Kawasaki syndrome (mucocutaneous lymph node syndrome). Am J Ophthalmol. 2000;129(1):101–2.
94. Choi HS, Lee SB, Kwon JH, Kim HS, Sohn S, Hong YM. Uveitis as an important ocular sign to help early diagnosis in Kawasaki disease. Korean J Pediatr. 2015;58(10):374–9.
95. Mobini N, Sarela A, Ahmed AR. Intravenous immunoglobulins in the therapy of autoimmune and systemic inflammatory disorders. Ann Allergy Asthma Immunol. 1995;74(2):119–28; quiz 28–33.
96. Becker MD, Rosenbaum JT. Current and future trends in the use of immunosuppressive agents in patients with uveitis. Curr Opin Ophthalmol. 2000;11(6):472–7.
97. Vucic S, Chong PS, Dawson KT, Cudkowicz M, Cros D. Thromboembolic complications of intravenous immunoglobulin treatment. Eur Neurol. 2004;52(3):141–4.
98. Rosenbaum JT. Myocardial infarction as a complication of immunoglobulin therapy. Arthritis Rheum. 1997;40(9):1732–3.
99. Ayliffe W, Haeney M, Roberts SC, Lavin M. Uveitis after antineutrophil cytoplasmic antibody contamination of immunoglobulin replacement therapy. Lancet. 1992;339(8792):558–9.
100. Vogele C, Andrassy K, Schmidbauer JM, Krastel H, Adler D, Ritz E. Retinal vasculitis and uveitis--an adverse reaction to intravenous immunoglobulins? Nephron. 1994;67(3):363.
101. Oh KT, Boldt HC, Danis RP. Iatrogenic central retinal vein occlusion and hyperviscosity associated with high-dose intravenous immunoglobulin administration. Am J Ophthalmol. 1997;124(3):416–8.
102. Erdem E, Kocabas E, Taylan Sekeroglu H, Ozgur O, Yagmur M, Ersoz TR. Crystalline-like keratopathy after intravenous immunoglobulin therapy with incomplete kawasaki disease: case report and literature review. Case Rep Ophthalmol Med. 2013;2013:621952.
103. Sobolewska B, Deuter C, Zierhut M. Current medical treatment of ocular mucous membrane pemphigoid. Ocul Surf. 2013;11(4):259–66.
104. Lim L, Suhler EB, Smith JR. Biologic therapies for inflammatory eye disease. Clin Experiment Ophthalmol. 2006;34(4):365–74.
105. https://aspe.hhs.gov/execsum/analysis-supply-distribution-demand-and-access-issues-associated-immune-globulin-intravenous-igiv.

11 Diagnostic Biopsies in the Management of Uveitis

Albert T. Vitale

Pearls

- The preoperative clinical impression and differential diagnosis are important in guiding the selection of diagnostic testing to be performed on intraocular specimens.
- PCR of aqueous and vitreous samples provides a highly sensitive and specific assay in the diagnosis of suspected infectious posterior uveitis or uncertain etiology and/or atypical presentation, allowing the differentiation of diverse potential microorganisms.
- Chorioretinal biopsies are preferred for uncertain disease processes primarily involving choroid in which the retina may be secondarily affected such as tuberculosis, sarcoidosis, PIOL, and cancer metastasis without evidence of systemic malignancy.

Diagnostic Vitreoretinal Surgery

Indications

In the vast majority of cases of posterior uveitis, a diagnosis may be reached by the combination of a comprehensive medical and ophthalmic history, review of systems, complete ocular examination, and directed laboratory investigations. The primary tissue level of intraocular inflammation (retinitis vs. choroiditis), the number (paucifocal vs. multifocal), location (posterior pole vs. periphery), and other lesion descriptors (color, size, shape), together with host factors (immunocompetence) are often sufficient to make a diagnosis based on "pattern recognition" in the correct clinical context [1]. For example, an area of focal retinitis adjacent to a hyperpigmented chorioretinal scar with accompanying vitritis in an otherwise healthy patient is suggestive of toxoplasmic retinochoroiditis, whereas typical multifocal wedges of hemorrhagic retinitis and scant vitreous cell in a profoundly immunosuppressed patient with HIV/AIDS evoke a diagnosis of CMV retinitis.

Diagnostic dilemmas arise when the clinical presentation is atypical (diffuse toxoplasmic retinochoroiditis in an immunocompromised patient resembling necrotizing herpetic retinitis), when the systemic work up in inconclusive, or where there has been inadequate response to or worsening of inflammation

A. T. Vitale (✉)
Ophthalmology and Visual Sciences, Uveitis and Vitreoretinal Divisions, John A. Moran Eye Center, University of Utah Hospital, Salt Lake City, UT, USA
e-mail: Albert.vitale@hsc.utah.edu

P. Lin, E. Suhler (eds.), *Treatment of Non-infectious Uveitis*,
https://doi.org/10.1007/978-3-030-22827-9_11

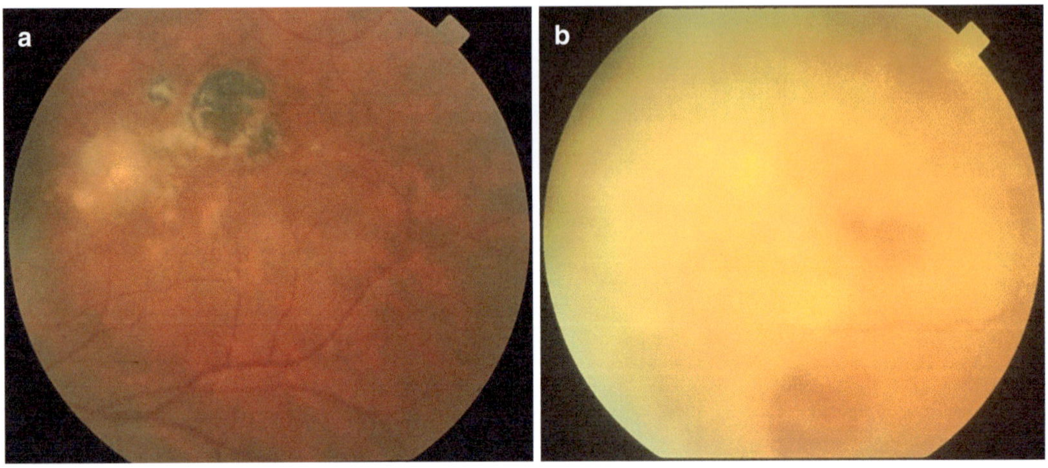

Fig. 11.1 (**a**) Classical toxoplasmic retinochoroiditis with an area of active focal retinitis adjacent to an old chorioretinal scar. (**b**) Diffuse toxoplasmic retinochoroiditis in an immunocompromised host. Funduscopic appearance inadequate to differentiate to this entity from herpetic necrotizing retinitis and syphilitic chorioretinitis

Table 11.1 Indications for diagnostic vitreoretinal surgery

Uveitis unknown etiology
Clinical presentation insufficient to make diagnosis
Atypical presentation
Systemic workup inconclusive
Inadequate response to conventional therapy
Suspected intraocular infection
Suspected intraocular malignancy
Biopsy has potential to alter management of uveitis and impact systemic health

with conventional therapy (unsuspected primary intraocular lymphoma or the treatment of infectious uveitis with corticosteroid monotherapy) (Fig. 11.1). In such cases, paracentesis to acquire aqueous fluid and vitreoretinal surgical techniques to obtain vitreous, retinal, subretinal, and/or chorioretinal biopsy specimens for directed laboratory analysis are essential in the differentiation of purely inflammatory from infectious and neoplastic etiologies and so allow the commencement of appropriate, specific therapy for these patients with severe, sight-threatening posterior uveitis (Table 11.1).

Anterior Chamber Paracentesis

Diagnostic anterior chamber paracentesis is a relatively safe procedure which may be performed in an outpatient setting and may serve as a useful adjunct in the diagnosis and monitoring of a variety of infectious and noninfectious uveitic entities as well as masquerade syndromes [2]. Among 361 patients undergoing this procedure, no major complications (endophthalmitis, cataract, keratitis) were reported [3] while in more recent retrospective study of 560 uveitic eyes, mild adverse events (anterior lens capsule touch, intracameral air, betadine allergy) were seen in only 4 (0.7%) cases [4].

While aqueous samples may be processed for microbiologic examination, such as Gram stain and culture in cases of suspected intraocular infection, they are typically sent for qualitative or real-time polymerase chain reaction (PCR) and/or local pathogen-specific antibodies with Goldmann-Witmer coefficient (GWC), the latter being more commonly employed in Europe. For PCR analysis, the aqueous is most useful when the differential diagnosis is narrow, as the maximum obtainable volume of aqueous is small

(300 μL), limiting the number of diagnostic tests that can be performed. For example, in patients presenting with the typical clinical feature of the acute retinal necrosis syndrome (ARN), PCR of the aqueous is usually sufficient to detect varicella zoster (VZV), herpes simplex (HSV), cytomegalovirus (CMV), or *Toxoplasma gondii* DNA and confirm the diagnosis [5]. The diagnostic yield can be increased by using PCR and the GWC together as these tests are complementary for the diagnosis of infectious uveitis [6]. While anterior paracentesis with PCR had little diagnostic utility and resulted in few management changes (13%) among patients with suspected infectious anterior uveitis [7], aqueous analysis with PCR and GWC for VZV, HSV, CMV and *Toxoplasma gondii* was positive in 29% of 152 cases of posterior uveitis but in none of 40 controls, resulting in a change of management in 24% of patients [8]. In the latter study, clinical features associated with a positive result included extensive retinitis and focal chorioretinitis, whereas multifocal chorioretinitis, retinal vasculitis, and neuroretinitis were rarely positive.

Cytologic analysis of aqueous specimens may be confirmatory in presumed phacogenic uveitis, revealing lipid-laden macrophages, and in suspected neoplastic masquerades, such as pseudohypopyon in the setting of acute myelogenous leukemic infiltration of the uveal tract [9].

Finally, measurement of IL-10 levels in the aqueous humor of patients suspected of primary intraocular lymphoma (PIOL) may be useful both as a screening tool and in monitoring the response to therapy. The mean IL-10 values were found to be significantly different between patients with PIOL and uveitis, with a cutoff of 50 pg/ml being both highly sensitive (89%) and specific (93%) [10].

Diagnostic Vitrectomy

Diagnostic vitrectomy is considered in patients with sight-threatening posterior uveitis in which the clinical presentation and initial noninvasive testing have failed to establish a pathoetiologic diagnosis and/or had been unresponsive to standard treatment. In this setting, vitreous biopsy analysis has the potential to significantly alter management by differentiating infectious, noninfectious and neoplastic uveitic masquerade processes. Specifically, diagnostic vitrectomy is employed in cases of suspected infectious posterior uveitis due to bacteria (acute and delayed onset postoperative endophthalmitis,), viruses (the herpetic necrotizing retinitides (ARN and progressive outer retinal necrosis or PORN)), protozoal and helminthic diseases (*Toxoplasma gondii* and *Toxocara* spp.), and fungi (endogenous endophthalmitis). Vitreous biopsy is an essential intervention in the diagnosis of masquerade syndromes such as PIOL and intraocular Whipple's disease [11].

Vitreous Tap/Biopsy

Vitreous biopsy techniques include a one-port approach using a 22–27-G needle on a 1 ml or 3 ml syringe inserted into the vitreous cavity through the pars plana (vitreous tap). Advantages of this approach include the convenience of the outpatient setting and the need for minimal equipment, and so, it may be ideally suited for cases in which a relatively small sample volumes are required (0.5–2.0 ml of intraocular fluid) and in which the differential diagnosis is narrow, such as in the setting of postoperative endophthalmitis, or when the exclusion or inclusion of only one or two diagnostic entities (e.g., necrotizing viral retinitis) is required. Disadvantages include smaller sample volumes limiting the number and type of potential diagnostic tests, especially when the differential diagnosis is broad, and the potential for iatrogenic complications associated with vitreous base traction and hypotony. In the setting of acute postoperative endophthalmitis, the endophthalmitis vitrectomy study (EVS) found no difference in outcomes between immediate tap/biopsy group and the three-port PPV group for patients with better than light perception vision at the study entry [12]. While there was a higher positive culture rate from vitreous samples as compared to those obtained from the aqueous, there were no differences in outcomes between the study groups with respect to vision, microbial yield, operative complications, or short-term retinal detachment [13]. Among 59 patients with posterior or panuveitis who underwent vitreous biopsy obtained either by vitreous tap or during standard three-port PPV, the initial diagnosis was confirmed or an infectious etiology excluded in 68% while the biopsy result altered management significantly in 12% of patients [14]. Complications were few and included one case each of hypotony and retinal detachment.

Pars Plana Vitrectomy (PPV)

A standard three-port PPV (20, 23, 25, and 27 G) is generally preferred when the differential diagnosis is broad as it allows larger sample volumes to be obtained in a controlled manner, and so, greater latitude in the scope of laboratory testing, as well as the opportunity to perform simultaneous therapeutic vitrectomy as needed (Fig. 11.2). Valved trocar smaller gauge (23, 25, and 27 G) transconjunctival, sutureless vitrectomy systems may be ideally suited for

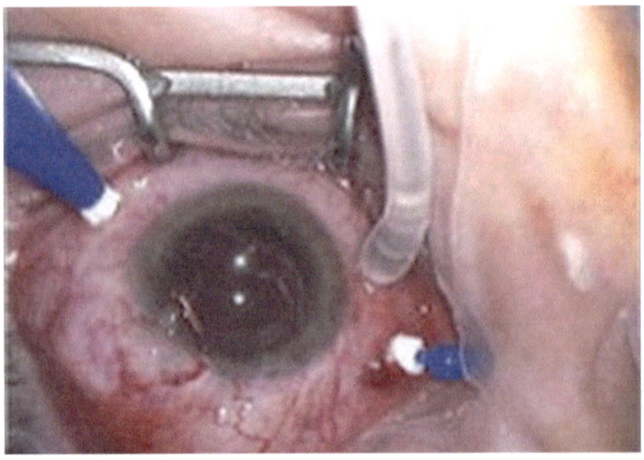

Fig. 11.2 Standard three-port 25 G pars plana vitrectomy

diagnostic purposes as well as therapeutically, when vitrectomy is required to clear the visual axis and/or in addressing vitreoretinal structural pathology. During diagnostic PPV, an undiluted (pure) vitreous specimen of up to 1.5 ml is obtained initially with the vitreous cutter connected directly to a 3 ml syringe under manual aspiration with the infusion line off until the eye softens. Larger volumes of undiluted vitreous (average of 2.4 ml) may be obtained using perfluorocarbon-perfused vitrectomy in which aspirated vitreous is replaced with perfluorocarbon liquid which is manually and simultaneously injected into the vitreous cavity through the infusion line connected to a syringe [15]. A dilute specimen is then obtained with the infusion line turned on, manually aspirating into a 20 ml syringe and/or by collecting the vitreous washings from the machine cassette. Depending on the suspected preoperative differential diagnosis, the undiluted sample is sent for PCR, cytologic and cytokine analysis, while the dilute specimen is processed for cell block preparation for cytologic analysis [hematoxylin-eosin (HE), periodic acid-Schiff (PAS) stains], immunohistochemistry (CD20, CD3, in situ hybridization for κ and λ light chains), flow cytometry, and microbiological analysis for cultures [16] (Table 11.2).

Subretinal, Endoretinal, and Chorioretinal Biopsy

Occasionally, analysis of the vitreous is either inappropriate or fails to provide useful diagnostic information. Uveitic masquerade syndromes such as PIOL presenting with subretinal or sub-RPE infiltration and certain infectious entities (i.e., atypical presentations of toxoplasmosis, necrotizing herpetic retinitis, syphilitic and candida retinitis), which are primarily located in the neurosensory retina or RPE, may require subretinal [17] or endoretinal biopsy [18–20] for definitive diagnosis (Fig. 11.3). In other instances, chorioretinal biopsy may be required for patients with progressive, medically unresponsive, sight-threatening infectious

Table 11.2 Vitreous sample processing

	Lymphoma	Infectious	Autoimmune inflammatory	Tumor metastasis
Undiluted vitreous	Cytologic analysis PCR: IgH gene rearrangements and TCR Cytokine analysis (IL-10 to IL-6 ratio) Myd88 L265P gene mutation	PCR: *Toxoplasma gondii,* HSV, VZV, TB complex, CMV	Cytologic analysis Cytokine analysis (IL-10 to IL-6 ratio)	Cytologic analysis
Diluted vitreous	Cell block preparation for cytologic analysis: HE and PAS stains Immunohistochemistry/flow cytometry (CD20 and CD3) In situ hybridization (κ and λ light chains and EBV)	Cell block preparation for cytologic analysis HE, PAS, fungal stains Microbiological analysis for cultures		Cell block preparation for cytologic analysis, immunohistochemistry

Adapted from: Mehta et al. [65]

CMV cytomegalovirus, *EBV* Epstein-Barr virus, *HE* hematoxylin-eosin, *HSV* herpes simplex virus, *IgH* heavy-chain immunoglobulin, *IL* interleukin, *PAP* Papanicolaou, *PAS* periodic acid-Schiff, *PCR* polymerase chain reaction, *TB* tuberculosis, *TCR* T-cell receptor, *VZV* varicella zoster virus

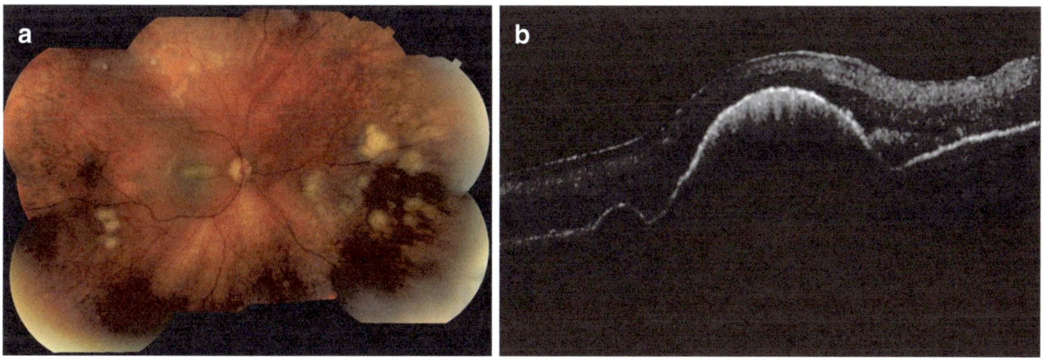

Fig. 11.3 (**a**) Color photograph of primary intraocular lymphoma presenting with subretinal infiltration. (**b**) SD-OCT of nasal retina showing both subretinal and sub-RPE infiltration

(tuberculosis), non-infectious (sarcoidosis), and masquerade (Whipple's disease) chorioretinal processes [21].

Fine-Needle Aspiration Biopsy (FNAB)

A variation of the vitreous biopsy technique is the fine-needle aspiration biopsy (FNAB) in which a 25–30 G, 1.5 inch (3.75 cm) needle is bent to an angle and connected to an aspirating syringe. The needle is passed into the eye via a pars plana incision and used to aspirate subretinal material under direct visualization with indirect ophthalmoscopy [22, 23]. As a vitrectomy is not performed with this technique, it carries a greater risk for vitreoretinal traction-related complications such as retinal detachment and does not allow for adequate gas tamponade postoperatively.

Subretinal Aspirate

Alternatively, infiltrative subretinal material may be sampled during the course of PPV following vitreous biopsy as described above, complete vitrectomy and removal of the posterior hyaloid. The biopsy site is usually selected at the edge of the lesion, at the junction of affected and normal retina, preferably in the superior hemiretina, to maximize the efficacy of postoperative gas tamponade. The biopsy site is then surrounded with endolaser and any vessels are diathermized. The intraocular pressure (IOP) is raised temporarily to greater than 50 mm Hg to reduce the risk of bleeding. A microvitreoretinal blade is used to incise the retina, and a 25-gauge, flexible, silicone cannula with the tip previously beveled is placed in the subretinal space; an assistant aspirates the biopsy specimen manually into a 3 ml syringe. The silicone-tipped cannula allows visualization of the cells flowing into the needle. Several such sites may be needed in order to obtain an adequate specimen and increase the yield. Fluid can be drawn from the mid-vitreous cavity to ensure that all the cells are in the syringe. A total volume of 0.5–1.0 ml within the syringe is usually adequate. Another maneuver to increase the yield is to enlarge the retinotomy, thus gaining access to a larger area of the subretinal space and obtaining a larger cellular aspirate. In some instances, material beneath the retina may be grasped with subretinal forceps and removed. After the intraocular specimen is removed, the intraocular pressure is lowered and hemostasis is confirmed. The peripheral retina is examined to exclude the presence of breaks or tears; an air-fluid exchange is performed, endolaser is applied around the retinotomy sites if not performed previously and the eye is insufflated with long-acting gas tamponade.

In the case of intraocular neoplasm and PIOL in particular, the aspirated material is more likely to have a higher concentration of viable cells than the adjacent intraocular fluid, reducing the chances of a false-negative cytologic result which occurs not infrequently following vitreous biopsy alone. Therefore, it is recommended that both vitreous biopsy and subretinal aspirate be performed during diagnostic PPV in suspected cases of PIOL which harbor characteristic subretinal lesions.

Endoretinal and Chorioretinal Biopsy

Judicious preoperative consideration of the differential diagnosis, careful biomicroscopic examination, multimodal imaging, and the disease course influence the choice of surgical procedure and so the biopsy site and depth. Endoretinal biopsy is ideal for the detection of intracellular pathogens such as HSV, VZV, CMV, and *Toxoplasma gondii* that spread by cell-to-cell contact within the retina, bacterial (syphilis) and fungal (candida) infections producing a retinitis and infiltrating processes (PIOL) located in the subretinal space and RPE in which the overlying vitreous may not be affected. Chorioretinal biopsies are preferred for uncertain disease processes primarily involving choroid in which the retina may be secondarily affected such as tuberculosis, sarcoidosis, PIOL, and cancer metastasis without evidence of systemic malignancy.

Endoretinal biopsy is performed during the course of PPV following vitreous biopsy, complete vitrectomy, and removal of the posterior hyaloid. As previously described with a subretinal aspirate, the biopsy site is usually selected at the junction of affected and normal retina, preferably in the superior hemiretina, to maximize the efficacy of postoperative gas tamponade, and surrounded with endolaser. If the retina is already detached, internal diathermy may be substituted and used to treat any vessels within the site. For cases in which the retina is attached, a 39 G cannula is used to inject saline under the neurosensory retina to create a small bleb. Again, the IOP is raised temporarily to greater than 50 mm Hg to reduce the risk of bleeding. An incision is then made in the retina using a needle knife, or MVR blade and vertical intraocular scissors are used to complete the neurosensory retinectomy to obtain at least a 2 mm by 2 mm biopsy specimen, left attached at one corner. The infusion should be temporarily turned off prior to removing the retinal sample to prevent turbulence and loss of the specimen. Broad-based forceps are then used to grasp the specimen and remove it from the eye.

Care should be taken not to lose the retinal biopsy sample as the forceps leave the eye at the sclerotomy site. Alternatively, the biopsy specimen may be manually aspirated through an 18-gauge needle into a 10 cc syringe and diluted to about 3 cc, visually confirming the specimen in the syringe. The plunger from the syringe is removed by the surgical assistant and the contents emptied onto a sterile petri dish, again confirming the presence of the specimen in the dish. After carefully aspirating excess fluid, the isolated specimen may be partitioned as described below. The peripheral retina is then examined, retinopexy applied to breaks if present, the retina is reattached with air-fluid exchange and long-acting non-expansile concentration of perfluoropropane (15%) or sulfahexafluoride (20%) is exchanged with the air.

Chorioretinal biopsy may be performed transclerally [21] or more commonly, by an ab interno approach [24]. As previously mentioned, FNAB may also be used to obtain retinal or choroidal tissue [25]. The majority of eyes undergoing ab interno chorioretinal biopsy have already undergone an inconclusive diagnostic vitrectomy and is described as follows [26]. If not previously performed, a vitreous biopsy, complete vitrectomy, and removal of the posterior hyaloid are achieved prior to delineating the intended biopsy site with endodiathermy or endolaser. Endodiathermy is preferred as this may achieve better retinal and choroidal hemostasis. After elevating the IOP to 50–60 mm HG, vertical scissors are used to incise the retina and choroid down to the sclera. The incision follows the outline of the diathermy nearly 360 degrees leaving the specimen hinged at one corner to prevent it from dislodging and floating freely in the vitreous cavity. While this procedure may be performed with 20–25 G vitrectomy systems, the access sclerotomy is usually 20 G and enlarged with an MVR blade prior to removal of the specimen. The chorioretinal tissue is then grasped near the hinge with a broad-platform forceps and removed rapidly from the eye to prevent hypotony and bleeding that may result from reduced intraocular pressure during this phase of the procedure. Bare sclera should be visualized within the biopsy site. The specimen is transferred to a specimen cup, partitioned as described below and the sclerotomy sutured immediately to its original size. Additional diathermy may be applied to the edge of the biopsy site and blood and/or residual tissue remnants removed with the vitreous cutter. Intraocular pressure is then slowly reduced and hemostasis verified. The peripheral retina is then examined, retinopexy applied to breaks if present, an air-fluid exchange is performed draining through the biopsy site which is then and surrounded with several rows of endolaser. A non-expansile concentration of perfluoropropane (15%) or silicone oil is employed as an extended tamponade.

Complications

The risks associated with intraocular biopsy procedures are congruent with those of vitreoretinal surgery in general. These include endophthalmitis, vitreous and choroidal hemorrhage, retinal breaks and detachment, proliferative vitreoretinopathy (PVR), elevated intraocular pressure (IOP), cataract progression, and exacerbation of underlying intraocular inflammation. In a recent retrospective review of 29 consecutive cases undergoing chorioretinal biopsy for suspected intraocular lymphoma over a 15 year period, no intraoperative complications were reported [14]. During the follow-up period, the complication rate was 14% and included two vitreous hemorrhages, both of which resolved spontaneously, and two late retinal detachments, each successfully repaired.

Sample Processing

The preoperative clinical impression and differential diagnosis are important in guiding the selection of diagnostic testing to be performed on intraocular specimens. Likewise, preoperative communication with respective laboratories is essential for effective sample processing.

Vitreous may be sent for cytopathology, flow cytometry, cytokine analysis, microbial culture, antibody testing, and molecular studies (PCR) (Table 11.2). Likewise, endoretinal and chorioretinal biopsy specimens are oriented and partitioned in the OR as follows: fresh tissue for microbiology, PCR, and cell culture media (RPMI); formalin fixation for paraffinization, immunohistochemistry, and/or in situ hybridization; and 4% glutaraldehyde for light and electron microscopy.

Cytology

Cytological evaluation may be performed on cells harvested from the vitreous, subretinal aspirate or chorioretinal biopsy specimen and requires immediate attention to prevent cellular degradation, especially in cases of suspected intraocular lymphoma, where rapid transport to the lab in tissue-culture medium (e.g., RPMI-1640S) may preserve cellular viability. While it remains the gold standard for the diagnosis of intraocular lymphoma, the sensitivity of vitreous cytopathology for this diagnosis has been historically low [27]. Samples are typically paucicellular, previous treatment with corticosteroids is cytolytic to lymphoma cells, and the presence of reactive T lymphocytes admixed with necrotic cells and debris may confound cytologic interpretation. Ultimately, cytologic evaluation may be limited by the skill of the cytopathologist and by its inability to immunophenotype (determine B-cell or T-cell origin) lymphocytes. Typical cytologic findings of PIOL on light microscopy (LM) with conventional stains (hematoxylin and eosin or Giemsa) include large lymphoid cells with scant basophilic cytoplasm and large, round-oval, indented or hypersegmented nuclei with prominent, frequently multiple nucleoli with mitotic figures [28] (Fig. 11.4). Tumor cells located between Bruch's membrane and the RPE is pathognomonic of PIOL [29].

Finally, in the appropriate clinical context, cytologic assessment of vitreous biopsy specimens has been shown to be of value in supporting the diagnosis of sarcoid-related posterior segment inflammation and in directing appropriate therapy [30].

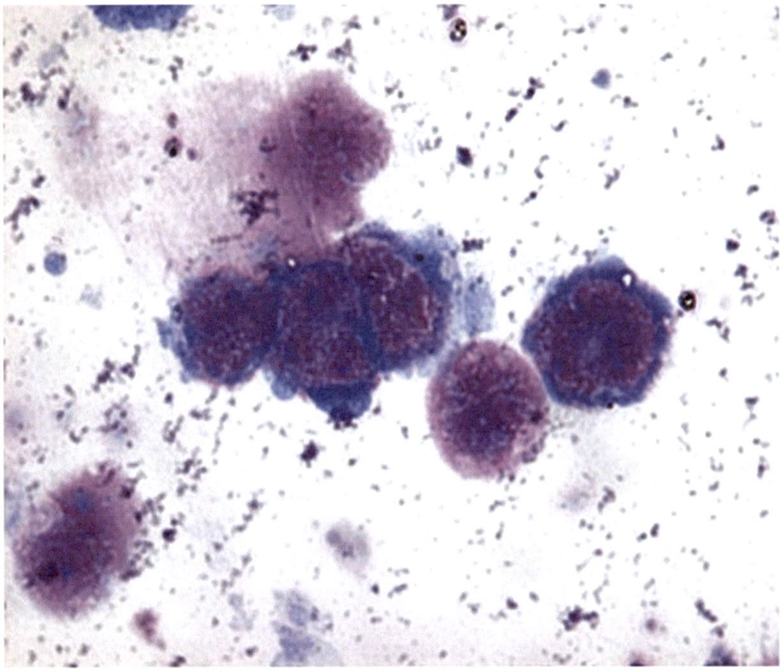

Fig. 11.4 Primary intraocular lymphoma: light microscopy with hematoxylin and eosin highlighting large lymphoid cells with scant basophilic cytoplasm and large, round-oval, indented or hypersegmented nuclei with prominent, frequently multiple nucleoli

Immunohistochemistry

Immunohistochemical techniques detect cell or tissue-bound antigens with monoclonal antibodies either by microscopic examination of immunofluorescence or by using fluorescence-activated cell sorters, otherwise known as flow cytometry (FCI). Both of these techniques permit the immunophenotyping of lymphocytes and so have been applied to the diagnosis of intraocular lymphoma and its differentiation from infectious and non-infectious uveitis [31, 32]. Specifically, most primary intraocular lymphomas consist of populations of monoclonal B lymphocytes that stain for specific B-cell markers (CD-19, CD-20, and CD-22) and have restricted expression of kappa or lambda chains, while in non-infectious posterior uveitis; there is a predominance of CD4+ helper or inducer T lymphocytes and elevated interleukin-2 receptor levels (CD-25) which is correlated with uveitis activity [33]. T-cell lymphomas, while much less common, can be identified by T-cell markers such as CD3 and DC8. In one study, FCI identified intraocular lymphoma in 7 or 10 patients as compared to only 3 diagnosed by cytology, [32] while in another, it provided corroborative support in 6 patients diagnosed by both modalities [34]. Davis and colleagues have reported that CD-22 + B lymphocytes comprising ≥20% of total cells on FCI had a positive predictive value of 88% for lymphoma while a CD4:CD8 T-lymphocyte ratio of ≥4 had a similarly positive predictive value of 70% for immunologically mediated uveitis [35].

Cytokine Analysis

Cytokine analysis of vitreous and/or aqueous samples from patients with suspected intraocular lymphoma may serve as a useful adjunct in distinguishing this entity from inflammatory posterior uveitis and in monitoring disease activity. Interleukin-10 (IL-10) is preferentially produced by malignant B lymphocytes in patients with intraocular lymphoma, whereas, interleukin-6 (IL-6) is found in high levels in patients with inflammatory uveitis [36]. Specifically, elevated vitreous levels of IL-10 and a ratio of IL-10 to IL-6 of >1 are suggestive of a diagnosis of PIOL [37, 38]. Likewise, IL-10 levels in the aqueous humor may be a useful biomarker for the diagnosis of PIOL and correlate with clinical response to local chemotherapy [10].

Microbiologic Analysis

While culture remains the gold standard for the diagnosis of intraocular infection, especially in cases of bacterial endophthalmitis, many intraocular microbes (viruses) are difficult to recover and identify by this method. It is important to hold bacterial specimens for a least 1 week and fungal cultures for 1 month as some organisms (*Propionibacterium acnes*) may require extended time periods to grow (Fig. 11.5).

Intraocular Antibody Analysis

Intraocular antibody production as a measure of the host response to a specific microbial pathogen can be computed utilizing the GWC: the ratio of specific antibody (aqueous or vitreous)/total IgG (aqueous or vitreous) to specific antibody (serum)/total IgG (serum) as measured by enzyme-linked immunosorbent assay (ELISA) or radioimmunoassay [39]. A ratio of greater than 4 is considered diagnostic of local antibody production [40]. Antibody testing of ocular fluids remains the gold standard for the diagnosis of ocular toxocarasis [41]. It has been used more widely in Europe than in the United States as an adjunct to the diagnosis of toxoplasmosis [42], necrotizing herpetic retinitis due to herpes simplex virus (HSV) and varicella zoster virus (VZV) while it is of little value in the diagnosis of cytomegalovirus (CMV) retinitis [43].

Molecular Analysis

PCR of aqueous and vitreous samples provides a highly sensitive and specific assay in the diagnosis of suspected infectious posterior uveitis or

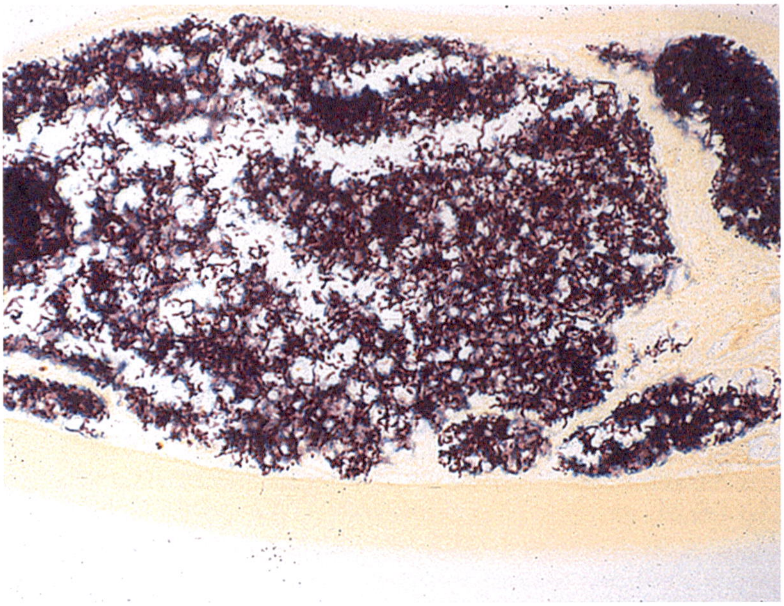

Fig. 11.5 Gram stain revealing a colony of gram-positive rods consistent with *Propionibacterium acnes*. Note the yellow lens capsule inferiorly. (Courtesy of Nick Mamalis, MD)

Table 11.3 PCR for intraocular infection

HSV I, VZV,CMV, EBV
Toxoplasma gondii
Mycobacterium tuberculosis
Borrelia burgdorferi
Propionibacterium
Leptospirosis
Tropheryma whipelli
Fungi (28s rDNA gene)
Bacteria (16s rDNA gene)
Metagenomics deep sequencing

uncertain etiology and/or atypical presentation, allowing the differentiation of diverse potential microorganisms (Table 11.3). Small volumes of fluid (0.1 ml) can be analyzed for the detection and differentiation of herpes family viruses (HSV 1, HSV 2, HSV-6, VZV, CMV, and EBV). While the test sensitivity is greater for the vitreous than the aqueous, in many cases of necrotizing retinitis, PCR and/or antibody determinations from the aqueous alone may provide sufficient substrate for analysis, obviating the need for vitrectomy [44].

PCR-based assays have also been developed for the detection of *Toxoplasma gondii*, bacteria, and fungi in cases of both acute and delayed-onset postoperative endophthalmitis. In one study using "universal" 16S rDNA primers, bacterial DNA was amplified in nearly all cases of acute postoperative endophthalmitis [45], while in the Endophthalmitis Vitrectomy Study, the reported rate of culture-positive cases was only 70% [46]. Similarly, diagnostic yields of up to 92% in cases of delayed-onset endophthalmitis due to *Propionibacterium acnes*, *Staphylococcus epidermidis*, or *Actinomyces israelii* [47] and fungi [48] have been reported, significantly improving the time to diagnosis over traditional techniques.

PCR screening of vitreous samples has proven invaluable in the diagnosis of medically unresponsive, atypical, or otherwise unusual causes of posterior uveitis, such as suspected Whipple's disease [49], Lyme disease [50], ocular tuberculosis [51], or cat-scratch disease [52].

Furthermore, the recent development by Doan and colleagues of an unbiased metagenomics deep sequencing approach to identify infectious organisms (fungi, parasites, DNA and RNA viruses) in otherwise idiopathic uveitis using small volumes of ocular fluid will likely change our concept of etiopathogenesis for many uveitic entities [53]. Finally, the diagnostic yield of PIOL may be improved by isolating cells with cytologic abnormalities with either laser capture or manual microdissection for PCR-based molecular assays to detect IgH, bcl-2, or T-cell receptor gamma gene rearrangements [54–56]. Furthermore, discovery of the myeloid differentiation primary response gene 88 (Myd88) mutation L265P in 86.7% of primary vitreoretinal lymphoma in one series might make PCR testing for this mutation highly sensitive in the diagnosis of PIOL. PCR testing for the Myd88 L265P mutation can be performed on paraffin-embedded blocks as well as live cells [57].

Outcomes

The reported yield following diagnostic PPV ranges from 20% to 92% [16, 31, 35, 58–62]. This variability is due in part to diverse definitions of the final diagnosis but more importantly to specific patient/case factors (preoperative clinical diagnostic suspicion and previous exposure to antimicrobial/anti-inflammatory therapy), vitreous sample processing (effective preoperative communication, time lag to testing, number and types of tests ordered, experience of cytopathologist), and surgical technique. In one series of 87 patients, the overall diagnostic yield in differentiating infectious from neoplastic disease in eyes with posterior uveitis was 39% [60]. A specific diagnosis was reached more often when an underlying infection was suspected preoperatively (42% of 65 eyes) as compared to intraocular malignancy (10% of 71 eyes). Intraocular antibody testing and PCR had the highest yields at 46% and 39%, respectively. In another study from the Bascom Palmer Eye Institute, vitreous analysis led to a diagnosis in 61% of 78 consecutive patients with 81% of patients having a final diagnosis that matched the indication for surgery [35]. When the initial and final clinical diagnoses were compared, the efficiency of the diagnostic procedure for cytology, flow cytometry, and bacterial/fungal culture were 67%, 79%, and 96%, respectively. The positive predictive value for cytologic evaluation for lymphoma was 100%, while the negative predictive value was 60.9%. For intraocular infection, the positive and negative predictive values for bacterial/fungal culture were 100% and 94.9%, respectively.

The diagnostic value of PCR from 105 aqueous and 38 vitreous specimens from among 133 patients with putative infectious chorioretinitis was reported from the same institution [63]. A definitive pathogen (HSV, VZV, CMV, EBV, *T. gondii*) was identified in 81% of 95 patients, leading to an alteration in treatment in 24% based on PCR alone. Clinical features associated with a positive result included early presentation (within a week of onset), extensive areas of retinitis, retinal vasculitis, and immunocompromised status.

Most recently, the largest data pool of reported cytologic diagnoses has been reviewed from among 5736 vitreous samples obtained during diagnostic and therapeutic vitrectomy from three teaching intuitions [16]. In eyes undergoing diagnostic PPV for suspected B-cell lymphoma, all 29 cases displayed cytologic atypia, whereas B-cell monoclonality by PCR analyses for IgH gene rearrangements was seen in 21 specimens. Cytologic analysis was likewise diagnostic in other patients suspected of malignancy including those with retinoblastoma, melanoma, and metastatic adenocarcinoma. The authors concluded that cytologic evaluation of vitrectomy samples provides valuable information in differentiating nonpathologic findings from infectious, inflammatory, and neoplastic conditions and stressed the importance of preoperative communication between the surgeon and pathologist.

There are no large-scale data on the diagnostic yield of trans pars plana subretinal aspiration, FNAB, endoretinal or chorioretinal biopsy as these procedures are performed relatively infrequently. In one series of 67 patients undergoing FNAB for melanoma, the adequate yield was obtained in 97% of eyes. In a retrospective review of 14 retinal, subretinal, retino-choroidal and choroidal biopsies taken for 13 eyes with uveitis of unclear etiology suspected of harboring infectious or malignant disease, the pathological diagnosis differed from the initial clinical diagnosis in 5 of 13 cases [64]. In seven, the tissue biopsy result directed specific treatment, while in 4, the biopsy excluded malignancy but failed to provide a specific diagnosis. In a recent retrospective review of 29 patients undergoing chorioretinal biopsy for suspected intraocular lymphoma, a definitive diagnosis was achieved in 59%, malignancy was effectively excluded in 31%, while in 10% a definitive diagnosis could not be reached [14]. Significant levels of vitritis appeared to be strongly predictive of a definitive biopsy result relative to lesser degrees of vitreal inflammation.

Summary

Diagnostic vitreoretinal surgery is an essential intervention for sight-threatening uveitis of unknown etiology in which the clinical presentation and systemic workup are either atypical or insufficient to make a diagnosis and/or when the response to conventional therapy is inadequate or paradoxical. This is especially important in cases of suspected intraocular infection or malignancy where intraocular fluid and/or tissue biopsy have the potential to significantly alter the management of uveitis and impact the systemic health of the patient.

References

1. Jabs DA, Busingye J. Approach to the diagnosis of the uveitides. Am J Ophthalmol. [Research Support, N.I.H., Extramural Research Support, Non--U.S. Gov't]. 2013;156(2):228–36.
2. Hunter RS, Lobo AM. Current diagnostic approaches to infectious anterior uveitis. Int Ophthalmol Clin. [Review]. 2011;51(4):145–56.
3. Van der Lelij A, Rothova A. Diagnostic anterior chamber paracentesis in uveitis: a safe procedure? Br J Ophthalmol. 1997;81(11):976–9.
4. Trivedi D, Denniston AK, Murray PI. Safety profile of anterior chamber paracentesis performed at the slit lamp. Clin Experiment Ophthalmol. [Comparative Study Research Support, Non-U.S. Gov't]. 2011;39(8):725–8.
5. Harper TW, Miller D, Schiffman JC, Davis JL. Polymerase chain reaction analysis of aqueous and vitreous specimens in the diagnosis of posterior segment infectious uveitis. Am J Ophthalmol. [Research Support, N.I.H., Extramural Research Support, Non--U.S. Gov't]. 2009;147(1):140–7.e2.
6. De Groot-Mijnes JD, Rothova A, Van Loon AM, Schuller M, Ten Dam-Van Loon NH, De Boer JH, et al. Polymerase chain reaction and Goldmann-Witmer coefficient analysis are complimentary for the diagnosis of infectious uveitis. Am J Ophthalmol. [Research Support, Non-U.S Gov't] 2006;141(2):313–8.
7. Anwar Z, Galor A, Albini TA, Miller D, Perez V, Davis JL. The diagnostic utility of anterior chamber paracentesis with polymerase chain reaction in anterior uveitis. Am J Ophthalmol. [Comparative Study Research Support, N.I.H., Extramural Research Support, Non-US Gov't; Research Support, US Gov't, Non-PHS] 2013;155(5):781–6.
8. Rothova A, de Boer JH, Ten Dam-van Loon NH, Postma G, de Visser L, Zuurveen SJ, et al. Usefulness of aqueous humor analysis for the diagnosis of posterior uveitis. Ophthalmology. [Research Support, Non--U.S. Gov't]. 2008;115(2):306–11.
9. Ayliffe W, Foster CS, Marcoux P, Upton M, Finkelstein M, Kuperwaser M, et al. Relapsing acute myeloid leukemia manifesting as hypopyon uveitis. Am J Ophthalmol. [Case Reports Research Support, Non-U.S. Gov't]. 1995;119(3):361–4.
10. Cassoux N, Giron A, Bodaghi B, Tran TH, Baudet S, Davy F, et al. IL-10 measurement in aqueous humor for screening patients with suspicion of primary intraocular lymphoma. Invest Ophthalmol Vis Sci. 2007;48(7):3253–9.
11. Rickman LS, Freeman WR, Green WR, Feldman ST, Sullivan J, Russack V, et al. Brief report: uveitis caused by Tropheryma whippelii (Whipple's bacillus). N Engl J Med. [Case Reports Research Support, Non-U.S. Gov't; Research Support, U.S. Gov't, P.H.S.] 1995;332(6):363–6.
12. Results of the Endophthalmitis Vitrectomy Study. A randomized trial of immediate vitrectomy and of intravenous antibiotics for the treatment of postoperative bacterial endophthalmitis. Endophthalmitis Vitrectomy Study Group. Arch Ophthalmol. [Clinical Trial Multicenter Study Randomized Controlled Trial Research Support, U.S. Gov't, P.H.S.]. 1995;113(12):1479–96.
13. Han DP, Wisniewski SR, Kelsey SF, Doft BH, Barza M, Pavan PR. Microbiologic yields and complication rates of vitreous needle aspiration versus mechanized vitreous biopsy in the Endophthalmitis Vitrectomy Study. Retina. [Clinical Trial Comparative Study Multicenter Study Randomized Controlled Trial Research Support, Non-U.S. Gov't Research Support, U.S. Gov't, P.H.S.] 1999;19(2):98–102.
14. Mastropasqua R, Thaung C, Pavesio C, Lightman S, Westcott M, Okhravi N, et al. The role of chorioretinal biopsy in the diagnosis of intraocular lymphoma. Am J Ophthalmol. 2015;160(6):1127–32.e1.
15. Quiroz-Mercado H, Rivera-Sempertegui J, Macky TA, Navarro-Lopez P, Griselda-Alvarez L, Ibarra-Ponce N, et al. Performing vitreous biopsy by perfluorocarbon-perfused vitrectomy. Am J Ophthalmol. 2005;140(6):1161–3.
16. Mehta M, Rasheed RA, Duker J, Reichel E, Feinberg E, Husain D, et al. Vitreous evaluation: a diagnostic challenge. Ophthalmology.. [Multicenter Study]. 2015;122(3):531–7.
17. Levy-Clarke GA, Byrnes GA, Buggage RR, Shen DF, Filie AC, Caruso RC, et al. Primary intraocular lymphoma diagnosed by fine needle aspiration biopsy of a subretinal lesion. Retina. 2001;21(3):281–4.

18. Freeman WR, Wiley CA, Gross JG, Thomas EL, Rao NA, Liggett PE. Endoretinal biopsy in immunosuppressed and healthy patients with retinitis. Indications, utility, and techniques. Ophthalmology. 1989;96(10):1559–65.
19. Rutzen AR, Ortega-Larrocea G, Dugel PU, Chong LP, Lopez PF, Smith RE, et al. Clinicopathologic study of retinal and choroidal biopsies in intraocular inflammation. Am J Ophthalmol. [Research Support, Non--U.S. Gov't Research Support, U.S. Gov't, P.H.S.]. 1995;119(5):597–611.
20. Freeman WR. Application of vitreoretinal surgery to inflammatory and infectious disease of the posterior segment. Int Ophthalmol Clin. [Research Support, Non-U.S. Gov't Research Support, U.S. Gov't, P.H.S. Review]. 1992;32(2):15–33.
21. Martin DF, Chan CC, de Smet MD, Palestine AG, Davis JL, Whitcup SM, et al. The role of chorioretinal biopsy in the management of posterior uveitis. Ophthalmology. 1993;100(5):705–14.
22. Palkovacs EM, Correa Z, Augsburger JJ, Eagle RC Jr. Acquired toxoplasmic retinitis in an immunosuppressed patient: diagnosis by transvitreal fine-needle aspiration biopsy. Graefes Arch Clin Exp Ophthalmol. 2008;246(10):1495–7.
23. Eide N, Walaas L. Fine-needle aspiration biopsy and other biopsies in suspected intraocular malignant disease: a review. Acta Ophthalmol. [Review]. 2009 Sep;87(6):588–601.
24. Cole CJ, Kwan AS, Laidlaw DA, Aylward GW. A new technique of combined retinal and choroidal biopsy. Br J Ophthalmol. 2008;92(10):1357–60.
25. Augsburger JJ, Shields JA. Fine needle aspiration biopsy of solid intraocular tumors: indications, instrumentation and techniques. Ophthalmic Surg. [Research Support, Non-U.S. Gov't]. 1984;15(1):34–40.
26. Elliot D. Transvitreal chorioretinal biopsy. In: Elliot DRP, editor. Surgical manafement of intraocular inflammation and infection. London: JP Medical; 2013. p. 62–4.
27. Davis JL. Diagnosis of intraocular lymphoma. Ocul Immunol Inflamm. 2004;12(1):7–16.
28. Whitcup SM, de Smet MD, Rubin BI, Palestine AG, Martin DF, Burnier M Jr, et al. Intraocular lymphoma. Clinical and histopathologic diagnosis. Ophthalmology. 1993;100(9):1399–406.
29. Barr CC, Green WR, Payne JW, Knox DL, Jensen AD, Thompson RL. Intraocular reticulum-cell sarcoma: clinico-pathologic study of four cases and review of the literature. Surv Ophthalmol. 1975;19(4):224–39.
30. Scott AW, Mruthyunjaya P, McCallum RM, Jaffe GJ. Diagnostic yield of vitreous biopsy in presumed sarcoidosis-related posterior segment inflammation. Graefes Arch Clin Exp Ophthalmol. [Case Reports Research Support, Non-U.S. Gov't]. 2012;250(9):1379–85.
31. Davis JL, Solomon D, Nussenblatt RB, Palestine AG, Chan CC. Immunocytochemical staining of vitreous cells. Indications, techniques, and results. Ophthalmology. 1992;99(2):250–6.
32. Davis JL, Viciana AL, Ruiz P. Diagnosis of intraocular lymphoma by flow cytometry. Am J Ophthalmol. 1997;124(3):362–72.
33. Deschenes J, Char DH, Freeman W, Nozik R, Garovoy M. Uveitis: lymphocyte subpopulation studies. Trans Ophthalmol Soc U K. 1986;105(Pt 2):246–51.
34. Zaldivar RA, Martin DF, Holden JT, Grossniklaus HE. Primary intraocular lymphoma: clinical, cytologic, and flow cytometric analysis. Ophthalmology. [Case Reports Research Support, Non-U.S. Gov't Research Support, U.S. Gov't, P.H.S.]. 2004;111(9):1762–7.
35. Davis JL, Miller DM, Ruiz P. Diagnostic testing of vitrectomy specimens. Am J Ophthalmol. 2005;140(5):822–9.
36. Chan CC, Whitcup SM, Solomon D, Nussenblatt RB. Interleukin-10 in the vitreous of patients with primary intraocular lymphoma. Am J Ophthalmol. 1995;120(5):671–3.
37. Chan CC. Molecular pathology of primary intraocular lymphoma. Trans Am Ophthalmol Soc. 2003;101:275–92.
38. Wolf LA, Reed GF, Buggage RR, Nussenblatt RB, Chan CC. Vitreous cytokine levels. Ophthalmology. 2003;110(8):1671–2.
39. Witmer RH. Antibody formation in rabbit eye studied with fluorescein-labeled antibody. AMA Arch Ophthalmol. 1955;53(6):811–6.
40. Dussaix E, Cerqueti PM, Pontet F, Bloch-Michel E. New approaches to the detection of locally produced antiviral antibodies in the aqueous of patients with endogenous uveitis. Ophthalmologica. 1987;194(2–3):145–9.
41. Benitez del Castillo JM, Herreros G, Guillen JL, Fenoy S, Banares A, Garcia J. Bilateral ocular toxocariasis demonstrated by aqueous humor enzyme-linked immunosorbent assay. Am J Ophthalmol. 1995;119(4):514–6.
42. Ronday MJ, Ongkosuwito JV, Rothova A, Kijlstra A. Intraocular anti-Toxoplasma gondii IgA antibody production in patients with ocular toxoplasmosis. Am J Ophthalmol. 1999;127(3):294–300.
43. de Boer JH, Verhagen C, Bruinenberg M, Rothova A, de Jong PT, Baarsma GS, et al. Serologic and polymerase chain reaction analysis of intraocular fluids in the diagnosis of infectious uveitis. Am J Ophthalmol. 1996;121(6):650–8.
44. Tran TH, Rozenberg F, Cassoux N, Rao NA, LeHoang P, Bodaghi B. Polymerase chain reaction analysis of aqueous humour samples in necrotising retinitis. Br J Ophthalmol. 2003;87(1):79–83.
45. Lohmann CP, Heeb M, Linde HJ, Gabel VP, Reischl U. Diagnosis of infectious endophthalmitis after cataract surgery by polymerase chain reaction. J Cataract Refract Surg. 1998;24(6):821–6.
46. Microbiologic factors and visual outcome in the endophthalmitis vitrectomy study. Am J Ophthalmol. [Clinical Trial Multicenter Study Randomized Controlled Trial Research Support, Non--U.S. Gov't Research Support, U.S. Gov't, P.H.S.]. 1996;122(6):830–46.

47. Lohmann CP, Linde HJ, Reischl U. Improved detection of microorganisms by polymerase chain reaction in delayed endophthalmitis after cataract surgery. Ophthalmology. 2000;107(6):1047–51; discussion 51–2.
48. Anand A, Madhavan H, Neelam V, Lily T. Use of polymerase chain reaction in the diagnosis of fungal endophthalmitis. Ophthalmology. [Comparative Study Evaluation Studies Research Support, Non--U.S. Gov't] 2001;108(2):326–30.
49. Rickman LS, Freeman WR, Green WR, Feldman ST, Sullivan J, Russack V, et al. Brief report: uveitis caused by Tropheryma whippelii (Whipple's bacillus). N Engl J Med. 1995;332(6):363–6.
50. Mikkila H, Karma A, Viljanen M, Seppala I. The laboratory diagnosis of ocular Lyme borreliosis. Graefes Arch Clin Exp Ophthalmol. 1999;237(3):225–30.
51. Ortega-Larrocea G, Bobadilla-del-Valle M, Ponce-de-Leon A, Sifuentes-Osornio J. Nested polymerase chain reaction for Mycobacterium tuberculosis DNA detection in aqueous and vitreous of patients with uveitis. Arch Med Res. 2003;34(2):116–9.
52. Kerkhoff FT, Bergmans AM, van Der Zee A, Rothova A. Demonstration of Bartonella grahamii DNA in ocular fluids of a patient with neuroretinitis. J Clin Microbiol. 1999;37(12):4034–8.
53. Doan T, Wilson MR, Crawford ED, Chow ED, Khan LM, Knopp KA, et al. Illuminating uveitis: metagenomic deep sequencing identifies common and rare pathogens. Genome Med. [Research Support, Non--U.S. Gov't Research Support, N.I.H., Extramural]. 2016;8(1):90.
54. Baehring JM, Androudi S, Longtine JJ, Betensky RA, Sklar J, Foster CS, et al. Analysis of clonal immunoglobulin heavy chain rearrangements in ocular lymphoma. Cancer. 2005;104(3):591–7.
55. Chan CC, Wallace DJ. Intraocular lymphoma: update on diagnosis and management. Cancer Control. 2004;11(5):285–95.
56. Wang Y, Shen D, Wang VM, Sen HN, Chan CC. Molecular biomarkers for the diagnosis of primary vitreoretinal lymphoma. Int J Mol Sci. [Research Support, N.I.H., Intramural]. 2011;12(9):5684–97.
57. Raja H, Salomao DR, Viswanatha DS, Pulido JS. Prevalence of Myd88 L265p mutation in histologically proven, diffuse large B-cell vitreoretinal lymphoma. Retina. [Research Support, Non-U.S. Gov't]. 2016;36(3):624–8.
58. Wittenberg LA, Maberley DA, Ma PE, Wade NK, Gill H, White VA. Contribution of vitreous cytology to final clinical diagnosis fifteen-year review of vitreous cytology specimens from one institution. Ophthalmology. 2008;115(11):1944–50.
59. Margolis R, Brasil OF, Lowder CY, Singh RP, Kaiser PK, Smith SD, et al. Vitrectomy for the diagnosis and management of uveitis of unknown cause. Ophthalmology. 2007;114(10):1893–7.
60. Mruthyunjaya P, Jumper JM, McCallum R, Patel DJ, Cox TA, Jaffe GJ. Diagnostic yield of vitrectomy in eyes with suspected posterior segment infection or malignancy. Ophthalmology. 2002;109(6):1123–9.
61. Green WR. Diagnostic cytopathology of ocular fluid specimens. Ophthalmology. 1984;91(6):726–49.
62. Stulting RD, Leif RC, Clarkson JG, Bobbitt D. Centrifugal cytology of ocular fluids. Arch Ophthalmol. 1982;100(5):822–5.
63. Harper TW, Miller D, Schiffman JC, Davis JL. Polymerase chain reaction analysis of aqueous and vitreous specimens in the diagnosis of posterior segment infectious uveitis. Am J Ophthalmol. 2009;147(1):140–7 e2.
64. Johnston RL, Tufail A, Lightman S, Luthert PJ, Pavesio CE, Cooling RJ, et al. Retinal and choroidal biopsies are helpful in unclear uveitis of suspected infectious or malignant origin. Ophthalmology. 2004;111(3):522–8.
65. Mehta M, et al. Vitreous evaluation: a diagnostic challenge. Ophthalmology. 2015;122(3):531–7.

Therapeutic Vitreoretinal Surgery for Noninfectious Intermediate, Posterior, and Panuveitis

12

Akbar Shakoor and Albert T. Vitale

Pearls

- Pars plana vitrectomy may improve inflammatory control and, potentially, refractory CME, noting that removal of vitreous will result in loss of the vitreous depot for intravitreally injected drugs.
- Pars plana vitrectomy with ERM +/− ILM removal may improve visual and anatomical outcomes in the management of medically refractory CME, but it is important to perform preoperative spectral domain OCT and, potentially, FA, to determine cases that might benefit from this surgery.
- Rarely, pars plana vitrectomy with silicone oil, with or without cyclitic membrane removal and/or FA implant placement, may be effective in maintaining IOP in hypotonous uveitic eyes.

With the advancement, over the last two decades, in surgical techniques, microsurgical instrumentation and the resultant reduction in perioperative surgical complications, the application of vitrectomy and adjunctive therapeutic vitreoretinal interventions have garnered greater interest in the management of ocular inflammatory disease (OID). There remains a general consensus that the management of uveitis is best achieved through medical intervention, but in the presence of structural complications and uncontrolled inflammation in both infectious and noninfectious disease, surgical management may be efficacious in limiting vision loss and preventing further structural disruption.

Indications for vitreoretinal procedures in OID (Table 12.1) include (1) achieving improved inflammatory control in eyes unresponsive to conventional immunomodulatory therapy (IMT) or regional glucocorticoid therapy; (2) the management of visually significant media opacity; (3) the management of structural complications such as tractional retinal detachment and epiretinal membrane (ERM); (4) the management of

Table 12.1 Indications for vitreoretinal surgery in uveitis

Inflammatory control in eyes unresponsive to conventional therapy
Visually significant media opacity
Structural complications such as retinal detachment and ERM
Uveitis-associated hypotony
Sustained-release drug delivery devices
Inflammatory disease due to infectious endophthalmitis and lens-induced uveitis
In association with cataract surgery

A. Shakoor (✉) · A. T. Vitale
Ophthalmology and Visual Sciences, Uveitis and Vitreoretinal Divisions, John A. Moran Eye Center, University of Utah Hospital, Salt Lake City, UT, USA
e-mail: Akbar.shakoor@hsc.utah.edu; Albert.vitale@hsc.utah.edu

P. Lin, E. Suhler (eds.), *Treatment of Non-infectious Uveitis*,
https://doi.org/10.1007/978-3-030-22827-9_12

uveitis-associated hypotony; (5) the placement of sustained-release drug delivery devices; (6) the management of acute inflammatory disease due to infectious endophthalmitis and lens-induced uveitis; and (7) in association with cataract surgery where pars plana vitrectomy (PPV), with or without lens implantation, may lead to better postoperative control of inflammation and a lower rate of structural complications of surgery.

Regardless of the indications for surgical intervention, perioperative control of inflammation is paramount. The use of perioperative steroid bursts is useful but true steroid sparing quiescence achieved through the use of IMT is preferred. For nonemergent procedures, it is certainly advisable to adequately suppress inflammatory activity utilizing topical, regional, and systemic steroids with or without systemic steroid-sparing IMT as necessary for a minimum of 3 months prior to surgery, particularly if cataract and intraocular lens (IOL) implantation is contemplated. In emergent surgical cases such as lens-induced uveitis or infectious endophthalmitis, where by their very nature, inflammatory control cannot be achieved prior to surgery, the risk of perioperative complications and poor outcomes increases. This can be mitigated in part by minimizing the scope of surgery and, in the case of lens-induced uveitis, considering the use of perioperative oral or intravenous steroids.

Preoperative imaging studies may be useful in planning the scope of vitreoretinal surgery in eyes with ocular inflammatory disease. Optical coherence tomography can demonstrate epimacular membranes [1] and cystoid macular edema [2–4] and allow the surgeon to gauge the relative impact of each on macular morphology. Wide-field fluorescein angiography may demonstrate areas of peripheral nonperfusion [5, 6], peripheral vascular leakage, neovascularization, and exudation that may be amenable to intraoperative treatment with laser photocoagulation or transscleral cryotherapy [7, 8]. Ultrasound of both the anterior segment and the posterior pole may demonstrate retinal detachment and tractional vitreoretinopathy where poor media precludes a comprehensive examination and may also demonstrate cyclitic membranes and ciliary body detachment that may be surgically addressed in hypotonus eyes [9].

Surgical Techniques

A standard three-port pars plana vitrectomy (PPV) is employed using 20-, 23-, 25-, or 27-gauge instrumentation. To avoid suprachoroidal or subretinal infusion, attention should be paid to the visualization of the infusion cannula by either utilizing a 6 mm infusion canula or infusing through the anterior segment until media opacity such as posterior synechiae, cataract, and cyclitic and vitreous membranes can be cleared.

Further interventions can include excision and peeling of macular or peripheral tractional preretinal membranes using manual or pneumatic scissors, end-grasping microsurgical forceps, membrane scrapers, or picks. The authors find that the design of the 25- and 27-gauge vitrectomy probes are particularly useful for the delamination and dissection of tractional membranes. Bimanual techniques can prove to be particularly useful in the dissection of cyclitic membranes and the membranes associated with proliferative vitreoretinopathy. An endoscopic approach through the pars plana has been used to directly visualize and dissect cyclitic membranes in the case of tractional ciliary body detachment in hypotonus eyes [10]. Visualizing agents such as triamcinolone acetonide (Kenalog) have been shown to be extremely useful in delineating the posterior hyaloid and facilitating its safe removal in patients with refractory uveitis undergoing PPV [11]. Should the vitreous be difficult to separate, high-flow aspiration, viscodissection, and/or retinal brushes, pics, and forceps may be necessary to elevate the posterior hyaloid. Similarly, indocyanine green (ICG) has been successfully employed to visualize the internal limiting membrane (ILM) in a subgroup of patients with uveitis undergoing PPV for persistent macular edema, with five of nine having significant visual improvement postoperatively [12].

In intermediate uveitis, peripheral neovascularization and nonperfusion may be treated with either endolaser photocoagulation or indirect laser photocoagulation. Neovascularization along snowbanks or exudation from a thickened snowbank may be treated with limited and local application of cryotherapy.

Sustained-release drug delivery devices may be either anchored via sutures to the pars plana as with the fluocinolone acetonide (FA) implant (Retisert, Bausch and Lomb, Rochester, NY) [13] or the now unavailable ganciclovir (Vitrisert, Bausch and Lomb, Rochester, NY) implant [13]. These implants require a 3–4 mm sclerostomy for insertion through the pars plana and, although generally well tolerated, may rarely be associated with postoperative complications such as hypotony, wound leakage, extrusion, vitreous hemorrhage, and endophthalmitis. Local side effects of the FA implant include high rates of cataract and glaucoma requiring surgery (to be covered in more detail in Chap. 12). Other sustained-release drug delivery systems may be placed in the vitreous through small gauge injectors in the clinic, including the intravitreal dexamethasone implant (Ozurdex, Allergan, Inc., Irvine, CA) [14], approved for the treatment of noninfectious uveitis, and the fluocinolone acetonide intravitreal insert (Illuvian, Alimera Sciences, Inc. Alpharetta, GA), approved currently for the treatment of diabetic macular edema for a period of up to 3 years after injection [15].

At the termination of vitreoretinal surgical procedures in uveitis, the peripheral retina should be viewed with scleral indentation and any iatrogenic breaks treated with either transscleral cryotherapy or laser photocoagulation. Sub-Tenon's or intravitreal steroids may then be administered unless otherwise contraindicated. Care should be taken especially in eyes in which an infectious etiology is suspected where regional, parenteral, or oral steroids should only be administered in conjunction with appropriate antimicrobial therapy or not at all.

Rationale for Vitreoretinal Procedures in OID

Inflammatory Control

Beyond the obvious role of PPV for the removal of media opacity from vitreous debris and hemorrhage (Fig. 12.1), there is some evidence to suggest that permanent removal of the vitreous may assist in the clearance of both antigenic material as well as inflammatory mediators. Increased levels of interleukin (IL)-1, IL-2, IL-6, and tumor necrosis factor alpha (TNF-α) have been found in the vitreous of eyes with active noninfectious posterior and intermediate uveitis. Increased IL-6, IL-8, soluble intercellular cell adhesion molecule

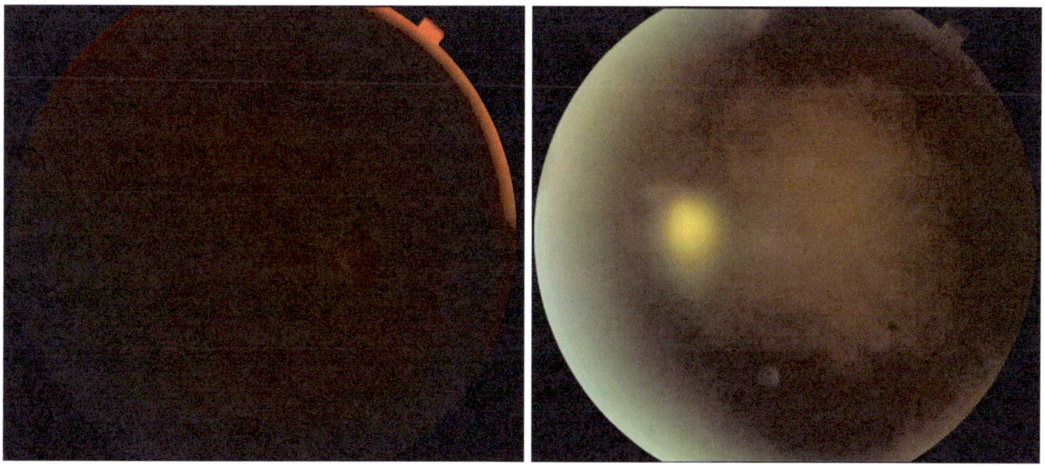

Fig. 12.1 A 45-year-old immunocompromised patient with histoplasma endogenous endophthalmitis and significant media opacity limiting vision and management

(sICAM), soluble vascular cell adhesion molecule (sVCAM), and interferon-inducible protein-10 were seen in the aqueous humor of eyes with active anterior uveitis compared to quiescent controls [16]. Autologous antigens such as type II collagen, found only in the vitreous and joint spaces, may produce uveitis and arthritis when introduced in animal models [17]. Opremcak and associates [18] detected T cells in the blood of patients with various uveitis syndromes that were reactive to type II collagen. The detection of antibodies to Rubella in the aqueous of patients with Fuchs' heterochromic uveitis [19] implies that antigens from infectious organisms, in some forms of uveitis, may serve as a source of immunoreactivity. It is hence plausible that PPV may permanently remove autoantigens from the posterior segment and hence modulate the immune response in eyes with uveitis.

Diamond and Kaplan, in 1978 [20], described the therapeutic benefit of PPV and lensectomy in 15 eyes. It was postulated that in the creation of a unicameral state, this procedure may alter the immunologic milieu of the eye, promoting improved inflammatory control [21]. These considerations, together with the notion that the penetration of systemically administered anti-inflammatory medications may be improved in vitrectomized eyes, may allow for a reduction in the dosage requirement of these drugs in controlling uveitis.

In a meta-analysis by Becker and Davis [22] of 44 interventional case series, cumulatively including 1762 eyes in 1575 patients, visual acuity improved in 708 eyes (68%), remained unchanged in 202 eyes (20%), and worsened in 124 eyes (12%). Data was included from 39 of the 44 series. The authors postulated that PPV is possibly relevant to the outcomes of improving vision and reducing inflammation and CME. Cumulatively, intermediate uveitis was present in nearly half (841) of these eyes. A decreased need for systemic medication postoperatively was noted by 25 of 44 authors. In addition, a reduction in the severity of inflammation and the frequency of recurrences among uveitis patients with diverse etiologies following PPV was noted in several cited studies [8, 23–33] with only a few reporting either no change in disease course or increased severity [34–36]. Scott and colleagues [29] reported a statistically significant decrease in the recurrence rate of intermediate, posterior, and panuveitis in 41 eyes of 38 patients after PPV. Similarly, Trittibach and associates [8] reported a statistically significant reduction in the percentage of eyes with uveitis relapses (15 eyes before, 7 after surgery) among 29 eyes of 23 pediatric patients with chronic uveitis following PPV.

The authors reported a fair to poor evidence rating on a number of the evaluated studies, citing low patient numbers and methodological weaknesses. They implied that randomized, controlled, collaborative trials or hypothesis-based case series with precise outcome measures that incorporate control groups would improve the quality of evidence supporting PPV as an adjunct to the medical treatment of uveitis [22].

Where PPV falls in the therapeutic stepladder is a question that remains to be adequately answered. While systemic and regional steroids are often a first line of therapy in posterior, intermediate, and panuveitis, whether IMT should be instituted concomitantly or prior to performing vitrectomy surgery is subject to further study. Kaplan [37] suggests that vitrectomy should take a place upstream of IMT in the management of chronic intermediate uveitis. Authors in favor of this approach cite a lower perioperative complication rate in association with newer, smaller-gauge vitrectomy instrumentation allowing patients to avoid prolonged systemic IMT and its associated morbidity with only minimal surgical risk. Arguments against using PPV as a primary therapeutic modality include the risks of surgical complications in an inflamed eye, the elimination of the vitreous as a depot for pharmacologic agents, as well as the contention that systemic IMT will address the causative immunopathology of inflammatory disease by targeting production of autoreactive T cells in extraocular locations.

In a small prospective, randomized pilot study, Quinones and colleagues [38] compared PPV to conventional IMT among 16 patients (18 eyes) with chronic intermediate uveitis

(IU) that was active despite therapy with periocular and/or systemic corticosteroids. Both groups demonstrated an improvement in visual acuity and vitreous inflammation. Owing to the small size of the study with only 11 eyes in patients randomized to PPV, no statistically significant differences in outcome were noted; however, resolution in all inflammatory indices was achieved in 82% of eyes in the PPV group compared with 42% of eyes randomized to IMT. Furthermore, 4 of 7 eyes randomized to IMT required PPV. At 6 months, the IMT group was noted to have more improvement in visual acuity compared to the PPV group; however, this trend was reversed at the 1-year and 18-month mark. While definitive recommendations cannot be made on the basis of this study, the superior inflammatory control achieved in the PPV group, without the use of IMT, is compelling. Furthermore, in a retrospective cohort study including 849 eyes, a subgroup analysis of the systemic immunosuppressive therapy for eye diseases (SITE) research group study found that one of the factors predictive of disease remission in intermediate uveitis was prior pars plana vitrectomy [39].

Avoiding the long-term institution of IMT is particularly relevant in the pediatric population. Giuliari and colleagues [7] reported retrospective outcomes with vitrectomy in the management of 28 eyes of 20 pediatric patients presenting with active uveitis with or without medical therapy at the time of surgery. Of note, six eyes presented with associated retinal vasculitis. At the termination of the study, inflammatory control had been achieved in 97% of the patients with or without medical adjuvant therapy, including 5 of 6 eyes with persistent retinal vasculitis. Visual acuity was improved in the majority of patients. The authors concluded that PPV was a useful adjunctive therapy in patients with medically recalcitrant uveitis even in a subgroup of patients with associated retinal vasculitis. It seems possible that PPV may allow a lower dose and a shorter duration of systemic IMT to achieve this end. This study also appears to highlight the importance of delineating retinal vasculitis by angiography in eyes with uveitis when contemplating surgical intervention and the prospective necessity for IMT. One caveat of this study was that systemic IMT was not compared to PPV.

Several other retrospective reports describe PPV as a safe and effective adjunctive or primary procedure in decreasing inflammation in childhood uveitis refractory to conventional IMT. PPV has been seen to be useful in managing complications of childhood uveitis in carefully selected cases and reducing the requirement for systemic IMT postoperatively [7, 8, 26, 40, 41].

Bacskulin and Eckardt [26] reported favorable outcomes with PPV in 19 eyes of 13 children with chronic uveitis with significant visual improvement in 63% and regression of CME in 7 of 8 cases following intervention. In a similar retrospective study by Trittibach and coworkers [8] of 22 eyes with chronic childhood intermediate uveitis and 7 with retinal vasculitis, there was a statistically significant improvement in log MAR VA (0.91–0.33) and a reduction in uveitic relapses and CME after PPV. Figueroa et al. [41] reported a reduction in the need for IMT, improved visual acuity, and inflammatory control in 7 eyes of 5 children with intermediate uveitis who underwent PPV and inferior transscleral cryotherapy.

Management of CME

CME may be seen in all forms of ocular inflammatory disease but is a prominent cause of vision loss in anterior, intermediate, and posterior uveitis. Left unmanaged, macular atrophy may ensue, rendering vision loss irreversible. It has been suggested that inflammatory mediators such as chemokines and cytokines present in the vitreous of eyes with uveitis may be implicated in the potentiation of vascular permeability. Furthermore, the presence of these mediators may result in firmer adhesion of the posterior hyaloid and internal limiting membrane (ILM) as well as the formation of epiretinal membranes that would create traction on the macula resulting in medically recalcitrant and chronic CME [42–44].

Indeed, PPV with separation of the posterior hyaloid may improve macular morphology in chronic uveitic CME by removing inflammatory mediators and autologous antigens that potentiate macular vascular leakage and reduce the anterior-posterior traction that an attached hyaloid may exert on the macula. Furthermore, PPV with peeling of ERM and ILM may improve visual and anatomical outcomes in the management of medically refractory CME.

It is of course critical to correctly select patients with uveitic CME for surgical management. Chronic CME with fixed or atrophic cysts and macular outer retinal atrophy or the presence of an enlarged foveal avascular zone may be less likely to respond to PPV. It is therefore important to adequately image the posterior pole with optical coherence tomography and fluorescein angiography prior to considering a vitreoretinal surgical procedure.

Data on the true efficacy of PPV for recalcitrant CME is not robust due in large part to low sample sizes and also to the paucity of data derived from randomized, controlled studies. The only randomized study on the effect of PPV for uveitic CME without concurrent macular pathology was a pilot trial conducted by Tranos and associates [45] which comprised 23 eyes of 23 patients with quiescent IU or posterior uveitis with CME unresponsive to 3 months of medical therapy with systemic corticosteroids or steroid-sparing IMT. The patients were randomly assigned to those undergoing PPV (12 patients) and those assigned to medical therapy including a variety of agents including systemic corticosteroid and IMT. Those assigned to surgery were administered a short course of oral prednisone which was tapered back to preoperative dosing 3–6 weeks after surgery. At 6 months, a statistically significant improvement in visual acuity was noted in the surgical group ($p = 0.01$) but not in the medically treated group ($p = 0.79$), with 5 of 12 eyes achieving visual acuity of 20/40 or better. Interestingly, improvement in visual acuity was not necessarily accompanied by angiographic improvement in CME. In fact, at the end of follow-up, there was no statistically significant difference in the appearance of CME by FA in either group from baseline. It is possible that improvement in VA was mediated by enhanced media clarity following PPV. While there was no statistically significant difference in the two groups with respect to AC inflammatory activity, vitritis was significantly less following surgical intervention. The problem with this study was that vitreous haze was not necessarily graded in a standardized fashion, nor was CME determined quantitatively using OCT, which would be expected to be more highly correlated with visual acuity than angiographic CME; the latter can persist despite complete resolution of CME on OCT.

Smaller nonrandomized clinical series have demonstrated some benefit in the management of medically recalcitrant CME with PPV. On the basis of their survey of the literature, Becker and Davis [22] found that a reduction in CME was felt to be a likely benefit of PPV in 19 publications and calculated the median reported percentage of patients per study with CME decreasing from 36% preoperatively to 18% postoperatively.

In a retrospective study by Wiechens and coworkers [46], refractory CME in 68 eyes either completely or partially resolved in 59% (25/42) of those with intermediate uveitis, 57.1% (8/14) with JIA-associated iridocyclitis, and 41.7% (5/12) with multifocal choroiditis with a significant increase in VA of 2 lines or more in 50%, 71.4%, and 41% of eyes, respectively.

Gutfleisch and colleagues [47] reported outcomes in PPV, ILM peeling, and intravitreal injection of 4 mg of triamcinolone acetonide (IVT) among 19 similar patients. CME improved in 58% of patients at 6 weeks postoperatively and in 44% at 12 months. A concomitant improvement in visual acuity was noted in 42% at 3 months and in 28% after 12 months.

Management of Structural Complications and Hypotony

Macular epiretinal membranes are a frequent complication of all forms of uveitis (Fig. 12.2.) [48]. They may result in a decrease in visual acuity, macular striae, and metamorphopsia and, along with vitreomacular adhesion, are a frequent factor in medically nonresponsive CME. Vitrectomy and membrane peeling in eyes

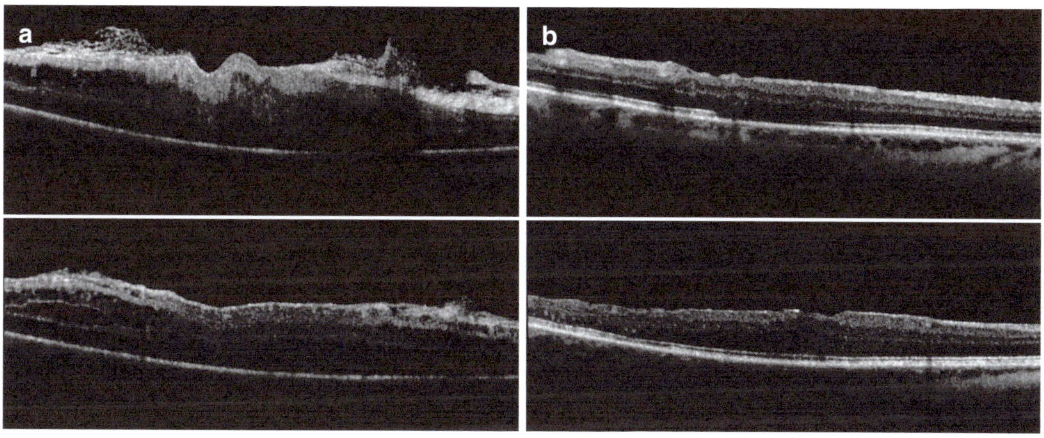

Fig. 12.2 Unilateral intermediate uveitis with significant epiretinal membrane in the right eye. (**a**) Preoperative optical coherence tomography of the superior and central macula. (**b**) Postoperative improvement of macular contour and vision improvement from 20/100 pre-op to 20/30 post-op at 3 months after pars plana vitrectomy, epiretinal membrane peel, and indocyanine green–assisted internal limiting membrane peel. A perioperative oral prednisone burst was administered

with uveitis may address CME by removal of inflammatory mediators, release of vitreomacular traction, as well as management of the epimacular membrane itself.

Gutfleisch and colleagues [47] reported outcomes in 19 patients with uveitic CME that was refractory to medical therapy undergoing PPV, ILM peeling, and intravitreal injection of 4 mg of triamcinolone acetonide. Central macular thickness and macular morphology was noted to improve in 58% of patients at 6 weeks, with further improvement in 44% at 12 months and worsening in 12%. Postoperative visual acuity improved in 42% at 3 months and in 28% after 12 months. Progression of cataract was noted in the majority of phakic patients after surgery.

In a retrospective case series with 6 months of follow-up, Tanawade et al. [49] demonstrated improvement in visual acuity in 5 of 16 eyes with CME, uveitis, and macular epiretinal membranes. Five eyes demonstrated no improvement in vision at all and visual acuity was noted to be worse than preoperative measurements in 6 out of 16 eyes. Worsening of visual acuity was attributed to worsening cataract postoperatively in two patients, persistent postoperative hypotony in one patient, and irreversible macular cicatricial pathology in the remainder. Peeling of the internal limiting membrane was performed in five of the six eyes that demonstrated improvement in acuity and in two and three of the eyes that had stable and worsened postoperative visual acuity, respectively.

Indeed, the efficacy of peeling the internal limiting membrane in addition to the ERM remains uncertain in the management of epiretinal membranes in general but also in the management of ERM in association with uveitis. Lee and associates [50] demonstrated improvement in macular thickness in both patients who underwent PPV with membrane peeling both with and without ILM peeling. However, the group of patients who did not undergo ILM peeling were noted to have a lower central macular thickness and were more likely to have an improved postoperative foveal contour. In this study, improvement in foveal contour and central macular thickness did not appear to correlate with visual acuity, and postoperative change in acuity between the two groups was not noted to be significantly different.

Conversely, a retrospective study by Park et al. [51] of 44 patients with uveitis who underwent PPV and membrane peeling, 20 of whom had the ILM removed as well, showed improvement or stability in both central macular thickness and visual acuity in 100% of patients in the ILM peeling group and only 79% of the patients in whom the ILM was not removed. The authors contend that there is a suggestion that ILM peeling may improve outcomes in uveitic ERM peeling surgery and that there are no ill effects from performing this additional peeling step.

Hypotony, although a less frequent complication than ocular hypertension, is noted in up to 10% of patients with uveitis [52]. It is more common in patients with anterior uveitis [53] and in the pediatric population [52], particularly in children with juvenile idiopathic arthritis-associated iridocyclitis. Hypotony in uveitis is associated with poor visual outcomes and typically results from chronic inflammatory loss of ciliary body function or from ciliary body detachment and disruption secondary to the formation of cyclitic membranes. Hypotony may lead to keratopathy with chronic corneal edema and scarring, maculopathy, optic neuropathy, and scleral collapse and with chronicity, loss of function, and eventual phthisis bulbi [10].

Vitrectomy with silicone oil tamponade has been suggested as a means of managing uveitis-associated hypotony in eyes with chronic hypotony that is not responsive to local or systemic immunomodulatory pharmacotherapy. De Smet and colleagues [54] reported outcomes in six patients with hypotony of duration of greater than 1 month undergoing vitrectomy surgery and dissection of ciliary body membranes. Silicone oil tamponade was performed only in eyes with atrophic ciliary processes. They showed a mean increase in intraocular pressure of 7 mmHg, and four of the six eyes demonstrated improved vision.

A similar retrospective case series of cyclitic membrane excision in four eyes of four patients with hypotony and juvenile idiopathic arthritis-associated uveitis [10] demonstrated an increase in intraocular pressure to normal in two patients at 1 month, and a gradual increase in mean intraocular pressure in all four patients such that IOP had normalized by 1 year. Silicone oil was utilized in only one eye in this study as a result of observed exudative maculopathy.

Morse and colleagues [55] reported sustained resolution of hypotony in four of five eyes that underwent vitrectomy and silicone oil tamponade without dissection of ciliary body membranes at a mean final follow-up period of 19 months. Conversely, in a series of 12 patients treated similarly, Kapur and associates [56] noted only a modest improvement in intraocular pressure with silicone oil tamponade. Seven of nine eyes followed to 1 year were able to maintain preoperative visual acuity. Dayani et al. showed that a combination of PPV, flucinolone acetonide implant, and silicone oil placement was effective in increasing mean IOP of 13 eyes from 11 patients with refractory uveitic hypotony significantly at 6 and 12 months. There were no intraoperative complications [57].

Sustained-Release Drug Delivery Implants

The first Federal Drug Administration (FDA)-approved sustained-release intravitreal drug delivery device for the management of uveitis was the ganciclovir 4.5 mg intravitreal implant Vitrasert (Bausch and Lomb, Rochester, NY) [58]. Although now, in the age of highly active antiretroviral therapy and other modern HIV management stratagems, it has been discontinued, the device proved to be efficacious in the management of cytomegalovirus retinitis in patients with HIV/AIDS.

The currently available nonbiodegradable, sustained-release intravitreal 0.59 mg fluocinolone acetonide (FA) implant Retisert (Bausch and Lomb, Rochester, NY) is approved by the Food and Drug Administration for the treatment of chronic noninfectious posterior uveitis. The Multicenter Uveitis Steroid Treatment (MUST) Trial [15] demonstrated significant reduction in uveitis recurrences, improvement in visual acuity, and prevention in uveitis-related complications sustained up to 5 years after implantation on par with conventional IMT. The FA implant appeared to have a more significant ability to control uveitis during these 5 years, and some patients who eventually were deemed refractory to IMT eventually crossed over to receive the FA implant. However, the not-yet-published 7-year data appear to favor visual outcomes in the IMT group compared to the FA implant group, given that relapses occurred in the FA implant group after 5 years.

As expected, almost all eyes after Retisert implantation require cataract surgery. Ocular hypertension was noted in 70% of Retisert-implanted eyes and 33.8% required incisional glaucoma surgery [13]. Other reported rare surgical complications include vitreous hemorrhage, hypotony, wound dehiscence, endophthalmitis, and extrusion of the implant.

Conclusions

A comprehensive review of the literature suggests a role for vitreoretinal surgical intervention in the management of uveitis and its structural complications. With careful patient selection and good preoperative medical management, vitrectomy alone may attenuate the inflammatory response in eyes by both reducing antigen load and reducing the levels of inflammatory mediators. Structural complications such as ERM, tractional retinal detachment, and cyclitic membranes leading to ciliary body failure and hypotony may also be addressed by PPV and adjunctive interventions such as membrane dissection and silicone oil tamponade with or without FA implant.

Given the paucity of randomized, controlled studies and the diversity in the uveitis syndromes, a true sense of the exact role of PPV in uveitis cannot be gleaned without further study. It is evident that critical assessment in well-designed, hypothesis-based, prospective, randomized, controlled, collaborative trials will be required to define exactly where vitreoretinal surgical intervention should be placed in the therapeutic algorithm. Whether IMT should be instituted prior to surgical intervention or if surgical intervention can in some cases supplant IMT is yet to be seen. Moreover, it will be important to determine if PPV can allow for a reduction in IMT dosing and duration in the management of uveitis and CME and, if so, in what particular anatomical categories. Until such questions can be answered, vitreoretinal surgical interventions should remain an adjunctive option in situations where conventional therapy with regional or systemic corticosteroids and IMT fail or are insufficient in the management of uveitis.

References

1. Nicholson BP, Zhou M, Rostamizadeh M, Mehta P, Agron E, Wong W, et al. Epidemiology of epiretinal membrane in a large cohort of patients with uveitis. Ophthalmology. 2014;121(12):2393–8.
2. Antcliff RJ, Stanford MR, Chauhan DS, Graham EM, Spalton DJ, Shilling JS, et al. Comparison between optical coherence tomography and fundus fluorescein angiography for the detection of cystoid macular edema in patients with uveitis. Ophthalmology. 2000;107(3):593–9.
3. Iannetti L, Accorinti M, Liverani M, Caggiano C, Abdulaziz R, Pivetti-Pezzi P. Optical coherence tomography for classification and clinical evaluation of macular edema in patients with uveitis. Ocul Immunol Inflamm. 2008;16(4):155–60.
4. Jittpoonkuson T, Garcia PM, Rosen RB. Correlation between fluorescein angiography and spectral-domain optical coherence tomography in the diagnosis of cystoid macular edema. Br J Ophthalmol. 2010;94(9):1197–200.
5. Hong BK, Nazari Khanamiri H, Rao NA. Role of ultra-widefield fluorescein angiography in the management of uveitis. Can J Ophthalmol. 2013;48(6):489–93.
6. Karampelas M, Sim DA, Chu C, Carreno E, Keane PA, Zarranz-Ventura J, et al. Quantitative analysis of peripheral vasculitis, ischemia, and vascular leakage in uveitis using ultra-widefield fluorescein angiography. Am J Ophthalmol. 2015;159(6):1161–8.e1.
7. Giuliari GP, Chang PY, Thakuria P, Hinkle DM, Foster CS. Pars plana vitrectomy in the management of paediatric uveitis: the Massachusetts Eye Research and Surgery Institution experience. Eye (Lond). 2010;24(1):7–13.
8. Trittibach P, Koerner F, Sarra GM, Garweg JG. Vitrectomy for juvenile uveitis: prognostic factors for the long-term functional outcome. Eye (Lond). 2006;20(2):184–90.
9. Roters S, Szurman P, Engels BF, Bartz-Schmidt KU, Krieglstein GK. Ultrasound biomicroscopy in chronic ocular hypotony: its impact on diagnosis and management. Retina. 2002;22(5):581–8.
10. Yu EN, Paredes I, Foster CS. Surgery for hypotony in patients with juvenile idiopathic arthritis-associated uveitis. Ocul Immunol Inflamm. 2007;15(1):11–7.
11. Sonoda KH, Enaida H, Ueno A, Nakamura T, Kawano YI, Kubota T, et al. Pars plana vitrectomy assisted by triamcinolone acetonide for refractory uveitis: a case series study. Br J Ophthalmol. 2003;87(8):1010–4.
12. Radetzky S, Walter P, Fauser S, Koizumi K, Kirchhof B, Joussen AM. Visual outcome of patients with macular edema after pars plana vitrectomy and indocyanine green-assisted peeling of the internal limiting membrane. Graefes Arch Clin Exp Ophthalmol. 2004;242(4):273–8.

13. Callanan DG, Jaffe GJ, Martin DF, Pearson PA, Comstock TL. Treatment of posterior uveitis with a fluocinolone acetonide implant: three-year clinical trial results. Arch Ophthalmol. 2008;126(9):1191–201.
14. Lowder C, Belfort R Jr, Lightman S, Foster CS, Robinson MR, Schiffman RM, et al. Dexamethasone intravitreal implant for noninfectious intermediate or posterior uveitis. Arch Ophthalmol. 2011;129(5):545–53.
15. Campochiaro PA, Brown DM, Pearson A, Chen S, Boyer D, Ruiz-Moreno J, et al. Sustained delivery fluocinolone acetonide vitreous inserts provide benefit for at least 3 years in patients with diabetic macular edema. Ophthalmology. 2012;119(10):2125–32.
16. van Kooij B, Rothova A, Rijkers GT, de Groot-Mijnes JD. Distinct cytokine and chemokine profiles in the aqueous of patients with uveitis and cystoid macular edema. Am J Ophthalmol. 2006;142(1):192–4.
17. Stuart JM, Cremer MA, Dixit SN, Kang AH, Townes AS. Collagen-induced arthritis in rats. Comparison of vitreous and cartilage-derived collagens. Arthritis Rheum. 1979;22(4):347–52.
18. Opremcak EMSD, Cowans AB. Cell mediated autoimmune mechanisms in uveitis. Assoc Res Vis Ophthalmol. 1993;34(4):1104.
19. Quentin CD, Reiber H. Fuchs heterochromic cyclitis: rubella virus antibodies and genome in aqueous humor. Am J Ophthalmol. 2004;138(1):46–54.
20. Diamond JG, Kaplan HJ. Lensectomy and vitrectomy for complicated cataract secondary to uveitis. Arch Ophthalmol. 1978;96(10):1798–804.
21. Streilein JW. Anterior chamber associated immune deviation: the privilege of immunity in the eye. Surv Ophthalmol. 1990;35(1):67–73.
22. Becker M, Davis J. Vitrectomy in the treatment of uveitis. Am J Ophthalmol. 2005;140(6):1096–105.
23. Freyler H, Velikay M. Vitrectomy in uveitis. Klin Monbl Augenheilkd. 1984;185(4):263–7.
24. Leuenberger PM. Importance of vitrectomy in the treatment of posterior uveitis. Klin Monbl Augenheilkd. 1984;184(5):445–8.
25. Eckardt C, Bacskulin A. Vitrectomy in intermediate uveitis. Dev Ophthalmol. 1992;23:232–8.
26. Bacskulin A, Eckardt C. Results of pars plana vitrectomy in chronic uveitis in childhood. Ophthalmologe. 1993;90(5):434–9.
27. Heiligenhaus A, Bornfeld N, Foerster MH, Wessing A. Long-term results of pars plana vitrectomy in the management of complicated uveitis. Br J Ophthalmol. 1994;78(7):549–54.
28. Verbraeken H. Therapeutic pars plana vitrectomy for chronic uveitis: a retrospective study of the long-term results. Graefes Arch Clin Exp Ophthalmol. 1996;234(5):288–93.
29. Scott RA, Haynes RJ, Orr GM, Cooling RJ, Pavesio CE, Charteris DG. Vitreous surgery in the management of chronic endogenous posterior uveitis. Eye (Lond). 2003;17(2):221–7.
30. Sikic J, Suic SP. Surgical treatment of uveitis. Coll Antropol. 2001;25 Suppl:71–6.
31. Soylu M, Demircan N, Pelit A. Pars plana vitrectomy in ocular Behcet's disease. Int Ophthalmol. 2001;24(4):219–23.
32. Stavrou P, Baltatzis S, Letko E, Samson CM, Christen W, Foster CS. Pars plana vitrectomy in patients with intermediate uveitis. Ocul Immunol Inflamm. 2001;9(3):141–51.
33. Ieki Y, Kiryu J, Kita M, Tanabe T, Tsujikawa A, Yamashiro K, et al. Pars plana vitrectomy for vitreous opacity associated with ocular sarcoidosis resistant to medical treatment. Ocul Immunol Inflamm. 2004;12(1):35–43.
34. Bovey EH, Gonvers M, Herbort CP. Pars plana vitrectomy in uveitis. Klin Monbl Augenheilkd. 1992;200(5):464–7.
35. Nolle B, Eckardt C. Vitrectomy in multifocal chorioretinitis. Ger J Ophthalmol. 1993;2(1):14–9.
36. Ozdemir O, Erkam N, Bakkaloglu A. Results of pars plana vitrectomy in Behcet's disease. Ann Ophthalmol. 1988;20(1):35, 38.
37. Kaplan HJ. Surgical treatment of intermediate uveitis. Dev Ophthalmol. 1992;23:185–9.
38. Quinones K, Choi JY, Yilmaz T, Kafkala C, Letko E, Foster CS. Pars plana vitrectomy versus immunomodulatory therapy for intermediate uveitis: a prospective, randomized pilot study. Ocul Immunol Inflamm. 2010;18(5):411–7.
39. Kempen JH, Gewaily DY, Newcomb CW, Liesegang TL, Kacmaz RO, Levy-Clarke GA, et al. Remission of intermediate uveitis: incidence and predictive factors. Am J Ophthalmol [Multicenter Study Research Support, N.I.H., Extramural Research Support, Non--U.S. Gov't]. 2016;164:110–7.e2.
40. Ulbig M, Kampik A. Pars plana vitrectomy in chronic uveitis in the child. Klin Monbl Augenheilkd. 1989;194(1):10–2.
41. Figueroa MS, Noval S, Contreras I, Arruabarrena C, Garcia-Perez JL, Sales M, et al. Pars plana vitrectomy as anti-inflammatory therapy for intermediate uveitis in children. Arch Soc Esp Oftalmol. 2010;85(12):390–4.
42. Schaal S, Tezel TH, Kaplan HJ. Surgical intervention in refractory CME – role of posterior hyaloid separation and internal limiting membrane peeling. Ocul Immunol Inflamm. 2008;16(5):209–10.
43. Ossewaarde-van Norel A, Rothova A. Clinical review: update on treatment of inflammatory macular edema. Ocul Immunol Inflamm. 2011;19(1):75–83.
44. Markomichelakis NN, Halkiadakis I, Pantelia E, Georgalas I, Chrysanthi K, Theodossiadis P, et al. Course of macular edema in uveitis under medical treatment. Ocul Immunol Inflamm. 2007;15(2):71–9.
45. Tranos P, Scott R, Zambarakji H, Ayliffe W, Pavesio C, Charteris DG. The effect of pars plana vitrectomy on cystoid macular oedema associated with chronic uveitis: a randomised, controlled pilot study. Br J Ophthalmol. 2006;90(9):1107–10.
46. Wiechens B, Reichelt JA, Urbat C, Nolle B. Pars plana vitrectomy in cystoid macular edema of

different forms of chronic uveitis. Ophthalmologe. 2003;100(1):33–43.
47. Gutfleisch M, Spital G, Mingels A, Pauleikhoff D, Lommatzsch A, Heiligenhaus A. Pars plana vitrectomy with intravitreal triamcinolone: effect on uveitic cystoid macular oedema and treatment limitations. Br J Ophthalmol. 2007;91(3):345–8.
48. Kempen JH, Altaweel MM, Holbrook JT, Jabs DA, Sugar EA. The multicenter uveitis steroid treatment trial: rationale, design, and baseline characteristics. Am J Ophthalmol. 2010;149(4):550–61.e10.
49. Tanawade RG, Tsierkezou L, Bindra MS, Patton NA, Jones NP. Visual outcomes of pars plana vitrectomy with epiretinal membrane peel in patients with uveitis. Retina. 2015;35(4):736–41.
50. Lee JW, Kim IT. Outcomes of idiopathic macular epiretinal membrane removal with and without internal limiting membrane peeling: a comparative study. Jpn J Ophthalmol. 2010;54(2):129–34.
51. Park DW, Dugel PU, Garda J, Sipperley JO, Thach A, Sneed SR, et al. Macular pucker removal with and without internal limiting membrane peeling: pilot study. Ophthalmology. 2003;110(1):62–4.
52. Sen HN, Drye LT, Goldstein DA, Larson TA, Merrill PT, Pavan PR, et al. Hypotony in patients with uveitis: The Multicenter Uveitis Steroid Treatment (MUST) Trial. Ocul Immunol Inflamm. 2012;20(2):104–12.
53. Aman R, Engelhard SB, Bajwa A, Patrie J, Reddy AK. Ocular hypertension and hypotony as determinates of outcomes in uveitis. Clin Ophthalmol. 2015;9:2291–8.
54. de Smet MD, Gunning F, Feenstra R. The surgical management of chronic hypotony due to uveitis. Eye (Lond). 2005;19(1):60–4.
55. Morse LS, BW MC 2nd. The use of silicone oil in uveitis and hypotony. Retina. 1991;11(4):399–404.
56. Kapur R, Birnbaum AD, Goldstein DA, Tessler HH, Shapiro MJ, Ulanski LJ, et al. Treating uveitis-associated hypotony with pars plana vitrectomy and silicone oil injection. Retina. 2010;30(1):140–5.
57. Dayani PN, Chow J, Stinnett SS, Jaffe GJ. Pars plana vitrectomy, fluocinolone acetonide implantation, and silicone oil infusion for the treatment of chronic, refractory uveitic hypotony. Am J Ophthalmol. 2011;152(5):849–56.e1.
58. Dhillon B, Kamal A, Leen C. Intravitreal sustained-release ganciclovir implantation to control cytomegalovirus retinitis in AIDS. Int J STD AIDS. 1998;9(4):227–30.

Local Drug Delivery for Noninfectious Uveitis

13

Xia Ni Wu and Lyndell Lim

Pearls

- Subconjunctival corticosteroids can provide respite from a frequent drop regimen and be combined with a mydriatic to minimize posterior synechiae formation
- There are now over two decades of experience demonstrating the safety and efficacy of subconjunctival triamcinolone in the treatment of nonnecrotizing noninfectious anterior scleritis
- The surgically implanted fluocinolone implant initially resulted in faster improvement of CME, with two to three times better inflammation control than systemic immunosuppressive therapy; however this initial benefit was lost by 5 years, with better visual outcomes in the systemic group seen at 7 years
- The principle behind utilizing anti-VEGF treatment for uveitic CME or inflammatory retinal or choroidal neovascularization is that control of inflammation with systemic immunosuppression or other means is concomitantly required and cannot be replaced by using anti-VEGF alone

Introduction

Target-specific drug delivery is the holy grail of modern medicine as it theoretically enables the use of smaller doses while minimizing the risk of systemic adverse events. Ocular inflammation lends itself to local therapies as both anterior and posterior segments of the eye are easily accessible and complications remain localized. Systemic treatment can then be reserved for chronic, more extensive inflammation, or inflammation associated with an underlying systemic disease. Topical therapy will be covered elsewhere in Chap. 2.

Local ocular injections are an integral part of the ophthalmologist's armamentarium and includes subconjunctival, periocular, and intravitreal routes. Periocular injections encompass sub-Tenon, peribulbar, orbital floor, and retrobulbar injections. Intraocular injections have the added advantage of allowing medications to directly bypass the blood-ocular barriers. Microinjections into the suprachoroidal space are currently being investigated [1, 2]. Corticosteroids remain the cornerstone of local treatment for uveitis although drugs such as methotrexate have shown encouraging results. A summary of the common

X. N. Wu
Lions Eye Institute, Nedlands, WA, Australia

L. Lim (✉)
Royal Victorian Eye and Ear Hospital, Centre for Eye Research Australia, University of Melbourne, East Melbourne, VIC, Australia
e-mail: limllp@unimelb.edu.au

P. Lin, E. Suhler (eds.), *Treatment of Non-infectious Uveitis*,
https://doi.org/10.1007/978-3-030-22827-9_13

Table 13.1 Local drug delivery routes

	Subconjunctival	Periocular	Intravitreal	Implantable
Common	Dexamethasone acetate Triamcinolone acetonide/ diacetate	Triamcinolone acetonide Triamcinolone diacetate	Triamcinolone acetonide Methotrexate Sirolimus	Ozurdex® (0.7 mg dexamethasone) Iluvien® (0.19 mg fluocinolone acetonide) Yutiq™ (0.18 mg fluocinolone) Retisert® (0.59 mg fluocinolone acetonide)
Less common	–	Dexamethasone Betamethasone Methylprednisolone	TNF-α inhibitor Anti-VEGF	–

TNF tumor necrosis factor, *VEGF* vascular endothelial growth factor

Table 13.2 Local corticosteroids

Drug	Periocular dosage	Intravitreal dosage	Relative potency	Half-life (hours)	Duration of action (days)
Hydrocortisone	–	–	1.0	8–12	1
Methylprednisolone sodium succinate	–	–	5.0	8–12	1–2
Triamcinolone acetonide/ diacetate	2–8 mg[a] 20–40 mg[b]	2–4 mg	5.0	18–36	60–120
Methylprednisolone acetate	–	–	5.0	18–36	60–120
Dexamethasone acetate/sodium phosphate	2–4 mg[a,b]	0.4 mg 0.7 mg[c]	25	36–54	7–10
Betamethasone acetate/ phosphate	–	–	25	36–54	7–10
Fluocinolone acetonide	–	0.59 mg[c] (0.5 mcg/day) 0.19 mg[c] (0.25 mcg/day)	–	–	–

[a]Subconjunctival
[b]Sub-Tenon/orbital floor
[c]Intravitreal implant

medications used for each of these local delivery routes is presented in Table 13.1.

Injection Methods

Injection methods for each of the various routes of local drug delivery can vary greatly. A detailed methodology, based upon the standard recommendations of the American Academy of Ophthalmology, is included in Appendix 13.1.

Local Corticosteroids

Corticosteroids are widely used in medicine and have well-documented systemic and local side effects. Commonly used corticosteroid preparations for regional injections include dexamethasone acetate/phosphate, triamcinolone acetonide/diacetate, and methylprednisolone (Table 13.2). Intraocular steroids have been used since 1974.

Subconjunctival Corticosteroids

Subconjunctival corticosteroid injections are largely limited to severe anterior uveitis and non-necrotizing noninfectious scleritis, with their use in the latter being relatively recent.

Anterior Uveitis

Short-acting corticosteroids such as dexamethasone are commonly used for anterior uveitis refractory to topical treatment [3, 4]. Subconjunctival corticosteroids can provide respite from a frequent drop regimen and can be combined with a mydriatic to minimize posterior synechiae formation. Despite this, there are few studies looking at this indication. Other short-acting corticosteroids such as methylprednisolone, betamethasone, and hydrocortisone are used less frequently. Subconjunctival dexamethasone sodium phosphate 0.4% has been demonstrated to achieve a peak concentration in the aqueous that is comparable to, or higher than, that attained by topical prednisolone acetate 1.0% [5, 6]. High concentrations are maintained for 24 hours [5]. Subconjunctival injection attained 6 times higher concentration in the vitreous compared to peribulbar delivery, and even more against topical drops [7, 8]. Time to peak intraocular concentration was 2.5–3 hours [7].

Subconjunctival injections of longer-acting corticosteroids act as depots with the additional advantage of prolonged action and easy access for removal if required. It has been used for moderate-to-severe chronic or recurrent anterior uveitis and, more recently, in nonnecrotizing anterior scleritis [3]. Triamcinolone, available in acetonide or diacetate forms, has a duration of action that lasts 6 weeks or more when injected locally [9]. Active drug depots can be present for up to 13 months after injection [10]. The most widely used preparation is Kenalog® (triamcinolone acetonide; Bristol-Meyers Squibb, New York, NY, USA).

Anterior Scleritis

Subconjunctival triamcinolone was traditionally avoided in scleritis management due to case reports of scleral necrosis and perforation dating back to the 1960s [11]. More recent case series demonstrated efficacy and safety in nonnecrotizing noninfectious anterior scleritis [12–17]. There is now over two decades of experience across multiple centers involving over 136 patients, with follow-up ranging up to 20 years and some patients receiving multiple injections [13].

Pharmacodynamics and Pharmacokinetics

Although the pharmacokinetics are not well understood, it is believed that subconjunctival corticosteroids enter the eye via some component of either transscleral, transcorneal, or hematogenous absorption [7, 18]. Studies suggest that aqueous and vitreous concentrations of dexamethasone were significantly higher with subconjunctival injections as compared to peribulbar injections, and higher still compared to oral corticosteroids [7]. Ocular levels far exceeded serum levels of 32.4 ng/mL although systemic absorption was noted to be considerable after both routes of injection. Physiological serum corticosteroid concentrations vary between 50 and 250 ng/mL during the day [8]. There is a paucity of pharmacokinetic studies on subconjunctival triamcinolone. Triamcinolone is minimally soluble and nonocular studies suggest that similar steroids are absorbed slower, thus maintaining drug levels for longer and impacting less on systemic levels [9].

Complications

The side effects of subconjunctival corticosteroids are primarily local with elevated intraocular pressure (IOP) being the most common. About one-third of patients treated with subconjunctival triamcinolone develop ocular hypertension, of which approximately 10% will require topical therapy and 10% will require surgical intervention [16, 17]. Onset of increased IOP varies from 1 week to 10 months [9, 10]. Removal of the triamcinolone deposit may be sufficient to revert the ocular hypertension [10, 19, 20]. Subconjunctival methylprednisolone acetate did not appear to increase IOP when given in lieu of topical drops after cataract surgery [21]. Scleral thinning or perforation is largely a theoretical risk with no reports in the past 40 years. Conjunctival necrosis was reported in 7 cases, 3 of whom received subconjunctival triamcinolone for anterior uveitis [22]. The remaining 4 cases received methylprednisolone and betamethasone for other conditions. Other adverse effects such as cataract progression and delayed wound healing have yet to be reported [9].

Periocular Corticosteroid (Posterior Sub-Tenon, Orbital Floor, Peribulbar)

Periocular injections, intravitreal injections, and surgical implants are considered for sight-threatening intermediate or posterior uveitis and in inflammatory cystoid macular edema (CME). Periocular injections have also been used for scleritis [23, 24]. Most of the published literature on the use of sub-Tenon or orbital floor injections have been with triamcinolone.

In the SITE (Systemic Immunosuppressive Therapy for Eye Diseases) Cohort Study, 73% of patients had complete resolution of inflammation within 6 months after the first periocular injection [25]. Visual acuity (VA) improved by ≥10 letters in 50% of the patients and CME improved in a third. Half of the eyes required multiple injections. Direct comparison is difficult across studies, however similar results have been reported from smaller studies [26–29]. Response rates range between 41–48% for inflammation control [28], 41–47% for improvement in CME [27, 29], and 33–57% halving their visual angle or gaining 2–3 lines of vision [26–28]. The POINT (PeriOcular vs. INTravitreal corticosteroids) trial reported an average 4.4 letter improvement at 8 weeks [29]. Recurrence occurs in 53–73% of patients in 4.6–7.6 months after injection [27, 28].

Pharmacodynamics and Pharmacokinetics

There are few prospective randomized-controlled trials (RCT) comparing the different formulations and routes of delivery. Sub-Tenon and orbital floor injections appear to have comparable effectiveness in two published RCTs, one of which compared triamcinolone to methylprednisolone [26, 30]. Triamcinolone was found to be more potent than methylprednisolone in nonhuman models, however results from human studies are conflicting [26]. Onset of effect is days to weeks and functional improvement is within weeks to months [26, 31, 32]. Duration of effect is approximately 2 months but can be up to 6 months [33, 34].

Periocular dexamethasone injections resulted in subretinal concentrations higher than serum levels, but lower than that with subconjunctival injections [35]. Triamcinolone was present at therapeutic levels in the vitreous and retinal pigment epithelium/choroid complex for at least 30 days after a single sub-Tenon injection in a rabbit model [36]. Low levels were also detected in the untreated fellow eye and in the serum. Systemic absorption is significant, with peribulbar injection of dexamethasone disodium phosphate 5 mg equivalent to a 50 mg oral dose of prednisolone [37].

Complications

Elevated IOP and cataract are commonly accepted complications of periocular corticosteroid injections [25]. A large multicenter retrospective cohort study found ocular hypertension rates of 34%, of whom approximately 7% required surgical intervention [25]. Smaller studies have reported rates between 8–35% [27, 29, 38–41]. Jea et al. noted that 44% of patients had a statistically significant rise of 5 mmHg compared to baseline IOP, with an average time to peak IOP ranging from 6–14 weeks [38, 42]. Ocular hypertension is more common with multiple injections but may be reversible if the corticosteroid depot is removed, even after a prolonged period [19, 43]. Cataract progression rates vary between 0.02/eye-year and 0.58/eye-year [27, 28, 40, 41].

Intravitreal Corticosteroid

Intravitreal injection of corticosteroid was originally reported in 1974 but has only recently gained significant traction, most notably for macular edema arising from vascular diseases [44]. Its application in ocular inflammation was limited initially to dexamethasone as an adjunct in endophthalmitis management, although depot formulations are now an established treatment for uveitic CME and inflammation of the posterior segment.

The use of intravitreal triamcinolone (IVTA) in uveitis is supported by two prospective RCTs and a small number of retrospective studies [29, 45–49]. Shin et al. noted faster improvement of CME after IVTA was used as an adjunct to systemic immunosuppression [45, 49]. Visual outcome however did not differ between the IVTA and sham injection groups, and did not improve significantly compared to baseline, possibly due to a ceiling effect. In contrast, POINT demonstrated a gain of 9.7 letters by 8 weeks [29]. There was an average of 39% reduction in central subfoveal thickness (CST) by 8 weeks and resolution of CME in 47% [29]. Previous smaller reports found 50–100% improvement of CME after 1 or more injections [45–48]. VA also improved in up to 75% of patients, although one-third reverted to baseline by 6–9 months [47, 48]. Visual function often did not correlate with anatomical improvement. This may reflect the chronicity of CME prior to treatment causing permanent structural damage and limiting visual recovery [48]. Patients with a shorter duration of CME, younger age, and better vision tended to do better [50]. Most studies show only a transient improvement of CME and VA with a single IVTA injection, highlighting the need for repeated injections or the addition of systemic treatment to limit disease activity and recurrences of secondary CME in chronic disease [29, 48, 49]. POINT demonstrated similar CME and VA outcomes for IVTA and the intravitreal dexamethasone implant Ozurdex®, and both were superior to periocular corticosteroids [29].

IVTA has also been found to reduce the need for systemic medication, with 54–88% of patients able to decrease or cease oral corticosteroids and/or second-line immunosuppressives [49, 50]. It can also be used to stabilize acute inflammation and, in some cases, allow institution of systemic therapy to decrease further recurrences [51, 52]. This is particularly useful in patients with unilateral active disease and those who are intolerant of high-dose oral prednisolone.

Pharmacodynamics and Pharmacokinetics

Triamcinolone 4 mg is almost used exclusively, having superseded dexamethasone due to the short therapeutic duration of the latter in the eye [53, 54]. Unsurprisingly, intravitreal injections achieve greater than sixfold concentration of corticosteroid in the vitreous than sub-Tenon injection [55]. Triamcinolone is confined to the eye and serum levels have been shown to be insignificant [56]. The mean half-life is 18.6 days in nonvitrectomized eyes and 3.2 days in vitrectomized [57]. Duration of effect is 3–4 months [57–61], however this is significantly less in vitrectomized eyes [57, 62].

Triamcinolone acetonide is commercially available as Kenalog-40® (Bristol-Meyers-Squibb, New York, NY, USA) which is preserved with benzyl alcohol, and Triesence® (Alcon Labs, Fort Worth, TX, USA) which is nonpreserved. Trivaris™ (Allergan Inc., Irvine, CA, USA) is another nonpreserved triamcinolone formulation that has recently entered the market. Triesence® and Trivaris™ are approved by the USA Food and Drug Administration (FDA) for intraocular use, while intraocular injections of Kenalog® are used off-label. Recent studies have shown that Triesence® has smaller particle sizes compared to Kenalog®, resulting in a greater number of particles for the same dosage [63, 64]; the impact this may have on the pharmacodynamics, pharmacodynamics, and potential complications are yet to be fully elucidated [63]. Animal models suggest that Triesence® has a longer therapeutic duration, however comparative human trials are yet to be performed [63, 65].

Complications

A recent meta-analysis reported an incidence of 32% of ocular hypertension associated with IVTA 4 mg injections [66]. Risk factors included preexisting glaucoma, higher baseline IOP, younger age, elevated IOP after a previous injection, uveitis, and higher dosage. Most required only topical treatment although cases requiring surgical intervention have been described [47, 67]. Rates of cataract progressing to surgery are up to 54% over 2 years [68, 69]. True incidence can be difficult to ascertain as the same complications can result from the primary ocular inflammation and the treatment thereof. Complications inherent to intravitreal injections include vitreous hemorrhage, lens penetration, retinal tears/detachment, and bacterial endophthalmitis. Reported rates have to be interpreted cautiously due to inconsistencies in definition and the retrospective nature of the case series reported.

Sterile endophthalmitis, a severe inflammatory response that typically develops 1 day after an intravitreal injection of triamcinolone, is an uncommon complication with rates of up to 9.3% with Kenalog® [70]. It is usually painless and can result in significantly decreased vision. There is good visual prognosis and resolution without further treatment [71]. The pathogenesis remains unclear and several hypotheses have been postulated. Potential inflammatory stimuli include endotoxins and apoptotic cells from "frustrated phagocytosis" of triamcinolone particles [64, 70, 72–74]. Triamcinolone particle size or the size of its aggregates have also been suggested to play a role [64]. The evidence base is currently small and conflicting.

Controversy: Kenalog® vs Triesence®

Triesence® was formulated on the back of concerns about benzyl alcohol being the cause of sterile endophthalmitis. This is not substantiated in the literature as the complication has occurred with both Triesence® and Kenalog® [64]. Our understanding of whether one formulation is more efficacious or safer than the other is limited by the lack of head-to-head clinical trials. The current standard of care relies on the clinician's experience and discretion until a gold standard can be established.

Implantable Corticosteroids

Sustained-release intravitreal corticosteroid implants have been recently developed to provide longer-term delivery to the posterior segment. Four devices are currently available: Retisert® (Bausch and Lomb, Rochester, NY, USA), Ozurdex® (Allergan, Inc., Irvine, California, USA), Iluvien® (Alimera Sciences, Alpharetta, GA, USA), and Yutiq™ (EyePoint Pharmaceuticals, Watertown, MA, USA).

Contraindications for the use of corticosteroid implants include patients with ocular infections and advanced glaucoma, unless a glaucoma drainage device has already been placed or can be simultaneously placed. The free-form pellets (Ozurdex®, Illuvien®) are also contraindicated in patients with aphakia or a posterior capsule breach due to the risk of implant migration into the anterior chamber [75]. There are currently no prospective studies that compare the safety of the three synthetic corticosteroid implants.

Retisert®

Retisert® was the first implantable corticosteroid to be developed. It is a nonbiodegradable implant containing 0.59 mg of fluocinolone in a polyvinyl acetate/silicone laminate. There are two components: the suture strut and the drug reservoir, measuring 2 mm wide, 1.5 mm thick, and 5 mm long. Retisert® is implanted surgically via a pars plana sclerotomy and secured by a scleral suture.

There are three prospective RCTs evaluating the efficacy of the fluocinolone implant [76–78]. The MUST (Multicenter Uveitis Steroid Treatment) trial reported comparable VA and CME outcomes between Retisert® and systemic immunosuppressive therapy through to 54 months [79]. The surgically implanted fluocinolone implant initially resulted in faster improvement of CME, with two to three times better inflammation control than systemic therapy [78, 79]. Reversal of this trend was noted thereafter with increased uveitis activity and CME, and loss of the initial VA gains in the implant group by 24 months, through to year 6 [80]. At the 7 year follow-up, systemic therapy was associated with a significant difference of 7.1 letters over the fluocinolone implant (+1.2 and −6.0 letters from baseline respectively) [80]. Both groups demonstrated approximately 20% decrease in macular thickness and resolution of inflammation in over 50%, although trends favored systemic therapy. It is thought that the uveitis relapses after the implants have been expended may have greater long-term sequelae than the relapses with systemic therapy, where there is usually a more graduated reduction in treatment. Previous studies have also reported three times fewer uveitis recurrences over the lifetime of the implant [76, 77]. The implant may reduce the need for adjunctive systemic or periocular treatments by up to 80% [76]. Given the practical constraints in reimplantation before future uveitis relapses, caution should be exercised if long-term monotherapy with local intraocular corticosteroid is being considered.

Pharmacodynamics and Pharmacokinetics

The Retisert® 0.59 mg implant was designed to release fluocinolone at an initial rate of 0.5 mcg/day and steady-state rate of 0.3–0.4 mcg/day over 1000 days. It has high potency and low solubility [81]. Aqueous levels of fluocinolone were 6.76 ng/mL at 1 month post-implantation and remained at a steady state of >6 ng/mL for over 12 months [82]. Longer follow-up was not available due to the limited study population. Animal models show concentrations of 11–18 ng/g in the vitreous and 42–87 ng/g in the retina, with minimal systemic absorption [83]. Clinical studies suggest a duration of effect of approximately 30 months, although MUST reported only a 10% replacement rate over 54 months [79].

Complications

As one would expect with all forms of long-acting intraocular steroid, there is a high rate of cataract and elevated IOP with Retisert®. Most studies report an 80–90% rate of cataract surgery within the first 24 months [76, 77, 84]. Three-quarters of patients required topical IOP-lowering drops and up to 45% required filtering surgery [80].

Complications specific to the implant itself include dissociation of the drug reservoir from the suture strut which usually requires surgical explantation [85]. Reported incidence is 5% over 6 years, with the earliest dissociation noted at 4.8 years [86]. Unfortunately, 40% of these patients had an associated decrease in VA. The implant model has since been redesigned and is under careful surveillance. Other complications include vitreous hemorrhage in up to 20%, with a third of patients having recurrent hemorrhages [78, 79]. The rate of hypotony was similarly high at 20%. Retinal detachment and endophthalmitis are rare, as were implant extrusions [77, 79]. Two cases of scleral thinning or melt have also been reported [77, 87]. Ocular discomfort, conjunctival hyperemia, and conjunctival hemorrhage were relatively common at 30–50%.

Ozurdex®

Ozurdex® is a biodegradable solid implant of dexamethasone 0.7 mg in a polylactic acid–glycolic acid matrix. It measures 0.46 mm in diameter and 6 mm in length and can be delivered via a preloaded 22 g injector through the pars plana, similar to an intravitreal injection. The implant contains no preservatives and metabolizes to form carbon dioxide and water.

The HURON (CHronic Uveitis evaluation of the intRavitreal dexamethasONe implant) trial was a phase II/III multicenter RCT of 229 eyes demonstrating the efficacy and safety of dexamethasone 0.7 and 0.35 mg implants in noninfectious intermediate or posterior uveitis [88]. There was a nonstatistically significant trend favoring the higher dosage implant and a similar safety profile between the two. Almost 50% had improved intraocular inflammation, and CST decreased by a mean of 99 μm at week 8. Rescue medication was required in 22–25% of treated patients compared to 38% in the sham group. POINT corroborated these findings, showing ≥20% improvement in CME in 84% and resolution in 61% by 8 weeks, and 9.5 letter gain [29]. The effects were attenuated at week 12 across all outcomes (67%, 37%, 7.2 letter gain, respectively). Similarly, the phase IV TAHOE (SusTained-release dexAmetHasone intravitreal implant fOr uveitic macular Edema) trial reported a mean 150 μm decrease in CST and 14.4 letter gain by 12 weeks, with 90% demonstrating complete resolution of CME at month 1 and 70% at month 3 [89]. Patients required an average of 2 injections over 12 months, and mean time to recurrence was 6.3 months [89]. Similar results have been reported in several longer-term retrospective studies with up to 50% showing an improvement in VA, inflammation, and CME within 2–6 months. Multiple injections over time were required in over 60% of patients, with the same or better clinical response seen with each repeated injection [75, 89–91]. POINT recently demonstrated the noninferiority of Ozurdex® to IVTA [29].

Pharmacodynamics and Pharmacokinetics

Ozurdex® has a biphasic drug release pattern whereby peak doses are released for 2 months followed by a lower maintenance dose for up to 6 months [92]. In a primate model, vitreous concentrations peaked at 213 ng/mL, significantly higher than serum levels of 1.11 ng/mL. No difference has been noted between vitrectomized and nonvitrectomized eyes [93]. Duration of effect in human eyes is approximately 4–6 months in uveitic CME, however this may be shorter in practice [75, 90].

Complications

Fragmentation of the Ozurdex® implant after injection has been described but is not thought to be clinically significant [94–96]. This has been supported by animal studies that found similar dissolution rates and intraocular levels between intact and fragmented implants [97].

The most frequent adverse effect is ocular hypertension. Contrary to initial reports of a lower risk of raised IOP [88], no difference was demonstrated between Ozurdex® and IVTA in the only prospective head-to-head trial to date [29]. Compared to periocular triamcinolone, Ozurdex® was 2.5 times more likely to cause ocular hypertension. POINT reported an absolute rise of ≥10 mmHg in 39% of cases and 34% required topical treatment [29]. Forty-one percent had IOP ≥ 24 mmHg, of whom 10% were ≥ 30 mmHg. No cases required surgical intervention. Time to peak IOP is 60 days with a return to baseline by 6 months and is reproducible and noncumulative with repeat injections [98, 99]. Cataract incidence is <10–15% although surgical rates are lower. Serious complications are infrequent with rates of <2% for vitreous hemorrhage, retinal detachment, hypotony, and implant dislocation [75, 88, 90, 99]. Endophthalmitis is rare [90]. Subconjunctival hemorrhage and ocular discomfort are common but benign [88, 100].

Iluvien® or Yutiq™

Iluvien® is a non-bioerodible implant containing 0.19 mg of fluocinolone acetonide, preloaded with a 25 g needle for intravitreal injection. The implant measures 3.5 mm length by 0.37 mm diameter and utilizes the same matrix of polyvinyl alcohol and silicone as Retisert®. It is approved in the United States and several European countries for diabetic macular edema. A nearly identical implant containing 0.18 mg fluocinolone acetonide called Yutiq™ was tested in an interventional investigator-sponsored new drug study and found at 2 years to reduce the number of inflammation recurrences [101]. However, glaucoma filtration surgery was required in 18%. Two phase III trials have since been completed, and both trials achieved their primary efficacy endpoint at 6 and 12 months of preventing recurrent uveitis flares. Yutiq™ was recently approved by the FDA for the treatment of noninfectious uveitis affecting the posterior segment.

Pharmacodynamics and Pharmacokinetics

Iluvien® and Yutiq™ was designed to release fluocinolone acetonide at a rate of 0.25 mcg/day for 36 months. Aqueous levels at 1 month post-injection were 2.17 ng/mL with steady-state levels of 0.5–1.0 ng/mL from 3 months onward [82]. Peak concentrations were reached at 1 week. Animal models have demonstrated consistently lower concentrations of fluocinolone in the various intraocular tissues with Iluvien® as compared to Retisert®, with minimal systemic absorption [102]. Clinical studies support these pharmacokinetic studies, with efficacy shown through 36 months [103].

Complications

As with all intraocular corticosteroids, cataract and glaucoma are common adverse effects. Cataracts are very common with 80% requiring cataract surgery during the diabetic macular edema trials for Iluvien® [103]. Ocular hypertension was present in about a third of patients, and filtration surgery was required in 4.8%. Vitreous floaters and conjunctival hemorrhage were common injection-related adverse effects. Posterior capsule opacification and ocular discomfort have also been noted.

> **Practice Points**
>
> The indications for periocular or intravitreal corticosteroids are nearly the same and there is currently no consensus regarding management algorithms. Periocular injections are typically used first line in anterior and intermediate uveitis and for complications such as CME in the context of controlled inflammation. IVTA is often used when prior periocular injections have been ineffectual or only partly effective, for more

severe cases when a rapid effect is required, or for chronic disease requiring a longer duration of effect (often in combination with the commencement of systemic immunosuppression). Since the POINT trial, there is an increasing move towards intraocular, rather than periocular, steroid use.

Implantable corticosteroids are a reasonable treatment option for patients with chronic unilateral noninfectious inflammation or those with unilateral or bilateral chronic disease who are intolerant of systemic treatment. Their use in patients with a prior vitrectomy is another indication, given that studies have shown that their duration of effect is unchanged by the lack of vitreous, unlike IVTA.

Anti-vascular Endothelial Growth Factor (VEGF)

VEGF has an important role in angiogenesis and the inflammatory cascade. In recent years, it has become a pivotal target for the intraocular treatment of choroidal and retinal vascular disease, in particular macular edema and neovascularization. Anti-VEGF agents available commercially include bevacizumab (Avastin®, Genentech, South San Francisco, CA, USA), ranibizumab (Lucentis®, Genentech, South San Francisco, CA, USA), aflibercept (Eylea, Regeneron, Tarrytown, NY, USA), and pegaptanib (Macugen, Gilead Sciences, Inc., San Dimas, CA, USA). All are currently used off-label in the treatment of uveitis and its complications. Bevacizumab 1.25 mg is the most commonly used followed by ranibizumab 0.5 mg as a distant second.

Elevated levels of VEGF have been found in the aqueous and vitreous of patients with uveitic CME and in inflammatory choroidal neovascular membranes (CNV) [104–106]. There is burgeoning research into the applicability of VEGF inhibition in inflammatory disorders [107–111]. Results are promising, though hampered by a lack of consistent protocols. The MINERVA study showed ranibizumab improved VA by 6.5 letters in 27 patients with post-inflammatory CNV by 2 months [112]. A mean of 5.8 injections over 12 months was required. The largest case series of 81 patients treated with bevacizumab reported a gain of 2.7 lines with a median of 3 injections over 3 years of follow-up [113].

Favorable effects of VEGF inhibition on uveitic CME and VA have also been described though the results have been mixed and less dramatic than the effect seen with IVTA [114–116]. A small randomized pilot trial comparing bevacizumab to triamcinolone reported improved VA with both agents over 36 weeks [115]. IVTA was found to have a greater effect on VA ($p = 0.007$) and resulted in a statistically significant improvement of CME. In contrast, there was a no significant improvement in CME with bevacizumab. Other case series, including one with follow-up of 1 year, have found an improvement in macular edema with bevacizumab, however repeated injections (range 2–3 over 4–12 months) were needed to facilitate a modest reduction in CME [114, 117]. Once present, the duration of effect can be prolonged, at up to 16 weeks for bevacizumab and 6 months for ranibizumab [116, 118]. Interestingly, there have been eight cases reported of a bilateral response from unilateral injection [119, 120]. The multicenter prospective MERIT (Macular Edema Ranibizumab versus Intravitreal anti-inflammatory Therapy) RCT is currently recruiting and will compare intravitreal methotrexate, ranibizumab, and Ozurdex® in macular edema refractory to intravitreal corticosteroid [111].

Pharmacodynamics and Pharmacokinetics

Anti-VEGF agents act by binding VEGF or its isoforms, thereby preventing it from binding to receptors on the endothelial cell surface. Mean vitreal concentration of VEGF in patients with uveitis was 82.75 pg/mL compared with diabetes (954.98 pg/mL) and age-related macular degeneration (AMD) (64 pg/mL) [106]. Control patients had levels below detection. Bevacizumab is a full-length recombinant humanized monoclonal antibody approved for use in systemic neoplasia. It binds to all isoforms of VEGF. Ranibizumab is a humanized antibody fragment that targets VEGF-A isoforms ($VEGF_{110}$, $VEGF_{125}$, and $VEGF_{165}$). Aflibercept is a synthetic fragment that binds VEGF-A and B and placental growth factor. Pegaptanib is a synthetic aptamer that targets $VEGF_{165}$ specifically. The latter three are produced for intravitreal use whereas bevacizumab requires post-production preparation.

Significant differences in the molecular structure of the anti-VEGF drugs result in very different pharmacokinetic profiles. In nonvitrectomized human eyes, the vitreous half-life is estimated at 9.8 days for bevacizumab and 7.2 days for ranibizumab [121, 122]. No data is available for aflibercept. Half-life was comparable in vitrectomized and nonvitrectomized rabbit eyes [123]. A recent pharmacokinetic study compared the systemic concentrations of VEGF and the anti-VEGF agents bevacizumab, ranibizumab, and aflibercept [124]. It is believed systemic clearance is related to the presence of the Fc region which protects against degradation. This domain is absent in ranibizumab but present in bevacizumab and aflibercept. Maximal serum concentration was reached 1 day after intravitreal injection of ranibizumab and aflibercept, and 7 days for bevacizumab. Ranibizumab appeared transiently in the systemic circulation, with minimal impact on systemic VEGF levels and no accumulation with repeat injection. Systemic exposure to bevacizumab was 35 times greater and serum levels appeared to accumulate with multiple injections. Bevacizumab was also associated with significantly reduced free VEGF in plasma. Aflibercept is the strongest suppressor of plasma VEGF levels; however, systemic exposure was actually lower than bevacizumab.

Complications

Knowledge of ocular and systemic adverse effects of the anti-VEGF agents are drawn largely from clinical trials in AMD. Studies in uveitis patients have reported only ocular and nonocular adverse effects [107, 115, 117, 125], with low rates of serious ocular complications such as endophthalmitis (0.02–0.04%) and retinal detachment (0.02%) [126, 127]. These rates may be even lower when evaluated against the number of injections rather than patients [128]. It is worth noting that anterior chamber inflammation can occur in up to 21% in uveitis patients [115].

Although anti-VEGF drugs appear less efficacious than IVTA for the treatment of uveitic CME, they are less likely to cause cataract progression and ocular hypertension. Raised IOP was noted in only 3.4–11.6% of treated patients, with <1% requiring incisional surgery [129]. Cataract progression has been described in 8% of those treated with ranibizumab and aflibercept compared with 17.3% of those treated with pegaptanib. Common but benign complications include blurred vision, conjunctival hemorrhage, vitreous floaters, and discomfort.

Anti-VEGF agents may also be a reasonable option when the patient has adverse reactions to local or systemic steroids such as concomitant central serous retinopathy or exquisite IOP steroid sensitivity. While anti-VEGF treatment for uveitic CME or inflammatory retinal or choroidal neovascularization is useful, control of inflammation with systemic immunosuppression or other means is concomitantly required and cannot be replaced by anti-VEGF monotherapy.

Systemic adverse effects have garnered close scrutiny given the morbidity and mortality risk found in the AMD studies. Incidence of serious side effects including vascular events such as stroke or myocardial infarcts, or mortality from any cause, is approximately 5%. The rate of thrombotic events was <4% for ranibizumab and aflibercept and 4.1% with bevacizumab [130]. The incidence ranged between 0.8 and 5% for thrombotic events and 2.8–4% for all-cause mortality [126]. It is difficult to ascertain the actual risk as the AMD study population are intrinsically at higher risk given their age and comorbidities. There is currently no consensus among the ophthalmic community as to the risk of systemic adverse effects or the comparative risk of each drug [131]. Added to this is the comparatively younger age of patients with uveitis, such that there are still unknown effects on fertility and the unborn fetus. Currently, all anti-VEGF agents have been assigned to pregnancy category C by the FDA. Polizzi and Mahajan reported a case series of three women who received intravitral bevacizumab while pregnant, including during organogenesis, who proceeded to have healthy full-term infants [132].

Methotrexate

Intravitreal methotrexate has been used in intraocular lymphoma associated with primary central nervous system lymphoma (PCNSL) since the late 1990s [133–135]. Its use in uveitis is relatively recent and has shown promise in improving inflammation and CME [136–139]. The usual dose is 400 mcg in 0.1 mL which has been demonstrated to not be retinotoxic in animal models [135]. Taylor et al. recently published the largest case series of 38 eyes with uveitis, showing 1 line visual gain and improved inflammation in 79% after a mean of 1.4 injections over 11.2 months [139]. There was a modest effect on CME. Meta-analysis including data from a previous smaller study from the same investigators showed an extended period of remission of up to 17 months. Relapses were seen in 17%, typically at 3 months, and the vast majority responded to a repeat injection. Smaller case series have reported similar findings and proposed additional visual gains with a more intensive intravitreal regime [136, 138].

Pharmacodynamics and Pharmacokinetics

Methotrexate is a competitive inhibitor of dihydrofolate reductase, resulting in decreased proliferation of B and T cells. The anti-inflammatory effects of intravitreal methotrexate are believed to be mediated by the release of adenosine and not via its known cytotoxic pathway [139]. Adenosine exerts inhibitory effects on neutrophils, macrophages, and T-cell activity. Methotrexate may also suppress interleukin-6 and interleukin-8 [138]. The half-life of intravitreal methotrexate is estimated to be 12.4–21.5 hours [140]. Drug clearance is expected to be accelerated in aphakic and/or vitrectomized eyes [141]. Therapeutic levels for lymphoma are widely considered to be 1 μM, and cytotoxic levels may be present for 2–5 days [141–143]. The dosage of 400 mcg is not believed to be retinotoxic and electroretinograms have not shown permanent changes [135, 141]. Serum levels of methotrexate were unchanged after intravitreal administration [140].

Complications

Superficial punctate keratopathy is the commonest ocular side effect of intravitreal methotrexate and can occur in up to 100% of patients [144]. It commonly appears after the third injection and subsides if the treatment interval is extended to 4 weeks. Folinic acid 0.003% eye drops and vitamin A eye ointment can be used concurrently to minimize this complication [136, 138, 139, 145]. One case of band keratopathy requiring surgery has been reported [144]. Sterile endophthalmitis has been reported in up to 10% [136, 146]. Cataract progression has been noted in a third of patients and glaucoma in up to 16%. Epiretinal membrane formation and unspecified maculopathy have also been reported [146]. Accurate estimation of risk is difficult due to the rarity of the conditions and the relatively new use of intravitreal methotrexate.

Sirolimus

Sirolimus is a macrolide antibiotic also known as rapamycin. It was originally isolated from *Streptomyces hygroscopicus* found on Easter Island (Rapa Nui). Sirolimus arrests cell-cycle progression in T cells, endothelial cells, and smooth muscle cells and additionally inhibits the production of antibodies [147]. It is FDA approved in renal transplant immunosuppression and in cardiac stents for ischemic heart disease.

Recent studies have examined the efficacy of subconjunctival and intravitreal sirolimus in ocular inflammation [148–151]. The SAVE (Sirolimus as a therapeutic Approach for uVEitis) study was a small prospective RCT comparing subconjunctival sirolimus 1320 mcg to intravitreal sirolimus 325 mcg in noninfectious uveitis. Improvement in inflammation was noted in 70%, however this did not correspond to improvements in VA or CME at 6 or 12 months [150]. There was no difference between the two modes of delivery. In those with active disease, 92% of patients were able to decrease systemic corticosteroid and 38% were able to completely cease treatment. Those with inactive disease at baseline were able to decrease the median prednisone dose from 9 to 2 mg/day by 12 months, but none were able to cease completely. Results from the phase III study, SAKURA (Sirolimus study Assessing double-masKed Uveitis tReAtment), showed significantly higher proportions of subjects in the low dose (440 mcg) group achieving vitreous haze score of 0–0.5+ by 6 months compared to an active control group (44 mcg), while the high dose group (880 mcg) did not achieve statistical significance [152]. Results from the follow-on study SAKURA 2 are yet to be published. Sirolimus has also been found to have antiangiogenic effects in animal models [153, 154].

Pharmacokinetics and Pharmacodynamics

Sirolimus aggregates to form vitreous depots when injected intravitreally [155]. Peak levels of 420 ng/mL were achieved at 6 hours post-injection of a 220 mcg dose in a rabbit model. Sirolimus remained detectable in the vitreous for 90 days after a single injection and in the retina/choroid for 8 weeks after repeated dosing. Clinical studies demonstrate an intraocular half-life of 7–8 days [155–157]. Ocular concentrations were minimal by 7–12 weeks even after repeated doses given 8 weeks apart. Systemic concentration was highest on day 2 at <2 ng/mL (352 mcg dose), well below the 5–15 ng/mL required for systemic immunosuppression. Intraocular concentration and duration of exposure appear to be dose-dependent.

Complications

Subconjunctival and intravitreal sirolimus are generally well-tolerated. Subconjunctival injections often cause moderate inflammation at the injection site which resolves spontaneously within 2 weeks. Vitreous floaters are also commonly reported, likely related to the rapid precipitation of the drug after injection. Serious complications appear to be dose-dependent. Sterile endophthalmitis was noted in 3.4% of patients receiving 880 mcg intravitreally and 0.9% in the 440 mcg group [147]. It is thought that the drug precipitates generate a nonspecific autoinflammatory response in already inflamed tissue, compounded by sirolimus having no immediate anti-inflammatory activity. Cataract incidence was 15% (880 mcg) and 7.2% (440 mcg). Ocular hypertension was noted in 16–20% and responded to topical treatment. No reports of systemic adverse effects have been reported.

Tumor Necrosis Factor Alpha Inhibitors

Tumor necrosis factor alpha (TNFα) is a pro-inflammatory cytokine. Systemic anti-TNFα agents are widely used to treat a variety of rheumatologic and uveitic conditions. Infliximab (Remicade®, Janssen Biotech, Inc., Horsham, PA, USA), adalimumab (Humira®, Abbott Laboratories, Abbott Park, IL, USA), and etanercept (Enbrel®, Pfizer Inc., New York, NY, USA) have recently been trialed as intravitreal injections, with equivocal results. Furthermore, concerns about a high rate of significant post-injection inflammation have resulted in calls for a moratorium on the intravitreal use of anti-TNFα drugs outside of carefully designed clinical trials [158–160]. A total of 122 patients have been reported in the literature to have received intravitreal injections of these agents, of which 37 had noninfectious uveitis or uveitic CME [161–164]. Results from up to 6 months of follow-up are conflicting although it is worth noting that there were no reports of worsening ocular inflammation in uveitic patients.

Pharmacodynamics and Pharmacokinetics

There is a dearth of studies regarding the behavior of intraocular anti-TNFα drugs, and therapeutic dose ranges are yet to be established. Animal studies have demonstrated retinotoxicity at ≥5 mg infliximab although lower dosages may paradoxically be more immunogenic [158, 165]. The half-life of infliximab is estimated to be 8.5 days [166]. No toxicity was noted for adalimumab 5 mg but follow-up was limited to 14 days. Etanercept levels peak immediately after injection in the vitreous and at 4 weeks in the retina and choroid, remaining detectable for over 8 weeks [167].

Complications

Intraocular inflammation ranging from anterior uveitis to panuveitis has been reported with infliximab, with some patients requiring vitrectomy [158, 160, 168]. Reports of other complications such as cataracts and ocular hypertension are few. No systemic adverse events from intraocular dosing of these agents have been reported.

Appendix 13.1: Summary of Local Ocular Drug Delivery Methods

Subconjunctival Injection (Anterior Sub-Tenon)

Method

- Anesthesia: topical anesthesia should be achieved with repeated applications of topical anesthetic such as proparacaine and oxybuprocaine. This can be augmented by placing a local anesthetic-soaked pledget on intended injection site for 5 minutes
- A 1 mL syringe with a 30 g needle is preferred; 27 g needle may be required for triamcinolone
- Insert the needle bevel toward the globe through the conjunctiva on the superior or inferior bulbar surface at a site that is usually covered by the upper or lower eyelid
- Inject up to 0.1 mL of medication (typically Kenalog®) to form a small bleb; injections may be placed at multiple sites, up to a total volume to 0.5–1.0 mL. A whitish deposit may be noted, hence the preference to place these injections at a site that would/will be covered by the eyelids

Subconjunctival administration offers an attractive alternative to peri- and intraocular injections as the needle tip is always visible and therefore theoretically safer. Consideration should be made to minimize cosmetic defects such as a visible deposit within the interpalpebral fissure and subconjunctival hemorrhage.

Periocular Triamcinolone (e.g. Kenalog®) Injection (Posterior Sub-Tenon, Orbital Floor, Peribulbar) [169]

There are several approaches to periocular injections. While each technique offers different advantages and risks, all aim to place the drug close to the post-equatorial globe. Retrobulbar injections are rarely performed, particularly in a clinic setting where treatment usually takes place. The most common usage is triamcinolone acetonide 20–40 mg given into the sub-Tenon or orbital floor space.

Anesthesia

Topical anesthesia is required for the sub-Tenon techniques. This can be augmented by the addition of a quick-acting local anesthetic mixed into the syringe containing the corticosteroid. Orbital floor and peribulbar injections typically do not require topical anesthesia.

- A 3 mL syringe is preferred
- All injections are given with the needle bevel facing the globe as to minimize engaging the sclera and inadvertent intraocular penetration

Posterior sub-Tenon injections can be delivered by either blunt cannula or sharp needle

(Nozik) technique. The technique aims to deposit the drugs close to the macula.

Sub-Tenon Injection (Blunt)

The specialized cannula is a blunt, curved 19 g needle 25 mm long.

- Ask the patient to look away from the intended site of injection, which is typically inferonasal
- Blunt curved scissors are used to make a small circumcorneal incision about 8 mm from the limbus
- Dissect onto bare sclera and into the sub-Tenon space
- Slide the cannula posteriorly along this track until the hilt is reached
- Inject the drug. Forceps can be used to provide counter traction and to hold the conjunctival opening closed

Difficulties can be encountered in accessing sub-Tenon space and in preventing regurgitation along injection track.

Sub-Tenon Injection (Nozik)

1. Use a 25- or 27 g 5/8″ needle
2. Ask the patient to look inferonasally
3. Insert the needle bevel toward the globe through the conjunctiva at a point 3–4 mm in front of the superotemporal fornix
4. Advance the needle to the hilt with lateral sweeping motions to maintain close contact with the globe while avoiding scleral penetration and inject up to 1 mL (40 mg)

This technique minimizes unsightly cosmetic blemishes but can result in ptosis [26, 31, 34, 170, 171]. This may result from disinsertion of the levator aponeurosis, direct needle trauma to the levator complex, or muscle fiber atrophy due to the triamcinolone [26, 170]. Subconjunctival hemorrhage and chemosis are rarely experienced.

Peribulbar Injection

Peribulbar injections can be approached transconjunctivally or transcutaneously through the lower eyelid.

1. Use a 25 g 1″ needle and 3 mL syringe
2. Ask the patient to look straight ahead as a gaze directed superonasally brings the optic nerve closer to the orbital rim
3. The needle is inserted at the meeting point between the lateral third and medial two-thirds of the lower orbital rim
4. Direct the needle slightly up-and-in with a side-to-side motion until the needle reaches its hilt
5. 1 mL of drug is deposited into the extraconal space

Orbital Floor Injection

Orbital floor injections are favored in some centers as it is believed they have a lower risk of globe perforation. Rarely, herniation of orbital fat following multiple orbital floor injections has been reported [172].

1. Use a 27 g 0.5″ or 1″ needle
2. Ask the patient to look straight ahead
3. The needle is inserted transcutaneously at the meeting point between the lateral third and medial two-thirds of the lower orbital rim
4. Advance the needle directly posteriorly
5. The drug is deposited on the orbital floor

All sharp-needle techniques carry an intrinsic risk of inadvertent globe perforation, which itself increases the risk of intraocular complications such endophthalmitis and retinal tears.

Intravitreal Injection of Triamcinolone [173]

Method

1. Anesthesia: topical anesthesia is required and can be augmented by placing a local anesthetic-soaked pledget on intended injection site for 5 minutes or by a subconjunctival injection of local anesthetic
2. A 1 mL syringe with a 27 g or 30 g 0.5″ needle is preferred
3. Instill povidone-iodine 5% into the conjunctival sac

4. Place an eyelid speculum
5. Ask the patient to look away from the intended site of injection, typically superotemporal
6. Mark the site of injection with calipers: 3.5 mm from the limbus in pseudophakic patients, 4.0 mm in phakic patients
7. Insert the needle approximately halfway into the vitreous cavity, directing the tip toward the optic nerve
8. Inject 0.05–0.1 mL of the medication
9. Check gross visual acuity or perform indirect ophthalmoscopy to ensure adequate central retinal artery circulation

Serious procedure-related complications occur infrequently at <1–5% and include retinal tears, vitreous hemorrhage, and endophthalmitis. Floaters, subconjunctival hemorrhage, and ocular surface irritation are common but benign.

References

1. Goldstein DA, Do D, Noronha G, Kissner JM, Srivastava SK, Nguyen QD. Suprachoroidal corticosteroid administration: a novel route for local treatment of noninfectious uveitis. Transl Vis Sci Technol. 2016;5(6):14.
2. Yeh S, Kurup SK, Wang RC, Foster CS, Noronha G, Nguyen QD, et al. Suprachoroidal injection of triamcinolone acetonide, CLS-TA, for macular edema due to noninfectious uveitis: a randomized, Phase 2 study (DOGWOOD). Retina. 2018;
3. Cunningham ETJ, Wender JD. Practical approach to the use of corticosteroids in patients with uveitis. Can J Ophthalmol. 2010;45(4):352–8.
4. Babu K, Mahendradas P. Medical management of uveitis – current trends. Indian J Ophthalmol. 2013;61(6):277–83.
5. Jain MR, Srivastava S. Ocular penetration of hydrocortisone and dexamethasone into the aqueous humour after subconjunctival injection. Trans Ophthalmol Soc U K. 1978;98(1):63–5.
6. McGhee CN, Watson DG, Midgley JM, Noble MJ, Dutton GN, Fern AI. Penetration of synthetic corticosteroids into human aqueous humour. Eye (Lond). 1990;4(Pt 3):526–30.
7. Weijtens O, Feron EJ, Schoemaker RC, Cohen AF, Lentjes EG, Romijn FP, et al. High concentration of dexamethasone in aqueous and vitreous after subconjunctival injection. Am J Ophthalmol. 1999;128(2):192–7.
8. Weijtens O, Schoemaker RC, Romijn FP, Cohen AF, Lentjes EG, van Meurs JC. Intraocular penetration and systemic absorption after topical application of dexamethasone disodium phosphate. Ophthalmology. 2002;109(10):1887–91.
9. Athanasiadis Y, Tsatsos M, Sharma A, Hossain P. Subconjunctival triamcinolone acetonide in the management of ocular inflammatory disease. J Ocul Pharmacol Ther. 2013;29(6):516–22.
10. Kalina PH, Erie JC, Rosenbaum L. Biochemical quantification of triamcinolone in subconjunctival depots. Arch Ophthalmol. 1995;113(7):867–9.
11. Sevel D, Abramson A. Necrogranulomatous scleritis treated by an onlay scleral graft. Br J Ophthalmol. 1972;56(11):791–9.
12. Tu EY, Culbertson WW, Pflugfelder SC, Huang A, Chodosh JC. Therapy of nonnecrotizing anterior scleritis with subconjunctival corticosteroid injection. Ophthalmology. 1995;102(5):718–24.
13. Croasdale CR, Brightbill FS. Subconjunctival corticosteroid injections for nonnecrotizing anterior scleritis. Arch Ophthalmol. 1999;117(7):966–8.
14. Zamir E, Read RW, Smith RE, Wang RC, Rao NA. A prospective evaluation of subconjunctival injection of triamcinolone acetonide for resistant anterior scleritis. Ophthalmology. 2002;109(4):798–805.
15. Albini TA, Zamir E, Read RW, Smith RE, See RF, Rao NA. Evaluation of subconjunctival triamcinolone for nonnecrotizing anterior scleritis. Ophthalmology. 2005;112(10):1814–20.
16. Roufas A, Jalaludin B, Gaskin C, McCluskey P. Subconjunctival triamcinolone treatment for non-necrotising anterior scleritis. Br J Ophthalmol. 2010;94(6):743–7.
17. Sohn EH, Wang R, Read R, Roufas A, Teo L, Moorthy R, et al. Long-term, multicenter evaluation of subconjunctival injection of triamcinolone for non-necrotizing, noninfectious anterior scleritis. Ophthalmology. 2011;118(10):1932–7.
18. Gaudio PA. A review of evidence guiding the use of corticosteroids in the treatment of intraocular inflammation. Ocul Immunol Inflamm. 2004;12(3):169–92.
19. Akduman L, Kolker AE, Black DL, Del Priore LV, Kaplan HJ. Treatment of persistent glaucoma secondary to periocular corticosteroids. Am J Ophthalmol. 1996;122(2):275–7.
20. Athanasiadis Y, Nithyanandrajah GA, Kumar B, Sharma A. Reversal of steroid induced raised intraocular pressure following removal of subconjunctival triamcinolone for cataract surgery. Cont Lens Anterior Eye. 2009;32(3):143–4.
21. Merkoudis N, Wikberg Matsson A, Granstam E. Comparison of peroperative subconjunctival injection of methylprednisolone and standard postoperative steroid drops after uneventful cataract surgery. Acta Ophthalmol. 2014;92(7):623–8.
22. Agrawal S, Agrawal J, Agrawal TP. Conjunctival ulceration following triamcinolone injection. Am J Ophthalmol. 2003;136(3):539–40.
23. Johnson KS, Chu DS. Evaluation of sub-Tenon triamcinolone acetonide injections in the treatment of scleritis. Am J Ophthalmol. 2010;149(1):77–81.

24. Beardsley RM, Suhler EB, Rosenbaum JT, Lin P. Pharmacotherapy of scleritis: current paradigms and future directions. Expert Opin Pharmacother. 2013;14(4):411–24.
25. Sen HN, Vitale S, Gangaputra SS, Nussenblatt RB, Liesegang TL, Levy-Clarke GA, et al. Periocular corticosteroid injections in uveitis: effects and complications. Ophthalmology. 2014;121(11):2275–86.
26. Ferrante P, Ramsey A, Bunce C, Lightman S. Clinical trial to compare efficacy and side-effects of injection of posterior sub-Tenon triamcinolone versus orbital floor methylprednisolone in the management of posterior uveitis. Clin Experiment Ophthalmol. 2004;32(6):563–8.
27. Leder HA, Jabs DA, Galor A, Dunn JP, Thorne JE. Periocular triamcinolone acetonide injections for cystoid macular edema complicating noninfectious uveitis. Am J Ophthalmol. 2011;152(3):441–48.e2.
28. Salek SS, Leder HA, Butler NJ, Gan TJ, Dunn JP, Thorne JE. Periocular triamcinolone acetonide injections for control of intraocular inflammation associated with uveitis. Ocul Immunol Inflamm. 2013;21(4):257–63.
29. Thorne JE, Sugar EA, Holbrook JT, Burke AE, Altaweel MM, Vitale AT, et al. Periocular triamcinolone vs. intravitreal triamcinolone vs. intravitreal dexamethasone implant for the treatment of uveitic macular edema: the PeriOcular vs. INTravitreal corticosteroids for uveitic macular edema (POINT) trial. Ophthalmology. 2019;126(2):283–95.
30. Venkatesh P, Kumar CS, Abbas Z, Garg S. Comparison of the efficacy and safety of different methods of posterior subtenon injection. Ocul Immunol Inflamm. 2008;16(5):217–23.
31. Tanner V, Kanski JJ, Frith PA. Posterior sub-Tenon's triamcinolone injections in the treatment of uveitis. Eye (Lond). 1998;12:679–85.
32. Jermak CM, Dellacroce JT, Heffez J, Peyman GA. Triamcinolone acetonide in ocular therapeutics. Surv Ophthalmol. 2007;52(5):503–22.
33. Riordan-Eva P, Lightman S. Orbital floor steroid injections in the treatment of uveitis. Eye (Lond). 1994;8:66–9.
34. Yoshikawa K, Kotake S, Ichiishi A, Sasamoto Y, Kosaka S, Matsuda H. Posterior sub-Tenon injections of repository corticosteroids in uveitis patients with cystoid macular edema. Jpn J Ophthalmol. 1995;39(1):71–6.
35. Weijtens O, Schoemaker RC, Lentjes EG, Romijn FP, Cohen AF, van Meurs JC. Dexamethasone concentration in the subretinal fluid after a subconjunctival injection, a peribulbar injection, or an oral dose. Ophthalmology. 2000;107(10):1932–8.
36. Nan K, Sun S, Li Y, Qu J, Li G, Luo L, et al. Characterisation of systemic and ocular drug level of triamcinolone acetonide following a single sub-Tenon injection. Br J Ophthalmol. 2010;94(5):654–8.
37. Weijtens O, van der Sluijs FA, Schoemaker RC, Lentjes EG, Cohen AF, Romijn FP, et al. Peribulbar corticosteroid injection: vitreal and serum concentrations after dexamethasone disodium phosphate injection. Am J Ophthalmol. 1997;123(3):358–63.
38. Helm CJ, Holland GN. The effects of posterior subtenon injection of triamcinolone acetonide in patients with intermediate uveitis. Am J Ophthalmol. 1995;120(1):55–64.
39. Iwao K, Inatani M, Kawaji T, Koga T, Mawatari Y, Tanihara H. Frequency and risk factors for intraocular pressure elevation after posterior sub-Tenon capsule triamcinolone acetonide injection. J Glaucoma. 2007;16(2):251–6.
40. Byun YS, Park YH. Complications and safety profile of posterior subtenon injection of triamcinolone acetonide. J Ocul Pharmacol Ther. 2009;25(2):159–62.
41. Roesel M, Gutfleisch M, Heinz C, Heimes B, Zurek-Imhoff B, Heiligenhaus A. Orbital floor triamcinolone acetonide injections for the management of active non-infectious uveitis. Eye (Lond). 2009;23(4):910–4.
42. Jea SY, Byon IS, Oum BS. Triamcinolone-induced intraocular pressure elevation: intravitreal injection for macular edema and posterior subtenon injection for uveitis. Korean J Ophthalmol. 2006;20(2):99–103.
43. Kawamura R, Inoue M, Shinoda H, Shinoda K, Itoh Y, Ishida S, et al. Incidence of increased intraocular pressure after subtenon injection of triamcinolone acetonide. J Ocul Pharmacol Ther. 2011;27(3):299–304.
44. Graham RO, Peyman GA. Intravitreal injection of dexamethasone. Treatment of experimentally induced endophthalmitis. Arch Ophthalmol. 1974;92(2):149–54.
45. Antcliff RJ, Spalton DJ, Stanford MR, Graham EM, Ffytche TJ, Marshall J. Intravitreal triamcinolone for uveitic cystoid macular edema: an optical coherence tomography study. Ophthalmology. 2001;108(4):765–72.
46. Young S, Larkin G, Branley M, Lightman S. Safety and efficacy of intravitreal triamcinolone for cystoid macular oedema in uveitis. Clin Experiment Ophthalmol. 2001;29(1):2–6.
47. Androudi S, Letko E, Meniconi M, Papadaki T, Ahmed M, Foster CS. Safety and efficacy of intravitreal triamcinolone acetonide for uveitic macular edema. Ocul Immunol Inflamm. 2005;13(2–3):205–12.
48. Roesel M, Gutfleisch M, Heinz C, Heimes B, Zurek-Imhoff B, Heiligenhaus A. Intravitreal and orbital floor triamcinolone acetonide injections in noninfectious uveitis: a comparative study. Ophthalmic Res. 2009;42(2):81–6.
49. Shin JY, Yu HG. Intravitreal triamcinolone injection for uveitic macular edema: a randomized clinical study. Ocul Immunol Inflamm. 2015;23(6):430–6.
50. Kok H, Lau C, Maycock N, McCluskey P, Lightman S. Outcome of intravitreal triamcinolone in uveitis. Ophthalmology. 2005;112(11):1916.e1–7.
51. Ozkiris A. Intravitreal triamcinolone acetonide injection for the treatment of posterior uveitis. Ocul Immunol Inflamm. 2006;14(4):233–8.

52. Park UC, Park JH, Yu HG. Long-term outcome of intravitreal triamcinolone acetonide injection for the treatment of uveitis attacks in Behcet disease. Ocul Immunol Inflamm. 2014;22(1):27–33.
53. Kwak HW, D'Amico DJ. Evaluation of the retinal toxicity and pharmacokinetics of dexamethasone after intravitreal injection. Arch Ophthalmol. 1992;110(2):259–66.
54. Tempest-Roe S, Joshi L, Dick AD, Taylor SR. Local therapies for inflammatory eye disease in translation: past, present and future. BMC Ophthalmol. 2013;13(1):39.
55. Inoue M, Takeda K, Morita K, Yamada M, Tanigawara Y, Oguchi Y. Vitreous concentrations of triamcinolone acetonide in human eyes after intravitreal or subtenon injection. Am J Ophthalmol. 2004;138(6):1046–8.
56. Andrade RE, Muccioli C, Farah ME, Nussenblatt RB, Belfort R Jr. Intravitreal triamcinolone in the treatment of serous retinal detachment in Vogt-Koyanagi-Harada syndrome. Am J Ophthalmol. 2004;137(3):572–4.
57. Beer PM, Bakri SJ, Singh RJ, Liu W, Peters GB 3rd, Miller M. Intraocular concentration and pharmacokinetics of triamcinolone acetonide after a single intravitreal injection. Ophthalmology. 2003;110(4):681–6.
58. Audren F, Tod M, Massin P, Benosman R, Haouchine B, Erginay A, et al. Pharmacokinetic-pharmacodynamic modeling of the effect of triamcinolone acetonide on central macular thickness in patients with diabetic macular edema. Invest Ophthalmol Vis Sci. 2004;45(10):3435–41.
59. Couch SM, Bakri SJ. Intravitreal triamcinolone for intraocular inflammation and associated macular edema. Clin Ophthalmol. 2009;3:41–7.
60. Jonas JB. Intraocular availability of triamcinolone acetonide after intravitreal injection. Am J Ophthalmol. 2004;137(3):560–2.
61. van Kooij B, Rothova A, de Vries P. The pros and cons of intravitreal triamcinolone injections for uveitis and inflammatory cystoid macular edema. Ocul Immunol Inflamm. 2006;14(2):73–85.
62. Chin HS, Park TS, Moon YS, Oh JH. Difference in clearance of intravitreal triamcinolone acetonide between vitrectomized and nonvitrectomized eyes. Retina. 2005;25(5):556–60.
63. Chen H, Sun S, Li J, Du W, Zhao C, Hou J, et al. Different intravitreal properties of three triamcinolone formulations and their possible impact on retina practice. Invest Ophthalmol Vis Sci. 2013;54(3):2178–85.
64. Dodwell DG, Krimmel DA, de Fiebre CM. Sterile endophthalmitis rates and particle size analyses of different formulations of triamcinolone acetonide. Clin Ophthalmol. 2015;9:1033–40.
65. Zacharias LC, Lin T, Migon R, Ghosn C, Orilla W, Feldmann B, et al. Assessment of the differences in pharmacokinetics and pharmacodynamics between four distinct formulations of triamcinolone acetonide. Retina. 2013;33(3):522–31.
66. Kiddee W, Trope GE, Sheng L, Beltran-Agullo L, Smith M, Strungaru MH, et al. Intraocular pressure monitoring post intravitreal steroids: a systematic review. Surv Ophthalmol. 2013;58(4):291–310.
67. Lasave AF, Zeballos DG, El-Haig WM, Diaz-Llopis M, Salom D, Arevalo JF. Short-term results of a single intravitreal bevacizumab (Avastin) injection versus a single intravitreal triamcinolone acetonide (Kenacort) injection for the management of refractory noninfectious uveitic cystoid macular edema. Ocul Immunol Inflamm. 2009;17(6):423–30.
68. Rechtman E, Danis RP, Pratt LM, Harris A. Intravitreal triamcinolone with photodynamic therapy for subfoveal choroidal neovascularisation in age related macular degeneration. Br J Ophthalmol. 2004;88(3):344–7.
69. Gillies MC, Sutter FK, Simpson JM, Larsson J, Ali H, Zhu M. Intravitreal triamcinolone for refractory diabetic macular edema: two-year results of a double-masked, placebo-controlled, randomized clinical trial. Ophthalmology. 2006;113(9):1533–8.
70. Jonisch J, Lai JC, Deramo VA, Flug AJ, Fastenberg DM. Increased incidence of sterile endophthalmitis following intravitreal preserved triamcinolone acetonide. Br J Ophthalmol. 2008;92(8):1051–4.
71. Roth DB, Chieh J, Spirn MJ, Green SN, Yarian DL, Chaudhry NA. Noninfectious endophthalmitis associated with intravitreal triamcinolone injection. Arch Ophthalmol. 2003;121(9):1279–82.
72. Jonas JB, Kreissig I, Spandau UH, Harder B. Infectious and noninfectious endophthalmitis after intravitreal high-dosage triamcinolone acetonide. Am J Ophthalmol. 2006;141(3):579–80.
73. Lorenzo-Carrero J, Gonzalez Barcia M, Perez Flores I. Sterile endophthalmitis after benzyl alcohol filtered triamcinolone acetonide injection. Arch Ophthalmol. 2008;126(1):142–3.
74. Roth D, Lee SS, Flynn HW, Moshfeghi DM. Inflammatory reactions after intravitreal triamcinolone acetonide: possible mechanisms and therapeutic options. Exp Rev Ophthalmol. 2010;5(3):273–6.
75. Tomkins-Netzer O, Taylor SR, Bar A, Lula A, Yaganti S, Talat L, et al. Treatment with repeat dexamethasone implants results in long-term disease control in eyes with noninfectious uveitis. Ophthalmology. 2014;121(8):1649–54.
76. Callanan DG, Jaffe GJ, Martin DF, Pearson PA, Comstock TL. Treatment of posterior uveitis with a fluocinolone acetonide implant: three-year clinical trial results. Arch Ophthalmol. 2008;126(9):1191–201.
77. Pavesio C, Zierhut M, Bairi K, Comstock TL, Usner DW. Evaluation of an intravitreal fluocinolone acetonide implant versus standard systemic therapy in noninfectious posterior uveitis. Ophthalmology. 2010;117(3):567–75, 75.e1.
78. Kempen JH, Altaweel MM, Holbrook JT, Jabs DA, Louis TA, Sugar EA, et al. Randomized com-

parison of systemic anti-inflammatory therapy versus fluocinolone acetonide implant for intermediate, posterior, and panuveitis: the Multicenter Uveitis Steroid Treatment trial. Ophthalmology. 2011;118(10):1916–26.
79. Kempen JH, Altaweel MM, Drye LT, Holbrook JT, Jabs DA, Sugar EA, et al. Benefits of systemic anti-inflammatory therapy versus fluocinolone acetonide intraocular implant for intermediate uveitis, posterior uveitis, and panuveitis: fifty-four-month results of the Multicenter Uveitis Steroid Treatment (MUST) trial and follow-up study. Ophthalmology. 2015;122(10):1967–75.
80. Kempen JH, Altaweel MM, Holbrook JT, Sugar EA, Thorne JE, Jabs DA, et al. Association between long-lasting intravitreous fluocinolone acetonide implant vs systemic anti-inflammatory therapy and visual acuity at 7 years among patients with intermediate, posterior, or panuveitis. JAMA. 2017;317(19):1993–2005.
81. Mikhail M, Sallam A. Novel intraocular therapy in non-infectious uveitis of the posterior segment of the eye. Med Hypothesis Discov Innov Ophthalmol. 2013;2(4):113–20.
82. Campochiaro PA, Nguyen QD, Hafiz G, Bloom S, Brown DM, Busquets M, et al. Aqueous levels of fluocinolone acetonide after administration of fluocinolone acetonide inserts or fluocinolone acetonide implants. Ophthalmology. 2013;120(3):583–7.
83. Driot JY, Novack GD, Rittenhouse KD, Milazzo C, Pearson PA. Ocular pharmacokinetics of fluocinolone acetonide after Retisert intravitreal implantation in rabbits over a 1-year period. J Ocul Pharmacol Ther. 2004;20(3):269–75.
84. Kempen JH, Altaweel MM, Drye LT, Holbrook JT, Jabs DA, Sugar EA, et al. Quality of life and risks associated with systemic anti-inflammatory therapy versus fluocinolone acetonide intraocular implant for intermediate uveitis, posterior uveitis, or panuveitis: fifty-four-month results of the Multicenter Uveitis Steroid Treatment trial and follow-up study. Ophthalmology. 2015;122(10):1976–86.
85. Akduman L, Cetin EN, Levy J, Becker MD, Mackensen F, Lim LL. Spontaneous dissociation and dislocation of Retisert pellet. Ocul Immunol Inflamm. 2013;21(1):87–9.
86. Holbrook JT, Sugar EA, Burke AE, Vitale AT, Thorne JE, Davis J, et al. Dissociations of the fluocinolone acetonide implant: the Multicenter Uveitis Steroid Treatment (MUST) trial and follow-up study. Am J Ophthalmol. 2016;164:29–36.
87. Georgalas I, Koutsandrea C, Papaconstantinou D, Mpouritis D, Petrou P. Scleral melt following Retisert intravitreal fluocinolone implant. Drug Des Devel Ther. 2014;8:2373–5.
88. Lowder C, Belfort R Jr, Lightman S, Foster CS, Robinson MR, Schiffman RM, et al. Dexamethasone intravitreal implant for noninfectious intermediate or posterior uveitis. Arch Ophthalmol. 2011;129(5):545–53.
89. Khurana RN, Bansal AS, Chang LK, Palmer JD, Wu C, Wieland MR. Prospective evaluation of a sustained-release dexamethasone intravitreal implant for cystoid macular edema in quiescent uveitis. Retina. 2017;37(9):1692–9.
90. Zarranz-Ventura J, Carreno E, Johnston RL, Mohammed Q, Ross AH, Barker C, et al. Multicenter study of intravitreal dexamethasone implant in noninfectious uveitis: indications, outcomes, and reinjection frequency. Am J Ophthalmol. 2014;158(6):1136–45.e5.
91. Tomkins-Netzer O, Talat L, Seguin-Greenstein S, Bar A, Lightman S. Outcome of treating pediatric uveitis with dexamethasone implants. Am J Ophthalmol. 2016;161:110–15.e2.
92. Chang-Lin JE, Attar M, Acheampong AA, Robinson MR, Whitcup SM, Kuppermann BD, et al. Pharmacokinetics and pharmacodynamics of a sustained-release dexamethasone intravitreal implant. Invest Ophthalmol Vis Sci. 2011;52(1):80–6.
93. Chang-Lin JE, Burke JA, Peng Q, Lin T, Orilla WC, Ghosn CR, et al. Pharmacokinetics of a sustained-release dexamethasone intravitreal implant in vitrectomized and nonvitrectomized eyes. Invest Ophthalmol Vis Sci. 2011;52(7):4605–9.
94. Rishi P, Mathur G, Rishi E. Fractured Ozurdex implant in the vitreous cavity. Indian J Ophthalmol. 2012;60(4):337–8.
95. Bourgault S, Albiani D. Re: Split Ozurdex implant: a caution. Can J Ophthalmol. 2013;48(3):218–9.
96. Roy R, Hegde S. Split Ozurdex implant: a caution. Can J Ophthalmol. 2013;48(1):e15–6.
97. Bhagat R, Zhang J, Farooq S, Li XY. Comparison of the release profile and pharmacokinetics of intact and fragmented dexamethasone intravitreal implants in rabbit eyes. J Ocul Pharmacol Ther. 2014;30(10):854–8.
98. Haller JA, Bandello F, Belfort R Jr, Blumenkranz MS, Gillies M, Heier J, et al. Randomized, sham-controlled trial of dexamethasone intravitreal implant in patients with macular edema due to retinal vein occlusion. Ophthalmology. 2010;117(6):1134–46.e3.
99. Boyer DS, Yoon YH, Belfort R Jr, Bandello F, Maturi RK, Augustin AJ, et al. Three-year, randomized, sham-controlled trial of dexamethasone intravitreal implant in patients with diabetic macular edema. Ophthalmology. 2014;121(10):1904–14.
100. Cebeci Z, Kir N. Role of implants in the treatment of diabetic macular edema: focus on the dexamethasone intravitreal implant. Diabetes Metab Syndr Obes. 2015;8:555–66.
101. Jaffe GJ, Lin P, Keenan RT, Ashton P, Skalak C, Stinnett SS. Injectable fluocinolone acetonide long-acting implant for noninfectious intermediate uveitis, posterior uveitis, and panuveitis: two-year results. Ophthalmology. 2016;123(9):1940–8.
102. Kane FE, Green KE. Ocular pharmacokinetics of fluocinolone acetonide following Iluvien implantation in the vitreous humor of rabbits. J Ocul Pharmacol Ther. 2015;31(1):11–6.

103. Campochiaro PA, Brown DM, Pearson A, Chen S, Boyer D, Ruiz-Moreno J, et al. Sustained delivery fluocinolone acetonide vitreous inserts provide benefit for at least 3 years in patients with diabetic macular edema. Ophthalmology. 2012;119(10):2125–32.
104. Fine HF, Baffi J, Reed GF, Csaky KG, Nussenblatt RB. Aqueous humor and plasma vascular endothelial growth factor in uveitis-associated cystoid macular edema. Am J Ophthalmol. 2001;132(5):794–6.
105. Shimada H, Yuzawa M, Hirose T, Nakashizuka H, Hattori T, Kazato Y. Pathological findings of multifocal choroiditis with panuveitis and punctate inner choroidopathy. Jpn J Ophthalmol. 2008;52(4):282–8.
106. Weiss K, Steinbrugger I, Weger M, Ardjomand N, Maier R, Wegscheider BJ, et al. Intravitreal VEGF levels in uveitis patients and treatment of uveitic macular oedema with intravitreal bevacizumab. Eye (Lond). 2009;23(9):1812–8.
107. Fine HF, Zhitomirsky I, Freund KB, Barile GR, Shirkey BL, Samson CM, et al. Bevacizumab (Avastin) and ranibizumab (Lucentis) for choroidal neovascularization in multifocal choroiditis. Retina. 2009;29(1):8–12.
108. Lott MN, Schiffman JC, Davis JL. Bevacizumab in inflammatory eye disease. Am J Ophthalmol. 2009;148(5):711–17.e2.
109. Cornish KS, Williams GJ, Gavin MP, Imrie FR. Visual and optical coherence tomography outcomes of intravitreal bevacizumab and ranibizumab in inflammatory choroidal neovascularization secondary to punctate inner choroidopathy. Eur J Ophthalmol. 2011;21(4):440–5.
110. D'Ambrosio E, Tortorella P, Iannetti L. Management of uveitis-related choroidal neovascularization: from the pathogenesis to the therapy. J Ophthalmol. 2014;2014:450428.
111. ClinicalTrials.gov [Internet]. Bethesda (MD): National Library of Medicine (US). 29 Feb 2000. Identifier NCT02623426, Macular Edema Ranibizumab v. Intravitreal anti-inflammatory Therapy Trial (MERIT); 7 Dec 2015 [cited 1 Nov 2018]; [about 8 screens]. Available from: https://clinicaltrials.gov/ct2/show/NCT02623426?term=merit+uveitis&rank=1.
112. Lai TYY, Staurenghi G, Lanzetta P, Holz FG, Melissa Liew SH, Desset-Brethes S, et al. Efficacy and safety of ranibizumab for the treatment of choroidal neovascularization due to uncommon cause: twelve-month results of the MINERVA study. Retina. 2018;38(8):1464–77.
113. Mansour AM, Arevalo JF, Fardeau C, Hrisomalos EN, Chan WM, Lai TY, et al. Three-year visual and anatomic results of administrating intravitreal bevacizumab in inflammatory ocular neovascularization. Can J Ophthalmol. 2012;47(3):269–74.
114. Cervantes-Castaneda RA, Giuliari GP, Gallagher MJ, Yilmaz T, MacDonell RE, Quinones K, et al. Intravitreal bevacizumab in refractory uveitic macular edema: one-year follow-up. Eur J Ophthalmol. 2009;19(4):622–9.
115. Soheilian M, Rabbanikhah Z, Ramezani A, Kiavash V, Yaseri M, Peyman GA. Intravitreal bevacizumab versus triamcinolone acetonide for refractory uveitic cystoid macular edema: a randomized pilot study. J Ocul Pharmacol Ther. 2010;26(2):199–206.
116. Bae JH, Lee CS, Lee SC. Efficacy and safety of intravitreal bevacizumab compared with intravitreal and posterior sub-tenon triamcinolone acetonide for treatment of uveitic cystoid macular edema. Retina. 2011;31(1):111–8.
117. Mackensen F, Heinz C, Becker MD, Heiligenhaus A. Intravitreal bevacizumab (Avastin) as a treatment for refractory macular edema in patients with uveitis: a pilot study. Retina. 2008;28(1):41–5.
118. Acharya NR, Hong KC, Lee SM. Ranibizumab for refractory uveitis-related macular edema. Am J Ophthalmol. 2009;148(2):303–9.e2.
119. Al-Dhibi H, Khan AO. Bilateral response following unilateral intravitreal bevacizumab injection in a child with uveitic cystoid macular edema. J AAPOS. 2009;13(4):400–2.
120. Acharya NR, Sittivarakul W, Qian Y, Hong KC, Lee SM. Bilateral effect of unilateral ranibizumab in patients with uveitis-related macular edema. Retina. 2011;31(9):1871–6.
121. Krohne TU, Eter N, Holz FG, Meyer CH. Intraocular pharmacokinetics of bevacizumab after a single intravitreal injection in humans. Am J Ophthalmol. 2008;146(4):508–12.
122. Krohne TU, Liu Z, Holz FG, Meyer CH. Intraocular pharmacokinetics of ranibizumab following a single intravitreal injection in humans. Am J Ophthalmol. 2012;154(4):682–86.e2.
123. Ahn SJ, Ahn J, Park S, Kim H, Hwang DJ, Park JH, et al. Intraocular pharmacokinetics of ranibizumab in vitrectomized versus nonvitrectomized eyes. Invest Ophthalmol Vis Sci. 2014;55(1):567–73.
124. Avery RL, Castellarin AA, Steinle NC, Dhoot DS, Pieramici DJ, See R, et al. Systemic pharmacokinetics following intravitreal injections of ranibizumab, bevacizumab or aflibercept in patients with neovascular AMD. Br J Ophthalmol. 2014;98(12):1636–41.
125. Mansour AM, Mackensen F, Mahendradas P, Khairallah M, Lai TY, Bashshur Z. Five-year visual results of intravitreal bevacizumab in refractory inflammatory ocular neovascularization. Clin Ophthalmol. 2012;6:1233–7.
126. Penedones A, Mendes D, Alves C, Batel Marques F. Safety monitoring of ophthalmic biologics: a systematic review of pre- and postmarketing safety data. J Ocul Pharmacol Ther. 2014;30(9):729–51.
127. Solomon SD, Lindsley K, Vedula SS, Krzystolik MG, Hawkins BS. Anti-vascular endothelial growth factor for neovascular age-related macular degeneration. Cochrane Database Syst Rev. 2014;(8):CD005139.
128. van der Reis MI, La Heij EC, De Jong-Hesse Y, Ringens PJ, Hendrikse F, Schouten JS. A systematic review of the adverse events of intravitreal anti-

vascular endothelial growth factor injections. Retina. 2011;31(8):1449–69.
129. Dedania VS, Bakri SJ. Sustained elevation of intraocular pressure after intravitreal anti-VEGF agents: what is the evidence? Retina. 2015;35(5):841–58.
130. Schmid MK, Bachmann LM, Fas L, Kessels AG, Job OM, Thiel MA. Efficacy and adverse events of aflibercept, ranibizumab and bevacizumab in age-related macular degeneration: a trade-off analysis. Br J Ophthalmol. 2015;99(2):141–6.
131. Biagi C, Conti V, Montanaro N, Melis M, Buccellato E, Donati M, et al. Comparative safety profiles of intravitreal bevacizumab, ranibizumab and pegaptanib: the analysis of the WHO database of adverse drug reactions. Eur J Clin Pharmacol. 2014;70(12):1505–12.
132. Polizzi S, Mahajan VB. Intravitreal anti-VEGF injections in pregnancy: case series and review of literature. J Ocul Pharmacol Ther. 2015;31(10):605–10.
133. Fishburne BC, Wilson DJ, Rosenbaum JT, Neuwelt EA. Intravitreal methotrexate as an adjunctive treatment of intraocular lymphoma. Arch Ophthalmol. 1997;115(9):1152–6.
134. Smith JR, Rosenbaum JT, Wilson DJ, Doolittle ND, Siegal T, Neuwelt EA, et al. Role of intravitreal methotrexate in the management of primary central nervous system lymphoma with ocular involvement. Ophthalmology. 2002;109(9):1709–16.
135. Velez G, Boldt HC, Whitcup SM, Nussenblatt RB, Robinson MR. Local methotrexate and dexamethasone phosphate for the treatment of recurrent primary intraocular lymphoma. Ophthalmic Surg Lasers. 2002;33(4):329–33.
136. Hardwig PW, Pulido JS, Erie JC, Baratz KH, Buettner H. Intraocular methotrexate in ocular diseases other than primary central nervous system lymphoma. Am J Ophthalmol. 2006;142(5):883–5.
137. Taylor SR, Habot-Wilner Z, Pacheco P, Lightman SL. Intraocular methotrexate in the treatment of uveitis and uveitic cystoid macular edema. Ophthalmology. 2009;116(4):797–801.
138. Bae JH, Lee SC. Effect of intravitreal methotrexate and aqueous humor cytokine levels in refractory retinal vasculitis in Behcet disease. Retina. 2012;32(7):1395–402.
139. Taylor SR, Banker A, Schlaen A, Couto C, Matthe E, Joshi L, et al. Intraocular methotrexate can induce extended remission in some patients in noninfectious uveitis. Retina. 2013;33(10):2149–54.
140. Nakauchi Y, Takase H, Sugita S, Mochizuki M, Shibata S, Ishiwata Y, et al. Concurrent administration of intravenous systemic and intravitreal methotrexate for intraocular lymphoma with central nervous system involvement. Int J Hematol. 2010;92(1):179–85.
141. Velez G, Yuan P, Sung C, Tansey G, Reed GF, Chan CC, et al. Pharmacokinetics and toxicity of intravitreal chemotherapy for primary intraocular lymphoma. Arch Ophthalmol. 2001;119(10):1518–24.
142. de Smet MD, Vancs VS, Kohler D, Solomon D, Chan CC. Intravitreal chemotherapy for the treatment of recurrent intraocular lymphoma. Br J Ophthalmol. 1999;83(4):448–51.
143. Ozkan EB, Ozcan AA, Alparslan N. Intravitreal injection of methotrexate in an experimental rabbit model: determination of pharmacokinetics. Indian J Ophthalmol. 2011;59(3):197–200.
144. Frenkel S, Hendler K, Siegal T, Shalom E, Pe'er J. Intravitreal methotrexate for treating vitreoretinal lymphoma: 10 years of experience. Br J Ophthalmol. 2008;92(3):383–8.
145. Taylor SR, Habot-Wilner Z, Pacheco P, Lightman S. Intravitreal methotrexate in uveitis. Ophthalmology. 2012;119(4):878–9.
146. Ma WL, Hou HA, Hsu YJ, Chen YK, Tang JL, Tsay W, et al. Clinical outcomes of primary intraocular lymphoma patients treated with front-line systemic high-dose methotrexate and intravitreal methotrexate injection. Ann Hematol. 2016;95(4):593–601.
147. Pleyer U, Thurau SR. Sirolimus for the treatment of noninfectious uveitis. Expert Opin Pharmacother. 2016;17(1):127–35.
148. Sen HN, Larson TA, Meleth AD, Smith WM, Nussenblatt RB. Subconjunctival sirolimus for the treatment of chronic active anterior uveitis: results of a pilot trial. Am J Ophthalmol. 2012;153(6):1038–42.
149. Bhatt N, Dalal M, Tucker W, Obiyor D, Nussenblatt R, Sen HN. Subconjunctival sirolimus in the treatment of autoimmune non-necrotizing anterior scleritis: results of a phase I/II clinical trial. Am J Ophthalmol. 2015;159(3):601–6.
150. Ibrahim MA, Sepah YJ, Watters A, Bittencourt M, Vigil EM, Do DV, et al. One-year outcomes of the SAVE study: Sirolimus as a therapeutic Approach for uVEitis. Transl Vis Sci Technol. 2015;4(2):4.
151. Merrill P, Nguyen QD, Clark WL, Wilson L, Valentine ME, Naor J, et al. The SAKURA study, a phase III, multicenter, randomized, double-masked, study of intravitreal injections of DE-109 for the treatment of active, noninfectious uveitis of the posterior segment: baseline ocular disease characteristics. Association for Research and Visual Science Annual Meeting; Orlando, FL, USA; 2014.
152. Nguyen QD, Merrill PT, Clark WL, Banker AS, Fardeau C, Franco P, et al. Intravitreal sirolimus for noninfectious uveitis: a phase III Sirolimus study Assessing double-masKed Uveitis tReAtment (SAKURA). Ophthalmology. 2016;123(11):2413–23.
153. Dejneka NS, Kuroki AM, Fosnot J, Tang W, Tolentino MJ, Bennett J. Systemic rapamycin inhibits retinal and choroidal neovascularization in mice. Mol Vis. 2004;10:964–72.
154. Yagasaki R, Nakahara T, Ushikubo H, Mori A, Sakamoto K, Ishii K. Anti-angiogenic effects of mammalian target of rapamycin inhibitors in a mouse model of oxygen-induced retinopathy. Biol Pharm Bull. 2014;37(11):1838–42.

155. Mudumba S, Bezwada P, Takanaga H, Hosoi K, Tsuboi T, Ueda K, et al. Tolerability and pharmacokinetics of intravitreal sirolimus. J Ocul Pharmacol Ther. 2012;28(5):507–14.
156. Dugel PU, Blumenkranz MS, Haller JA, Williams GA, Solley WA, Kleinman DM, et al. A randomized, dose-escalation study of subconjunctival and intravitreal injections of sirolimus in patients with diabetic macular edema. Ophthalmology. 2012;119(1):124–31.
157. Petrou PA, Cunningham D, Shimel K, Harrington M, Hammel K, Cukras CA, et al. Intravitreal sirolimus for the treatment of geographic atrophy: results of a phase I/II clinical trial. Invest Ophthalmol Vis Sci. 2015;56(1):330–8.
158. Giganti M, Beer PM, Lemanski N, Hartman C, Schartman J, Falk N. Adverse events after intravitreal infliximab (Remicade). Retina. 2010;30(1):71–80.
159. Pulido JS, Pulido JE, Michet CJ, Vile RG. More questions than answers: a call for a moratorium on the use of intravitreal infliximab outside of a well-designed trial. Retina. 2010;30(1):1–5.
160. Wu L, Hernandez-Bogantes E, Roca JA, Arevalo JF, Barraza K, Lasave AF. Intravitreal tumor necrosis factor inhibitors in the treatment of refractory diabetic macular edema: a pilot study from the Pan-American Collaborative Retina Study Group. Retina. 2011;31(2):298–303.
161. Androudi S, Tsironi E, Kalogeropoulos C, Theodoridou A, Brazitikos P. Intravitreal adalimumab for refractory uveitis-related macular edema. Ophthalmology. 2010;117(8):1612–6.
162. Farvardin M, Afarid M, Shahrzad S. Long-term effects of intravitreal infliximab for treatment of sight-threatening chronic noninfectious uveitis. J Ocul Pharmacol Ther. 2012;28(6):628–31.
163. Markomichelakis N, Delicha E, Masselos S, Sfikakis PP. Intravitreal infliximab for sight-threatening relapsing uveitis in Behcet disease: a pilot study in 15 patients. Am J Ophthalmol. 2012;154(3):534–41.e1.
164. Hamam RN, Barikian AW, Antonios RS, Abdulaal MR, Alameddine RM, El Mollayess G, et al. Intravitreal adalimumab in active noninfectious uveitis: a pilot study. Ocul Immunol Inflamm. 2016;24(3):319–26.
165. Theodossiadis PG, Liarakos VS, Sfikakis PP, Charonis A, Agrogiannis G, Kavantzas N, et al. Intravitreal administration of the anti-TNF monoclonal antibody infliximab in the rabbit. Graefes Arch Clin Exp Ophthalmol. 2009;247(2):273–81.
166. Giansanti F, Ramazzotti M, Vannozzi L, Rapizzi E, Fiore T, Iaccheri B, et al. A pilot study on ocular safety of intravitreal infliximab in a rabbit model. Invest Ophthalmol Vis Sci. 2008;49(3):1151–6.
167. Fauser S, Kalbacher H, Alteheld N, Koizumi K, Krohne TU, Joussen AM. Pharmacokinetics and safety of intravitreally delivered etanercept. Graefes Arch Clin Exp Ophthalmol. 2004;242(7):582–6.
168. Arias L, Caminal JM, Badia MB, Rubio MJ, Catala J, Pujol O. Intravitreal infliximab in patients with macular degeneration who are nonresponders to antivascular endothelial growth factor therapy. Retina. 2010;30(10):1601–8.
169. Flaxel C. Posterior sub-Tenon's injections. In: Dunn JP, Langer PD, editors. Basic techniques of ophthalmic surgery. San Francisco: American Academy of Ophthalmology; 2009. p. 225–8.
170. Ideta S, Noda M, Kawamura R, Shinoda K, Suzuki K, Ishida S, et al. Dehiscence of levator aponeurosis in ptosis after sub-Tenon injection of triamcinolone acetonide. Can J Ophthalmol. 2009;44(6):668–72.
171. Lafranco Dafflon M, Tran VT, Guex-Crosier Y, Herbort CP. Posterior sub-Tenon's steroid injections for the treatment of posterior ocular inflammation: indications, efficacy and side effects. Graefes Arch Clin Exp Ophthalmol. 1999;237(4):289–95.
172. Smith JR, George RK, Rosenbaum JT. Lower eyelid herniation of orbital fat may complicate periocular corticosteroid injection. Am J Ophthalmol. 2002;133(6):845–7.
173. Bhagat N, Zarbin MA. Intravitreal injections. In: Dunn JP, Langer PD, editors. Basic techniques of ophthalmic surgery. San Francisco: American Academy of Ophthalmology; 2009. p. 229–32.

Novel Approaches to the Treatment of Noninfectious Uveitis

14

Justine R. Smith

Pearls

- Treatment with biologic drugs that target various leukocyte functions or inflammatory cytokines is an active area of research in clinical uveitis.
- Harnessing immunomodulatory cells of the immune system – including regulatory T cells, regulatory B cells, or mesenchymal stem/stromal cells – is a potential new therapeutic approach for intraocular inflammation.
- Antibody-based blockade of selected integrins, which mediate leukocyte transendothelial migration, has been associated with risk of progressive multifocal leukoencephalopathy in patients, but alternative methods of limiting the migration process may prove useful for the treatment of noninfectious uveitis.
- Drugs directed at the complement pathway may have a role in the management of noninfectious uveitis, but additional experimental data are needed before this approach can be considered for the clinic.

Introduction

Patients with vision-threatening noninfectious autoimmune or autoinflammatory uveitis are frequently treated with immunosuppression [1]. Some of these individuals will respond to treatment with conventional immunosuppressive drugs (e.g., antimetabolites covered in Chap. 4 or alkylating agents covered in Chap. 6), tumor necrosis factor (TNF) blockers (Chap. 7), or the interferons (Chap. 10). For a substantial number of patients, however, these drugs will not be effective and/or there will be contraindications or side effects that limit use. Thus, there is considerable interest in the development of alternative therapeutic agents for these patients, targeted to pathogenic mechanisms of the disease [2]. There are multiple potential groups of biological drug targets. This chapter contains a discussion of selected promising targets that are on the horizon for treatment of severe noninfectious uveitis, either in clinical trials or in preclinical testing: leukocytes, adhesion molecules, inflammatory cytokines, the complement system, and oxidative stress.

Dr. Smith is supported by an Australian Research Council Future Fellowship (FT130101648).

J. R. Smith (✉)
Flinders University College of Medicine and Public Health, Adelaide, SA, Australia
e-mail: justine.smith@flinders.edu.au

P. Lin, E. Suhler (eds.), *Treatment of Non-infectious Uveitis*,
https://doi.org/10.1007/978-3-030-22827-9_14

Leukocytes as Drug Targets

Noninfectious uveitis is defined by a mixed leukocyte infiltration of the eye [3]. Studies in the rodent model of immune-mediated uveitis, experimental autoimmune uveoretinitis (EAU), have identified $CD4^+$ T helper cells – Th17 and/or Th1 subsets – as initiators of the inflammation [4]. Infiltrating monocytes give rise to macrophages, which mediate the tissue destruction that accompanies the inflammation [5, 6]. B cells are also present in the inflamed eye; their pathogenic role in uveitis is uncertain, but may include secretion of antibody, local presentation of antigen to T cells, production of inflammatory cytokines, and support of T cell survival [7].

Targeting T Cells

The CD4+ T cell was the target of the first biologic treatment for uveitis. In the early 1990s, Thurau and colleagues [8] successfully treated a young adult with posterior uveitis that had not responded to conventional systemic immunosuppression with a series of intravenous infusions of cM-T412, a murine–human anti-CD4 antibody. However, this antibody was found to produce an extended reduction in CD4+ T cells and was never marketed. A more selective therapeutic approach that is currently under investigation for uveitis is blockade of costimulation. Cytotoxic T lymphocyte-associated antigen (CTLA)-4 modulates the interaction between CD28 and CD80 or CD86, inhibiting costimulation. Abatacept is a recombinant human CTLA-4-Fc fusion protein. To date, the published literature on the use of this biologic for uveitis is limited but, unfortunately, suggests effectiveness may be short term: the Multinational Interdisciplinary Working Group for Uveitis in Childhood found sustained effect over 12 months in just 14% of 21 patients treated for juvenile idiopathic arthritis-associated uveitis [9].

Targeting Monocytes

The eye contains resident macrophages, but tissue damage in uveitis is caused by macrophages derived from monocytes that migrate into the eye from the circulation during the disease. [5, 10] There are no treatments in clinical use for uveitis that target the mononuclear phagocytes specifically. However, when mice with EAU are treated with anti-CCR2 antibody to deplete blood monocytes, entry of these cells into the eye is reduced and structural damage within the eye is prevented [11]; this experimental study suggests the possibility of targeting monocytes as a treatment for uveitis. An interesting translational investigation of peripheral blood monocytes from patients with uveitis shows treatment with corticosteroid is associated with enrichment of the $CD14^{++}CD16^{+}$ monocyte population, which are restricted in their ability to drive T cell responses [12], offering another approach to therapeutic monocyte manipulation.

Targeting B Cells

The basic mechanisms of B cell involvement in uveitis remain to be clarified and are likely a larger contributor than previously described. Meanwhile, the B cell-depleting drug rituximab has been reported to be highly effective for treatment of different forms of uveitis in the clinic [7]. Descriptions of successful treatment include single cases and small series of patients with undifferentiated and juvenile idiopathic arthritis-associated chronic anterior uveitis, diffuse subretinal fibrosis uveitis syndrome, and Vogt–Koyanagi–Harada disease [11, 13–17]. One small, randomized clinical trial demonstrated superiority of rituximab over cyclophosphamide, in combination with antimetabolite in patients with Behçet disease [18].

Immunomodulatory Cell Therapy

There is considerable interest in the possibility of using immunomodulatory cells to treat uveitis. The effectiveness of administering regulatory T cells has been demonstrated in mouse EAU, using antigen-specific Treg cells [19], but also polyclonal Treg cells [20], which would be more readily translated to clinical use to suppress inflammation. Other studies in EAU have identified a role for regulatory B cells in control of intraocular inflammation [21], suggesting future use of these immunomodulatory cells to treat uveitis. Finally, infusion of mesenchymal stem/stromal cells reduces the severity of EAU by promoting the systemic generation of regulatory monocytes that induce nonspecific innate immune tolerance [22], suggesting yet another opportunity for immunomodulatory cell therapy.

Adhesion Molecules as Drug Targets

Passage of leukocytes across the wall of a blood vessel, from the circulation to the tissue, is strictly controlled by the vascular endothelial cells that line the blood vessel. Proteins expressed on the endothelial surface coordinate "stages" of leukocyte migration that include rolling, firm adhesion, spreading and crawling, and transmigration [23]. Common protein families are involved in leukocyte transendothelial migration throughout the body, although the involvement of individual family members depends on the specific molecular phenotype of the local vascular endothelial cell population [24].

Key adhesion molecules expressed by the endothelium include the selectins and immunoglobulin superfamily members [23]. P- and E-selectin interact with leukocyte glycoproteins, such as PSGL-1, in the early stages of leukocyte migration. Immunoglobulin superfamily adhesion molecules participate throughout extravasation: intercellular adhesion molecule (ICAM)-1, vascular cell adhesion molecule (VCAM)-1, and activated leukocyte adhesion molecule (ALCAM) interact with integrins expressed on leukocytes. Endothelial junctional proteins, including CD144, the junctional adhesion molecule (JAM) family, and claudins, are important for the later stages of leukocyte migration.

Previous studies using scanner laser ophthalmoscopy [25] and recent work using multimodal imaging [26] have demonstrated that during EAU, leukocytes migrate from the bloodstream into the posterior eye via the retinal vasculature. Consistently, there is increased expression of selectins and immunoglobulin superfamily molecules – especially P-selectin and ICAM-1 – by the retinal endothelium as the inflammation begins [27]. Histopathological studies of human eyes with anterior or posterior uveitis have demonstrated increased expression of these groups of adhesion molecules on the iris or retinal vascular endothelium, respectively [28–30]. Soluble forms of the selectins and immunoglobulin superfamily molecules rise in the blood during active uveitis [31–33]. Interestingly, adhesion molecule genetic polymorphisms are associated with some forms of uveitis [34].

The therapeutic potential of adhesion molecule blockade in uveitis has been investigated in EAU. Antibody blockade of the interactions between P- and E- selectin, ICAM-1, and VCAM-1, and their respective ligands, has been shown to reduce inflammation in this model [34–37]. Translational in vitro studies, using the transwell migration assay, in which cells move between chambers separated by a simulated endothelium, have demonstrated the importance of ICAM-1 in CD4+ T cell migration into the human retina [38]. Antibody blockade of ICAM-1 during transwell migration significantly reduces the number of Th1- or Th17-polarized cells that move through the transwell for a majority of human leukocyte donors; in contrast, VCAM-1 and ALCAM blockade reduces movement in a minority of donors. However, the utilization of adhesion molecules is also leukocyte subset dependent; in independent studies using the same transwell system, VCAM-1 and ALCAM join ICAM-1 in mediating migration of activated dendritic cells into the eye [39].

Biologics have already been developed to target integrins for treatment of inflammatory diseases outside the eye. Efalizumab is a humanized monoclonal antibody directed against αL integrin, which prevents interactions with ICAM-1. Alicaforsen is an antisense ICAM-1 oligonucleotide, formulated as an enema. Both drugs are effective in inflammatory bowel disease [40], and efalizumab is also therapeutic for psoriasis [41]. Natalizumab is a humanized monoclonal antibody directed against α4 integrin, which inhibits interactions with VCAM-1. This drug is effective in multiple sclerosis [42] and inflammatory bowel disease [40]. In one case report, a patient with undifferentiated autoimmune uveitis, who had persistent macular edema despite systemic treatment with corticosteroid and mycophenolate mofetil, experienced disease remission following a 9-month course of efalizumab [43].

Clearly, there is a large body of experimental and clinical evidence for the important role of adhesion molecules in the development of uveitis, and biologic drugs are already available. Unfortunately, a major hurdle to progress in this area has come with recognition that anti-integrin antibody therapy carries a high risk of progressive multifocal leukoencephalopathy. For this reason, efalizumab has been withdrawn from the market, and the use of natalizumab is restricted. The risk of this fatal viral disease has been quantified for natalizumab to be approximately 1 in 250, although it may be reduced by careful patient selection [44]. As an alternative to integrins, targeting immunoglobulin superfamily members on the vascular endothelium holds promise as a future treatment of noninfectious uveitis.

Inflammatory Cytokines as Drug Targets

Cytokines are small proteins that mediate intercellular communication. Multiple inflammatory and immunomodulatory cytokines have been implicated in the progression and control of uveitis, respectively, in experimental and clinical studies dating back to the 1990s. Thus, inflammatory cytokines are obvious drug targets. Indeed, drugs that specifically inhibit the activity of master inflammatory cytokine, tumor necrosis factor (TNF)-α, have become the standard second-line treatment for noninfectious uveitis [45]. Drugs targeted to other inflammatory cytokines have reached the clinic more recently, including drugs that block the activities of interleukin (IL)-1, IL-2, IL-6, IL-17, and IL-23.

Interleukin-1 exists in α and β forms, which act via a common receptor that is blocked by the naturally occurring IL-1 receptor antagonist (IL-1RA) [46]. Macrophages are the usual common source of IL-1β, which acts on many cells to induce expression of multiple inflammatory molecules: other cytokines including chemokines, adhesion molecules, eicosanoids, and enzymes that catalyze the formation of reactive oxygen and nitrogen species. It is also a growth factor for T cells and B cells. Several drugs have been used in patients to manipulate IL-1 activity. Multiple case reports and small series describe the effective use of human anti-IL-1β antibody, canakinumab, and recombinant IL-1RA, anakinra, in uveitis associated with juvenile idiopathic arthritis, Behçet disease, and cryopyrin-associated periodic syndrome [47]. However, with one of the large randomized controlled clinical trials of the human anti-IL-1β antibody, gevokizumab, failing to reach its primary end point, the future for IL-1β therapeutic blockade in uveitis is uncertain.

Interleukin-2 is a critical signal for the proliferation and activation of CD4+ T cells [48]. Daclizumab is a chimeric mouse–human antibody directed against the α subunit of the IL-2 receptor. In uveitis patients in particular, an important mechanism of action of this drug is the induction of $CD56^{(bright)}$ regulatory natural killer cells that secrete IL-10, which is an immunomodulatory cytokine [49]. At least 8 US-based studies have evaluated the use of daclizumab in up to 39 patients with different uveitis subsets, including birdshot retinochoroidopathy, Behçet uveitis, juvenile idiopathic arthritis-associated uveitis, and undifferentiated uveitis [50]. The value of daclizumab appears to be reduction in the use of other immunosuppressive medications. At this time, daclizumab is not marketed, and thus, it is no longer available to treat patients with uveitis. It remains under study for multiple sclerosis [42], however, and no doubt results of those trials will determine future availability.

Interleukin-6 is a downstream inflammatory cytokine that is produced by multiple cell populations and induces proliferation, differentiation, and trafficking of T and B cells, neutrophils, and monocytes [51]. This cytokine acts via a complex of the IL-6 receptor binding domain and gp130 signal transduction domain. Two monoclonal antibodies directed against the human IL-6 receptor are presently under study for treatment of noninfectious uveitis: tocilizumab and sarilumab. Published case reports and series have described successful treatment of uveitis and cystoid macular edema with tocilizumab in patients with birdshot retinochoroidopathy, Behçet uveitis, juvenile idiopathic arthritis-associated uveitis, and undifferentiated uveitis [52–55]. No information has been published on sarilumab for uveitis to date, but a phase II clinical trial is presently in progress: "a randomized, double-masked and placebo-controlled study to evaluate the efficacy and safety of sarilumab administered subcutaneously every 2 weeks in patients with noninfectious, intermediate, posterior or pan-uveitis."

Interleukin-17A is an inflammatory cytokine, produced by CD4+ Th17 cells; it induces cytokine, chemokine, and eicosanoid production by multiple cell populations, including endothelial cells, neutrophils, macrophages, epithelial cells, and fibroblasts [56]. Secukinumab is an anti-human IL-17 antibody that has been evaluated as a treatment for noninfectious uveitis in a series of clinical trials. The first "proof of concept" phase II clinical trial included 16 subjects with the full spectrum of noninfectious uveitis, who were treated intravenously with secukinumab; vision or inflammation improved, or corticosteroid dose was reduced in two-thirds of subjects [57]. Subsequently, three phase III clinical trials, involving 274 patients suffering from uveitis based in the posterior eye or associated with Behçet disease who were treated with a subcutaneous form of the biologic, failed to meet primary efficacy end points [58]. A later dose-ranging phase II clinical trial, which included 37 patients with intermediate, posterior, or pan uveitis, showed a higher response rate for the intravenous versus the subcutaneous formulation, possibly explaining the lack of efficacy of secukinumab in the phase III studies [59]. Differences in activities of IL-17, homeostatic Th17 cells, and pathogenic Th17 cells are another consideration that may be relevant to the effectiveness of IL-17 blockade in patients with uveitis.

Interleukin-23 is key signal for the conversion of naïve CD4+ T cells to pathogenic Th17 cells [60]. Interleukin-23-deficient mice are resistant to EAU, and increased serum levels of IL-23 have been measured in patients with spondyloarthropathy and uveitis, Vogt–Koyanagi–Harada uveitis, Behçet uveitis, and birdshot retinochoroidopathy [61–64]. Despite the literature supporting IL-23 as a therapeutic target in noninfectious uveitis, the most clinically effective method for blocking IL-23 or its receptor treatment is uncertain. Ustekinumab is an IL-12/IL-23 p40 neutralizing antibody that is administered subcutaneously. A phase II clinical trial of the drug did not benefit patients with relapsing-remitting multiple sclerosis, but the drug is effective for moderate-to-severe psoriasis [65, 66]. Results from a clinical trial that has enrolled patients with Behçet uveitis are pending.

Complement System as a Drug Target

The complement system is an important component of the innate immune network [67, 68]. The system consists of a group of circulating proteins that interact cascade fashion to opsonize apoptotic cells or microbes, marking them for phagocytosis, and to directly lyse foreign pathogens. In addition, complement anaphylatoxins – C3a and C5a – induce immune cell activation. It is well established that the anterior and posterior segments of the normal human eye have low levels of complement activity [69, 70]. The eye also contains complement regulatory proteins [71, 72].

There is good evidence from human studies that complement components play a role in uveitis. Genetic polymorphisms of multiple components have been associated with different uveitis subsets including anterior uveitis, multifocal choroiditis, and sarcoidosis-associated uveitis: C2, C4, factor H, factor B, and factor I [34]. Importantly, activation of complement within the eye has been measured in the aqueous of patients with anterior uveitis [73] and in the vitreous of patients with intermediate uveitis [74].

Studies from the laboratory also support a role for complement system in the pathogenesis of uveitis, although specific involvements are debated. Suppression of complement regulatory proteins exacerbates murine experimental autoimmune anterior uveitis [75], and treatment of rats with recombinant complement regulatory protein, Crry, inhibits the inflammation [76]. Work from one group has demonstrated that systemically or locally administered anti-C5a antibody reduces the severity of mouse EAU by limiting C5a-mediated macrophage activation [77]. In contrast, studies from an independent group have indicated that C5a- and C5a receptor gene-deficient mice experience no reduction in EAU, while C3 gene-deficient mice develop significantly less severe EAU than wild-type animals [78, 79]. Separately, EAU and endotoxin-induced uveitis in mice have been attenuated by intravitreal injection of a viral vector-encoded complement inhibitor domain derived from C3b/C4b receptor [80].

Given the data supporting the involvement of the complement system in uveitis, consideration of complement blockade as a therapy is appropriate. Many complement-targeted agents are in development. The most studied agent is eculizumab, which is a humanized mouse anti-C5a antibody that is used to treat patients with paroxysmal nocturnal hemoglobinuria and hemolytic uremic syndrome [81]. However, apart from the contradictory results in mouse EAU, this agent is extremely expensive. There is also a concern that targeting complement components may be associated with high risk of infectious complications, although human studies conducted to date suggest that this is practically only a concern in childhood.

Oxidative Stress as a Drug Target

Oxidative stress reflects an imbalance in the activity of reactive oxygen or nitrogen species and the body's antioxidative mechanisms [82]. In addition to direct toxicity, reactive oxygen/nitrogen species induce the production of cytokines, chemokines, and other inflammatory mediators. Rao and colleagues [83] first drew attention to oxidative stress in uveitis almost 30 years ago, in studies of guinea pig EAU, which at that time was termed experimental allergic uveitis. Treatment of animals with antioxidants, including superoxide dismutase, catalase, and sodium benzoate, resulted in marked attenuation of the intraocular inflammation.

Multiple studies in EAU and other rodent uveitis models have linked reduction in severity and/or tissue damage to reduced oxidative stress [84]. Interestingly, in EAU, onset of oxidative stress precedes the infiltration by leukocytes; this early stress has been localized to retina photoreceptors and reflects TNF-α-induced mitochondrial oxidative stress [85]. Once EAU is established, infiltrating macrophages and neutrophils are major sources of reactive oxygen and nitrogen species [86].

Over 30 studies have reported evidence of oxidative stress in Behçet disease on the basis of examination of serum or leukocytes (e.g., [87–89]). A small number of studies have implicated oxidative stress in other forms of uveitis, including sympathetic ophthalmia [90] and anterior uveitis [91, 92]. However, the few clinical studies of antioxidant drugs for uveitis have yielded limited information or been negative. A study of curcumin for chronic anterior uveitis enrolled 53 patients, but 40% subject dropout was reported and clinical improvement was not defined [93]. A randomized, controlled trial of vitamin C and vitamin E for acute anterior uveitis involved 145 subjects: no impact on anterior chamber cells was observed, although visual acuity at 8 weeks was superior in the treated group [94]. A randomized, controlled trial of vitamin E for uveitic macular edema halted the planned 80-person enrollment at 17 individuals due to lack of benefit [95].

Despite long-standing and solid experimental evidence of the involvement of oxidative stress in uveitis and the availability of antioxidant agents, treatment of uveitis directed at this basic disease mechanism has not progressed far toward clinical application. No doubt the situation in part reflects the lack of conclusive clinical studies. In addition, there is difficulty in dissecting mechanisms of action of many antioxidants, which often have other activities. In addition, the active ingredient in many over-the-counter preparations is not known, and such formulations may not be pure. With the development of agents under regulatory bodies, however, this is expected to be an area of growth for uveitis therapies in the coming decade.

Conclusion

Many novel therapeutic agents, targeting different mediators of noninfectious uveitis, are at various stages of translation to the clinic. In addition to the potential and realized drug targets covered in this discussion, other options include chemokines, growth factors, eicosanoids, matrix metalloproteinases, the ubiquitin–proteasome system, and inflammasomes. Patients with uveitis frequently have associated systemic diseases, and the direction in this field will be led not only by ophthalmology but also by other medical specialties, including rheumatology, gastroenterology, dermatology, and neurology. Since complications related to suppression of the systemic immune response will be an ongoing concern for the majority of systemically delivered biologics, the possibility of invasive or noninvasive local drug delivery is an important consideration for treatment of intraocular inflammatory disease. This is an exciting time for patients who suffer from noninfectious uveitis and the medical practitioners who manage their disease.

References

1. de Smet MD, Taylor SR, Bodaghi B, et al. Understanding uveitis: the impact of research on visual outcomes. Prog Retin Eye Res. 2011;30(6):452–70.
2. Lin P, Suhler EB, Rosenbaum JT. The future of uveitis treatment. Ophthalmology. 2014;121(1):365–76.
3. Van Ginderdeuren R, Van Calster J, Stalmans P, Van den Oord J. A new and standardized method to sample and analyse vitreous samples by the Cellient automated cell block system. Acta Ophthalmol. 2014;92(5):e388–92.
4. Caspi RR. Understanding autoimmune uveitis through animal models. The Friedenwald Lecture. Invest Ophthalmol Vis Sci. 2011;52(3):1872–9.
5. Kezic J, McMenamin PG. The monocyte chemokine receptor CX3CR1 does not play a significant role in the pathogenesis of experimental autoimmune uveoretinitis. Invest Ophthalmol Vis Sci. 2010;51(10):5121–7.
6. Zhao J, Chen M, Xu H. Experimental autoimmune uveoretinitis (EAU)-related tissue damage and angiogenesis is reduced in CCL2(−)/(−) CX(3)CR1gfp/gfp mice. Invest Ophthalmol Vis Sci. 2014;55(11):7572–82.
7. Smith JR, Stempel AJ, Bharadwaj AS, Appukuttan B. Involvement of B cells in non-infectious uveitis. Clin Transl Immunology. 2016;5:e63.
8. Thurau SR, Wildner G, Reiter C, Riethmuller G, Lund OE. Treatment of endogenous uveitis with anti-CD4 monoclonal antibody: first report. Ger J Ophthalmol. 1994;3(6):409–13.
9. Tappeiner C, Miserocchi E, Bodaghi B, et al. Abatacept in the treatment of severe, longstanding, and refractory uveitis associated with juvenile idiopathic arthritis. J Rheumatol. 2015;42(4):706–11.
10. London A, Benhar I, Mattapallil MJ, Mack M, Caspi RR, Schwartz M. Functional macrophage heterogeneity in a mouse model of autoimmune central nervous system pathology. J Immunol. 2013;190(7):3570–8.
11. Heiligenhaus A, Miserocchi E, Heinz C, Gerloni V, Kotaniemi K. Treatment of severe uveitis associated with juvenile idiopathic arthritis with anti-CD20 monoclonal antibody (rituximab). Rheumatology. 2011;50(8):1390–4.
12. Liu B, Dhanda A, Hirani S, et al. CD14++CD16+ monocytes are enriched by glucocorticoid treatment and are functionally attenuated in driving effector T cell responses. J Immunol. 2015;194(11):5150–60.
13. Tappeiner C, Heinz C, Specker C, Heiligenhaus A. Rituximab as a treatment option for refractory endogenous anterior uveitis. Ophthalmic Res. 2007;39(3):184–6.
14. Miserocchi E, Pontikaki I, Modorati G, Bandello F, Meroni PL, Gerloni V. Rituximab for uveitis. Ophthalmology. 2011;118(1):223–4.
15. Cornish KS, Kuffova L, Forrester JV. Treatment of diffuse subretinal fibrosis uveitis with rituximab. Br J Ophthalmol. 2015;99(2):153–4.
16. Caso F, Rigante D, Vitale A, et al. Long-lasting uveitis remission and hearing loss recovery after rituximab in Vogt-Koyanagi-Harada disease. Clin Rheumatol. 2015;34(10):1817–20.
17. Umran RMR, Shukur ZYH. Rituximab for sight-threatening refractory pediatric Vogt-Koyanagi-Harada disease. Mod Rheumatol. 2018;28(1):197–9.
18. Davatchi F, Shams H, Rezaipoor M, et al. Rituximab in intractable ocular lesions of Behcet's disease;

randomized single-blind control study (pilot study). Int J Rheum Dis. 2010;13(3):246–52.
19. Terrada C, Fisson S, De Kozak Y, et al. Regulatory T cells control uveoretinitis induced by pathogenic Th1 cells reacting to a specific retinal neoantigen. J Immunol. 2006;176(12):7171–9.
20. Gregoire S, Terrada C, Martin GH, et al. Treatment of uveitis by in situ administration of ex vivo-activated polyclonal regulatory T cells. J Immunol. 2016;196(5):2109–18.
21. Wang RX, Yu CR, Dambuza IM, et al. Interleukin-35 induces regulatory B cells that suppress autoimmune disease. Nat Med. 2014;20(6):633–41.
22. Ko JH, Lee HJ, Jeong HJ, Kim MK, Wee WR, Yoon SO, Choi H, Prockop DJ, Oh JY. Mesenchymal stem/stromal cells precondition lung monocytes/macrophages to produce tolerance against allo- and autoimmunity in the eye. Proc Natl Acad Sci U S A. 2016;113(1):158–63.
23. Ley K, Laudanna C, Cybulsky MI, Nourshargh S. Getting to the site of inflammation: the leukocyte adhesion cascade updated. Nat Rev Immunol. 2007;7(9):678–89.
24. Nolan DJ, Ginsberg M, Israely E, et al. Molecular signatures of tissue-specific microvascular endothelial cell heterogeneity in organ maintenance and regeneration. Dev Cell. 2013;26(2):204–19.
25. Parnaby-Price A, Stanford MR, Biggerstaff J, et al. Leukocyte trafficking in experimental autoimmune uveitis in vivo. J Leukoc Biol. 1998;64(4):434–40.
26. Chen X, Kezic JM, Forrester JV, et al. In vivo multimodal imaging of experimental autoimmune uveoretinitis in transgenic reporter mice reveals the dynamic nature of inflammatory changes during disease progression. J Neuroinflammation. 2015;12:17.
27. Crane IJ, Liversidge J. Mechanisms of leukocyte migration across the blood-retina barrier. Semin Immunopathol. 2008;30(2):165–77.
28. Kuppner MC, Liversidge J, McKillop-Smith S, Lumsden L, Forrester JV. Adhesion molecule expression in acute and fibrotic sympathetic ophthalmia. Curr Eye Res. 1993;12(10):923–34.
29. Wakefield D, McCluskey P, Palladinetti P. Distribution of lymphocytes and cell adhesion molecules in iris biopsy specimens from patients with uveitis. Arch Ophthalmol. 1992;110(1):121–5.
30. Whitcup SM, Chan CC, Li Q, Nussenblatt RB. Expression of cell adhesion molecules in posterior uveitis. Arch Ophthalmol. 1992;110(5):662–6.
31. Haznedaroglu E, Karaaslan Y, Buyukasik Y, et al. Selectin adhesion molecules in Behcet's disease. Ann Rheum Dis. 2000;59(1):61–3.
32. Lee MT, Hooper LC, Kump L, et al. Interferon-beta and adhesion molecules (E-selectin and s-intracellular adhesion molecule-1) are detected in sera from patients with retinal vasculitis and are induced in retinal vascular endothelial cells by Toll-like receptor 3 signalling. Clin Exp Immunol. 2007;147(1):71–80.
33. Zaman AG, Edelsten C, Stanford MR, et al. Soluble intercellular adhesion molecule-1 (sICAM-1) as a marker of disease relapse in idiopathic uveoretinitis. Clin Exp Immunol. 1994;95(1):60–5.
34. Yang MM, Lai TY, Luk FO, Pang CP. The roles of genetic factors in uveitis and their clinical significance. Retina. 2014;34(1):1–11.
35. Whitcup SM, DeBarge LR, Caspi RR, Harning R, Nussenblatt RB, Chan CC. Monoclonal antibodies against ICAM-1 (CD54) and LFA-1 (CD11a/CD18) inhibit experimental autoimmune uveitis. Clin Immunol Immunopathol. 1993;67(2):143–50.
36. Uchio E, Kijima M, Tanaka S, Ohno S. Suppression of experimental uveitis with monoclonal antibodies to ICAM-1 and LFA-1. Invest Ophthalmol Vis Sci. 1994;35(5):2626–31.
37. Xu H, Manivannan A, Jiang HR, et al. Recruitment of IFN-gamma-producing (Th1-like) cells into the inflamed retina in vivo is preferentially regulated by P-selectin glycoprotein ligand 1:P/E-selectin interactions. J Immunol. 2004;172(5):3215–24.
38. Bharadwaj AS, Schewitz-Bowers LP, Wei L, Lee RW, Smith JR. Intercellular adhesion molecule 1 mediates migration of Th1 and Th17 cells across human retinal vascular endothelium. Invest Ophthalmol Vis Sci. 2013;54(10):6917–25.
39. Furtado JM, Bharadwaj AS, Ashander LM, Olivas A, Smith JR. Migration of toxoplasma gondii-infected dendritic cells across human retinal vascular endothelium. Invest Ophthalmol Vis Sci. 2012;53(11):6856–62.
40. Mosli MH, Rivera-Nieves J, Feagan BG. T-cell trafficking and anti-adhesion strategies in inflammatory bowel disease: current and future prospects. Drugs. 2014;74(3):297–311.
41. Frampton JE, Plosker GL. Efalizumab: a review of its use in the management of chronic moderate-to-severe plaque psoriasis. Am J Clin Dermatol. 2009;10(1):51–72.
42. Straus Farber R, Harel A, Lublin F. Novel agents for relapsing forms of multiple sclerosis. Annu Rev Med. 2016;67:309–21.
43. Wang J, Ibrahim M, Turkcuoglu P, et al. Intercellular adhesion molecule inhibitors as potential therapy for refractory uveitic macular edema. Ocul Immunol Inflamm. 2010;18(5):395–8.
44. Baldwin KJ, Hogg JP. Progressive multifocal leukoencephalopathy in patients with multiple sclerosis. Curr Opin Neurol. 2013;26(3):318–23.
45. Levy-Clarke G, Jabs DA, Read RW, Rosenbaum JT, Vitale A, Van Gelder RN. Expert panel recommendations for the use of anti-tumor necrosis factor biologic agents in patients with ocular inflammatory disorders. Ophthalmology. 2014;121(3):785–796.e783.
46. Schett G, Dayer JM, Manger B. Interleukin-1 function and role in rheumatic disease. Nat Rev Rheumatol. 2016;12(1):14–24.
47. Willermain F, Rosenbaum JT, Bodaghi B, et al. Interplay between innate and adaptive immunity in the development of non-infectious uveitis. Prog Retin Eye Res. 2012;31(2):182–94.

48. Bachmann MF, Oxenius A. Interleukin 2: from immunostimulation to immunoregulation and back again. EMBO Rep. 2007;8(12):1142–8.
49. Li Z, Lim WK, Mahesh SP, Liu B, Nussenblatt RB. Cutting edge: in vivo blockade of human IL-2 receptor induces expansion of CD56(bright) regulatory NK cells in patients with active uveitis. J Immunol. 2005;174(9):5187–91.
50. Wroblewski K, Sen HN, Yeh S, et al. Long-term daclizumab therapy for the treatment of noninfectious ocular inflammatory disease. Can J Ophthalmol. 2011;46(4):322–8.
51. Lin P. Targeting interleukin-6 for noninfectious uveitis. Clin Ophthalmol. 2015;9:1697–702.
52. Deroux A, Chiquet C, Bouillet L. Tocilizumab in severe and refractory Behcet's disease: four cases and literature review. Semin Arthritis Rheum. 2016;45:733–7.
53. Deuter CM, Zierhut M, Igney-Oertel A, et al. Tocilizumab in uveitic macular edema refractory to previous immunomodulatory treatment. Ocul Immunol Inflamm. 2016:1–6.
54. Mesquida M, Molins B, Llorenc V, Sainz de la Maza M, Adan A. Long-term effects of tocilizumab therapy for refractory uveitis-related macular edema. Ophthalmology. 2014;121(12):2380–6.
55. Papo M, Bielefeld P, Vallet H, et al. Tocilizumab in severe and refractory non-infectious uveitis. Clin Exp Rheumatol. 2014;32(4 Suppl 84):S75–9.
56. Korn T, Bettelli E, Oukka M, Kuchroo VK. IL-17 and Th17 cells. Annu Rev Immunol. 2009;27:485–517.
57. Hueber W, Patel DD, Dryja T, et al. Effects of AIN457, a fully human antibody to interleukin-17A, on psoriasis, rheumatoid arthritis, and uveitis. Sci Transl Med. 2010;2(52):52ra72.
58. Dick AD, Tugal-Tutkun I, Foster S, et al. Secukinumab in the treatment of noninfectious uveitis: results of three randomized, controlled clinical trials. Ophthalmology. 2013;120(4):777–87.
59. Letko E, Yeh S, Foster CS, et al. Efficacy and safety of intravenous secukinumab in noninfectious uveitis requiring steroid-sparing immunosuppressive therapy. Ophthalmology. 2015;122(5):939–48.
60. Gaffen SL, Jain R, Garg AV, Cua DJ. The IL-23-IL-17 immune axis: from mechanisms to therapeutic testing. Nat Rev Immunol. 2014;14(9):585–600.
61. Przepiera-Bedzak H, Fischer K, Brzosko M. Extra-articular symptoms in constellation with selected serum cytokines and disease activity in spondyloarthritis. Mediators Inflamm. 2016;2016:7617954.
62. Chi W, Yang P, Li B, Wu C, Jin H, Zhu X, Chen L, Zhou H, Huang X, Kijlstra A. IL-23 promotes CD4+ T cells to produce IL-17 in Vogt-Koyanagi-Harada disease. J Allergy Clin Immunol. 2007;119(5):1218–24.
63. Chi W, Zhu X, Yang P, Liu X, Lin X, Zhou H, Huang X, Kijlstra A. Upregulated IL-23 and IL-17 in Behcet patients with active uveitis. Invest Ophthalmol Vis Sci. 2008;49(7):3058–64.
64. Yang P, Foster CS. Interleukin 21, interleukin 23, and transforming growth factor beta1 in HLA-A29-associated birdshot retinochoroidopathy. Am J Ophthalmol. 2013;156(2):400–406.e2.
65. Segal BM, Constantinescu CS, Raychaudhuri A, Kim L, Fidelus-Gort R, Kasper LH, Ustekinumab MS Investigators. Repeated subcutaneous injections of IL12/23 p40 neutralising antibody, ustekinumab, in patients with relapsing-remitting multiple sclerosis: a phase II, double-blind, placebo-controlled, randomised, dose-ranging study. Lancet Neurol. 2008;7(9):796–804.
66. Chen Z, Gong Y, Shi Y. Novel biologic agents targeting interleukin-23 and interleukin-17 for moderate-to-severe psoriasis. Clin Drug Investig. 2017;37(10):891–9.
67. Merle NS, Church SE, Fremeaux-Bacchi V, Roumenina LT. Complement system part I – molecular mechanisms of activation and regulation. Front Immunol. 2015;6:262.
68. Merle NS, Noe R, Halbwachs-Mecarelli L, Fremeaux-Bacchi V, Roumenina LT. Complement system part II: role in immunity. Front Immunol. 2015;6:257.
69. Mondino BJ, Rao H. Complement levels in normal and inflamed aqueous humor. Invest Ophthalmol Vis Sci. 1983;24(3):380–4.
70. Mondino BJ, Sidikaro Y, Sumner H. Anaphylatoxin levels in human vitreous humor. Invest Ophthalmol Vis Sci. 1988;29(7):1195–8.
71. Lass JH, Walter EI, Burris TE, et al. Expression of two molecular forms of the complement decay-accelerating factor in the eye and lacrimal gland. Invest Ophthalmol Vis Sci. 1990;31(6):1136–48.
72. Mondino BJ, Sumner H. Complement inhibitors in normal cornea and aqueous humor. Invest Ophthalmol Vis Sci. 1984;25(4):483–6.
73. Mondino BJ, Glovsky MM, Ghekiere L. Activated complement in inflamed aqueous humor. Invest Ophthalmol Vis Sci. 1984;25(7):871–3.
74. Mondino BJ, Sidikaro Y, Mayer FJ, Sumner HL. Inflammatory mediators in the vitreous humor of AIDS patients with retinitis. Invest Ophthalmol Vis Sci. 1990;31(5):798–804.
75. Jha P, Sohn JH, Xu Q, et al. Suppression of complement regulatory proteins (CRPs) exacerbates experimental autoimmune anterior uveitis (EAAU). J Immunol. 2006;176(12):7221–31.
76. Manickam B, Jha P, Hepburn NJ, et al. Suppression of complement activation by recombinant Crry inhibits experimental autoimmune anterior uveitis (EAAU). Mol Immunol. 2010;48(1–3):231–9.
77. Copland DA, Hussain K, Baalasubramanian S, et al. Systemic and local anti-C5 therapy reduces the disease severity in experimental autoimmune uveoretinitis. Clin Exp Immunol. 2010;159(3):303–14.
78. Read RW, Szalai AJ, Vogt SD, McGwin G, Barnum SR. Genetic deficiency of C3 as well as CNS-targeted expression of the complement inhibitor sCrry ameliorates experimental autoimmune uveoretinitis. Exp Eye Res. 2006;82(3):389–94.
79. Read RW, Vogt SD, Barnum SR. The complement anaphylatoxin receptors are not required for the

development of experimental autoimmune uveitis. J Neuroimmunol. 2013;264(1–2):127–9.
80. Li Y, Zhu P, Verma A, Prasad T, Deng H, Yu D, Li Q. A novel bispecific molecule delivered by recombinant AAV2 suppresses ocular inflammation and choroidal neovascularization. J Cell Mol Med. 2017;21(8):1555–71.
81. Ricklin D, Lambris JD. Complement in immune and inflammatory disorders: therapeutic interventions. J Immunol. 2013;190(8):3839–47.
82. Rahal A, Kumar A, Singh V, et al. Oxidative stress, prooxidants, and antioxidants: the interplay. Biomed Res Int. 2014;2014:761264.
83. Rao NA, Sevanian A, Fernandez MA, et al. Role of oxygen radicals in experimental allergic uveitis. Invest Ophthalmol Vis Sci. 1987;28(5):886–92.
84. Yadav UC, Kalariya NM, Ramana KV. Emerging role of antioxidants in the protection of uveitis complications. Curr Med Chem. 2011;18(6):931–42.
85. Nguyen AM, Rao NA. Oxidative photoreceptor cell damage in autoimmune uveitis. J Ophthalmic Inflamm Infect. 2011;1:7–13.
86. Kerr EC, Raveney BJ, Copland DA, Dick AD, Nicholson LB. Analysis of retinal cellular infiltrate in experimental autoimmune uveoretinitis reveals multiple regulatory cell populations. J Autoimmun. 2008;31(4):354–61.
87. Bozkurt M, Yuksel H, Em S, et al. Serum prolidase enzyme activity and oxidative status in patients with Behcet's disease. Redox Rep. 2014;19(2):59–64.
88. Korkmaz S, Erturan I, Naziroglu M, Uguz AC, Cig B, Ovey IS. Colchicine modulates oxidative stress in serum and neutrophil of patients with Behcet disease through regulation of Ca(2)(+) release and antioxidant system. J Membr Biol. 2011;244(3):113–20.
89. Ozyazgan S, Andican G, Erman H, et al. Relation of protein oxidation parameters and disease activity in patients with Behcet's disease. Clin Lab. 2013;59(7–8):819–25.
90. Parikh JG, Saraswathy S, Rao NA. Photoreceptor oxidative damage in sympathetic ophthalmia. Am J Ophthalmol. 2008;146(6):866–875.e862.
91. Lan C, Tam PO, Chiang SW, et al. Manganese superoxide dismutase and chemokine genes polymorphisms in chinese patients with anterior uveitis. Invest Ophthalmol Vis Sci. 2009;50(12):5596–600.
92. Turk A, Aykut M, Akyol N, et al. Serum anti-carbonic anhydrase antibodies and oxidant-antioxidant balance in patients with acute anterior uveitis. Ocul Immunol Inflamm. 2014;22(2):127–32.
93. Lal B, Kapoor AK, Asthana OP, et al. Efficacy of curcumin in the management of chronic anterior uveitis. Phytother Res. 1999;13(4):318–22.
94. van Rooij J, Schwartzenberg SG, Mulder PG, Baarsma SG. Oral vitamins C and E as additional treatment in patients with acute anterior uveitis: a randomised double masked study in 145 patients. Br J Ophthalmol. 1999;83(11):1277–82.
95. Nussenblatt RB, Kim J, Thompson DJ, et al. Vitamin E in the treatment of uveitis-associated macular edema. Am J Ophthalmol. 2006;141(1):193–4.

Special Considerations: Treatment of Pediatric Uveitis

15

Himanshu K. Banda and Steven Yeh

Pearls

- Diagnosis of uveitis in children may be delayed and difficult, and children will therefore often present with advanced disease with structural complications.
- Topical steroids should be utilized as first line for anterior uveitis but chronic use should be limited to 2–3 drops a day or less to avoid the complications of cataracts or elevated intraocular pressure.
- Local steroids may be utilized as adjunctive or bridge therapy for acute disease.
- Systemic immunomodulation is often indicated for chronic inflammatory disease from entities such as JIA; methotrexate is the most commonly utilized first-line systemic agent.
- Biologic drugs are gaining increasing use and have demonstrated benefit in numerous inflammatory diseases affecting children, but do not have first-line status as yet due to expense and limited long-term follow-up.

Introduction

Pediatric uveitis is a relatively rare condition that poses unique diagnostic and treatment challenges. Though children constitute only 5–10% of patients with uveitis [1, 2], severe vision loss may result in an estimated 25–33% of pediatric uveitis cases [3, 4]. Morbidity and poor visual outcomes in children may be greater than in the adult population due to delays in diagnosis and establishing ocular pathology [5, 6]. In adults, uveitis presents with symptoms such as ocular redness, photosensitivity, pain, and increased lacrimation. Posterior uveitis may present as blurred vision, scotomata, or increasing floaters. Uveitis in the pediatric population may be difficult to recognize early in its course, as pediatric-aged patients may not verbalize their symptoms; in some patients, leukocoria or strabismus may be the early findings, as inflammation has been longstanding. The risk of severe vision loss and ocular morbidity is thought to be higher in children than in adults, potentially due to unique disease presentations, difficulty in performing a comprehensive eye exam, medication adherence, and limited approved medical and surgical treatment options. [7] Studies published provide considerable information concerning new drugs and treatment strategies for pediatric uveitis.

H. K. Banda · S. Yeh (✉)
Department of Ophthalmology, Uveitis and Vasculitis Service, Emory Eye Center, Emory University School of Medicine, Atlanta, GA, USA

P. Lin, E. Suhler (eds.), *Treatment of Non-infectious Uveitis*,
https://doi.org/10.1007/978-3-030-22827-9_15

General Approach for Treatment of Pediatric Uveitis

Early diagnosis and proper classification of uveitis are important first steps toward better long-term prognosis of pediatric uveitis. Classification can be based on etiology (infectious, noninfectious, or as a manifestation of a masquerade syndrome), or via anatomic location based on the International Uveitis Study Group [8]. The preferred treatment strategy for most types of noninfectious uveitis is the "step-ladder approach" [9, 10]. With anterior segment involving inflammatory disease, topical therapy is usually administered as initial therapy. Topical cycloplegics are administered to prevent formation of synechiae by dilating the pupil and posteriorly mobilizing the lens/iris diaphragm. With anterior segment inflammation, topical corticosteroids are initiated as first-line treatment when noninfectious uveitis is suspected. In patients in whom an infectious etiology is suspected, topical corticosteroids may be used as adjunctive therapy once appropriate antimicrobial therapy is initiated. It is important to realize that even in the context of well-controlled inflammatory disease, chronic use of topical corticosteroids may result in the complications of cataract formation and pressure elevation, both of which are particularly unwelcome in children. In a study of 75 children with well-controlled JIA, chronic use of topical prednisolone at doses of four drops daily or higher was associated with the formation of 0.16 cataracts per eye-year, roughly equivalent odds of one in six per year of therapy. The same study reported a reduction in cataract risk to 0.01 per eye-year with three drops a day, and zero cataracts per eye-year with BID administration or less. Hence, most clinicians will move on to systemic therapy in chronic anterior uveitis patients requiring more than 2–3 drops of prednisolone daily [11]. It is further important for the clinician to remember the above is specific to prednisolone therapy and that more potent formulations such as difluprednate will lead to similar complications with shorter durations and frequency of use; hence, these drugs should be used only under the closest of supervision and for the shortest time period possible [12]. If topical treatment as outlined above is inadequate, local corticosteroid injections may be utilized cautiously for proven noninfectious disease, although cataract and ocular hypertension warrant monitoring, and younger children may require anesthesia for administration. Systemic steroid treatment can also be implemented cautiously, as serious systemic side effects such as delayed attainment of axial height or growth retardation related to premature closure of epiphyseal plates, adrenal suppression, osteoporosis, infection, mood instability and/or exacerbation of existing psychiatric disease, weight gain, and hyperglycemia require monitoring, as well as collaborative management with pediatric specialists [13]. In cases of intermediate, posterior uveitis or panuveitis, regional or systemic therapy may also be considered due to improved penetrance to the vitreous and posterior pole as bridging therapy; however, patients with chronic inflammatory disease should be considered candidates for systemic immunosuppression to avoid the side effects of chronic topical therapy or repeated local administration of corticosteroids.

Many of the same agents utilized in adults for treatment of chronic systemic inflammatory diseases are utilized in the treatment of children with uveitis. In Table 15.1, we list many of the agents, and their comparative dosing in adults and in children, as well as any specific toxicity or monitoring that is necessary in the pediatric population [14]. The disease-specific evidence for use of some of these drugs will be described in the sections below.

Anterior Uveitis

Juvenile Idiopathic Arthritis

Juvenile idiopathic arthritis (JIA) is the most commonly known systemic disease associated with pediatric anterior uveitis, and as such, much of the evidence in treating chronic uveitis in children is derived from experience in this disease indication. Approximately 50–80% of uveitis cases in children are secondary to JIA [15]. Using

Table 15.1 Agents and their comparative dosing in adults and children and specific toxicity or monitoring in the pediatric population

Medication	Adult dosage	Pediatric dosage	Pediatric side effects/toxicity
Prednisone	1–2 mg/kg (starting), maximum dosage 80 mg/day PO[a]	1–2 mg/kg (starting)[a]	Growth retardation, weight gain, hypertension, osteoporosis. Cushingoid features
Methotrexate	15–20 mg/week (maximum 25 mg/week)	10–15 mg/m^2 (maximum 30 mg/m^2 if given SC)	GI toxicity (oral ulcers, nausea, vomiting), hepatorenal toxicity
Mycophenolate mofetil	2–3 grams/day divided BID	600 mg/m^2 twice daily; adult doses for older children[b]	Hair loss, GI discomfort, leukopenia
Cyclosporine	2.5–5 mg/kg divided BID	2.5–5 mg/kg/day divided BID; children may metabolize more quickly than adults	Nephrotoxicity, hypertension, hirsutism, hyperlipidemia
Adalimumab (Humira)	40 mg q 2 weeks	< 30 kg (20 mg q 2 weeks) ≥30 kg (40 mg q 2 weeks)	Increased susceptibility to infections, reactivation of tuberculosis
Infliximab (Remicade)	3–5 mg/kg typical starting; maximum dosage: 10 mg/kg; dosing q4–8w after loading	3–5 mg/kg monthly typical starting; 10–20 mg/kg monthly usage has been reported in refractory uveitis	Reactivation of latent tuberculosis, anti-TNF antibodies, lupus-like syndrome, infusion reactions

[a]Consider IV Solu-Medrol (i.e., adults, 500–1000 mg; pediatric, 15–30 mg/kg or 1000 mg) if high-dose oral prednisone >80 mg/day is needed

[b]Renal transplant recipients

the criteria based on the International League of Associations for Rheumatology, JIA is divided into subtypes based on the number of joints involved within the first 6 months of the disease, along with the presence or absence of systemic findings, such as fever. This categorization is further subdivided by the presence or absence of certain biological markers such as rheumatoid factor (RF) and antinuclear antibodies (ANA) [16]. The particular subtype of JIA directly impacts the risk of developing uveitis.

If JIA-associated anterior uveitis is not treated effectively with judicious monitoring of inflammation and secondary structural complications, this chronic disease process may confer significant visual morbidity. Studies have shown that in the high-risk group of oligoarthritis-associated uveitis (representing 30–40% of patients with JIA), approximately 10–30% suffer from anterior uveitis [17–19]. Approximately 30% of the patients have ocular complications at the time of the diagnosis [20].

Treatment strategy of JIA patients is to reduce active inflammation in the anterior chamber as much as possible with aggressive topical corticosteroids as first line, with attention to the potential attendant complications of chronic steroid eye drop use described above. Monitoring intraocular pressure (IOP) while on topical steroid drops is recommended as one-third of patients may have increased IOP after 4–6 weeks of therapy. Five percent of patients can be "high responders," with elevations of IOP greater than 15 mm Hg from baseline and total IOP greater than 31 mm Hg [21]. In complex cases, intravenous methylprednisone or oral prednisone has been shown to be useful (dose of 15–30 mg/kg to a maximum of 1 g, repeated daily for 1–3 doses) [22]; however, high-dose corticosteroids alone in controlling JIA-associated uveitis are of limited value [20]. Oral prednisone may also be used with similar caveats to that noted above, with typical starting dose in children of 1–2 mg/kg daily for severe disease. Side effects of long-term systemic glucocorticoid use mandate weaning these agents with the early introduction of disease-modifying antirheumatic drugs (DMARDs). Systemic immunosuppression with one of the DMARDs is recommended if inadequate control of inflammation is demonstrated after 3 months of topical treatment, particularly with >3 drops daily [23]. Disease recurrence when weaning topical glucocorticoids is another indication for initiated DMARDs. Evidence comes predominantly from retrospective case series since controlled clinical trials of the drugs in JIA uveitis have not been undertaken.

Methotrexate (MTX) is typically used as the first-line steroid-sparing agent. MTX is indicated after 12 weeks of topical glucocorticoid if there is no improvement in anterior chamber (AC) cell grade ≤0.5+ or sooner if >2 drops are required, if there is worsening inflammation or if ocular complications develop. The dose of 15 mg/m^2 once weekly is most commonly used, with a maximum of 20 mg orally or 25 mg by subcutaneous injection, although some investigators have utilized weekly subcutaneous doses as high as 30–40 mg/weekly (ref S. Angeles-Han). In a systematic review, improvements in intraocular inflammation were seen in 73% (95% CI 67–81%) [24]. Adverse events, most commonly gastrointestinal discomfort, nausea, and elevated liver enzymes, were experienced in 19.6% of patients where data were available. Additional common side effects that require careful monitoring include fatigue or malaise for one or more days after MTX administration, which in some cases may be treatment limiting, and hair loss, which is reversible with dose reduction or discontinuation. Older children should be counseled on the risks of concomitant alcohol consumption and teratogenic side effects. MTX treatment was associated with a reduced need for cataract extraction, required in 29% of treated patients compared with 64% of those never receiving MTX [25]. Current recommendations indicate MTX be continued for at least 12 months once uveitis is inactive and for 24 months in those with poor visual prognosis. [26]

DMARDs including mycophenolate mofetil (MMF), tacrolimus, azathioprine, leflunomide, and cyclosporine are used infrequently in JIA-associated uveitis [27]. In one retrospective study, leflunomide, when compared to MTX, has been associated with more frequent uveitis flares [28].

Adding a biologic agent is recommended if there is worsening of disease or failure to achieve AC cell grade 0 after 3–4 months on MTX [26]. A double-blinded, placebo-controlled randomized controlled trial (RCT) demonstrated a positive effect of adalimumab in treating JIA-associated uveitis, with adalimumab patients experiencing a 75% risk reduction of flare when compared to placebo (should reference Sycampre study by Ramanan here) [29]. Adalimumab is dosed at 40 mg every 2 weeks in children weighing more than 30 kg, while children weighing less than 30 kg are typically started on 20 mg every 2 weeks. In patients with incomplete response, weekly administration has been shown to convey additional anti-inflammatory effect [30]. Case series have also demonstrated a positive effect of infliximab in children, although doses as high as 10–20 mg/kg/dose may be required [31]. Etanercept, in contrast, is not recommended in JIA uveitis as a double-blinded RCT demonstrated no difference in uveitis control when compared to placebo [32]. As in the adult population, monoclonal antibodies such as infliximab and adalimumab are both recommended over etanercept, with relatively little published experience with the newer agents golimumab and certolizumab. Treatment duration is not certain; however, there is a generalized consensus to continue treatment for 24 months after disease activity has been well controlled and after successful discontinuation of corticosteroids [26]. Other agents with published benefit in the treatment of JIA uveitis include tocilizumab, in whom a Spanish open label study reported 19 of 25 patients in remission after 1 year and additional substantial improvements reported in patients with concomitant uveitis macular edema [33–35]. Selected patients have shown benefit with the T-cell costimulation blocker abatacept (Orencia); however, larger studies have had relatively poor results, with only 3 of 21 patients with active uveitis and arthritis showing sustained ocular benefit [36].

Juvenile Ankylosing Spondylitis

Though juvenile spondyloarthropathies represent clinical entities separate from adult disease, the course of uveitis seen in children is similar to adults. Chronic anterior uveitis and HLA-B27 positivity may develop in as many as 15% of children with juvenile spondyloarthropathies such as ankylosing spondylitis (AS) [37].

The modified New York criteria is used for diagnosis of AS; HLA-B27 positivity is not required for the diagnosis [38]. The anterior uveitis in AS usually begins after the first decade of life. It is typically nongranulomatous, acute, unilateral, and recurrent. Compared to JIA, uveitis associated with seronegative spondyloarthropathies is often symptomatic with acute painful attacks. Therapy typically includes frequent intensive topical steroids and cycloplegic agents. Oral steroids or even local steroid injections may be used in cases refractory to topical steroid administration. Some sources suggest that nonsteroidal anti-inflammatory drugs (NSAIDs) may be used long term in recurrent cases. In patients with chronic disease or recurrent disease with secondary complications, however, anti-tumor necrosis factor inhibitors have demonstrated efficacy and proven beneficial for uveitis associated with juvenile spondyloarthropathies (Fig. 15.1).

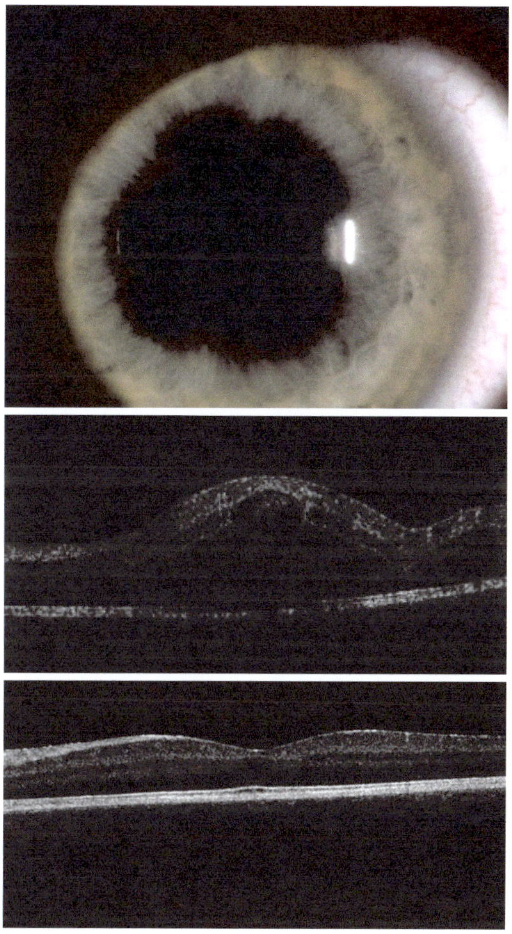

Fig. 15.1 Slit lamp photograph of an HLA-B27-positive patient with anterior and intermediate uveitis shows posterior synechiae from recurrent disease exacerbations (left). A spectral domain optical coherence tomography scan (upper right) shows macular edema while the patient was on methotrexate and prednisone. Following initiation of infliximab and a prednisone taper, the cystoid macular edema has resolved (lower right)

Sarcoidosis and Blau/Jabs disease

Sarcoidosis is rare in children. Two subsets of pediatric sarcoidosis are described in the literature. Children between 8 and 15 years of age typically present with universal lung involvement, with eye, skin, liver, and spleen involvement in 20–40% of cases. Cases of uveitis in less than 5 years of age are not distinguished by pulmonary involvement, but a triad of uveitis, arthropathy, and skin rash [39].

Ocular manifestations are similar to those seen in adults. Anterior uveitis is the most common ocular manifestation in the younger and older subsets. The sequelae of anterior uveitis, including glaucoma, cataracts, and band keratopathy, were the most common cause of visual morbidity in untreated or inadequately treated ocular sarcoidosis [40]. Sarcoidosis may also affect the retinal vasculature or choroid.

Biopsy of extraocular sites (i.e., involving skin, lymph node) is highly preferred in the diagnostic workup [41]. Angiotensin-converting enzyme (ACE) levels may play some role in diagnosis. Though ACE levels tend to be more elevated in children than adults, when compared to age-matched controls, ACE levels in pediatric sarcoidosis patients are higher. ACE levels are not specific for sarcoid and may be elevated in diseases affecting the lungs and liver, as well as in normal growing children [42].

Steroids are the primary treatment for the ocular manifestations of sarcoidosis, especially in the setting of multisystem involvement. Not all children with ocular sarcoidosis respond to topical, periocular, or oral steroids. Low-dose MTX may be useful and safe [43]. Further studies are warranted related to the efficacy of biologics for pediatric ocular sarcoidosis.

Many children who were once diagnosed with granulomatous uveitis thought to be due to sarcoidosis are now known to have Blau/Jabs syndrome, a genetic autoinflammatory syndrome caused by a mutation in the NOD2/CARD15 gene. Blau/Jabs disease is inherited in an autosomal dominant fashion and typically presents in the younger childhood years with granulomatous uveitis, dermatitis, and arthritis, with skeletal abnormalities such as syndactyly and camptodactyly also commonly observed. Positive experience has been reported treating this and other autoinflammatory diseases with anakinra, an IL-1receptor antagonist, and more recently with tocilizumab [44, 45].

Tubulointerstitial Nephritis and Uveitis (TINU)

Uveitis may occur in patients with tubulointerstitial uveitis. With a female predominance, the median age of TINU is 15 years. Though typically anterior in location, uveitis associated with TINU may be intermediate, posterior, or a panuveitis. While episodes of TINU are typically self-limited, pediatric patients tend to have a more chronic course of uveitis compared to adults. In one tertiary referral population, 32% of patients under the age of 20 with bilateral sudden-onset anterior uveitis were found to have TINU [46].

Diagnosis of TINU may include urine testing for the beta-2 microglobulin molecule, which is typically elevated in nephritic conditions and in the context of typical ocular inflammatory disease may be considered diagnostic [47]. Serological testing for renal function by measurement of blood urea nitrogen (BUN) and creatinine levels is of obvious import for staging of renal disease. Renal biopsy, when performed, reveals inflammatory cell infiltration and secondary edema and inflammatory cells. Prognosis of ocular involvement is typically favorable, and treatment with topical corticosteroids is often adequate. In refractory cases, or those involving the posterior segment, systemic or periocular corticosteroids may be used. Immunomodulatory therapy may be required in patients who do not respond to steroids or who manifest a more chronic course [48].

Intermediate Uveitis

Pars Planitis

Intermediate uveitis is inflammation involving the peripheral retina, pars plana, and vitreous base [49]. This entity may represent one-fifth to one-quarter of pediatric uveitis cases. Pars planitis presents clinically with complaints of floaters and blurred vision. Conjunctival injection, pain, and photophobia are less common presentations. Vitreous cells are a hallmark diagnostic finding. The presence of snowballs, which represent active inflammatory cells, and snowbanks, which are inactive acellular debris, can be seen on depressed peripheral examination [50]. Distinguishing between active and inactive material may be challenging for many clinicians. Other harbingers for active disease include sheathing of the venules and retinal arterioles resulting from an associated vasculitis.

Given the relative asymptomatic course of pediatric pars planitis, complications related to sequelae of inflammation may be more advanced at presentation. Posterior subcapsular cataract is the most common type of cataract described in pars planitis, related to both corticosteroid use and uncontrolled inflammation.

Cystoid macular edema, secondary glaucoma, band keratopathy, exudative and rhegmatogenous retinal detachments, and neovascularization secondary to retinal ischemia tend to be more common in children with pars planitis than adults (Fig. 15.2). Optic nerve involvement may be seen more often in children than adults as well [51]. Although rarely observed in children, pars planitis with optic neuritis may be associated with multiple sclerosis (MS). Human leukocyte antigen (HLA) testing should be considered in female patients with bilateral pars planitis. The relationship between HLA-DR15, pars planitis, and MS has been documented [52].

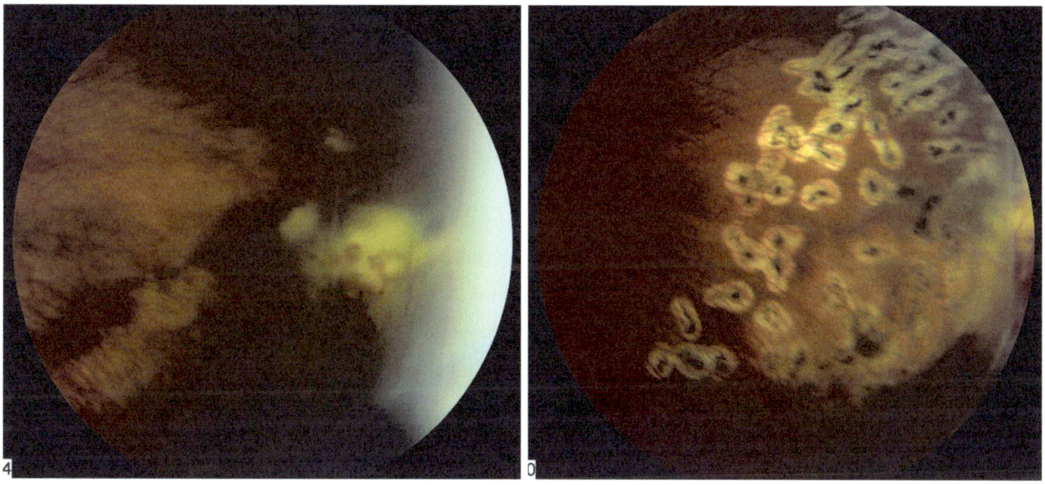

Fig. 15.2 Fundus photograph of the left eye shows active pars plana snow bank with overlying retinal neovascularization (left). Following initiation of immunosuppression with methotrexate and prednisone in addition to local therapy with a periocular corticosteroid injection, laser photocoagulation, and cryotherapy, the pars plana and retinal neovascularization have regressed (right)

The diagnosis of pars planitis is based on clinical manifestations, and a thorough review of systems and history should be gathered to exclude medical illness that may affect the patient's health directly and particularly if immunosuppression is being considered. Diagnostic testing to rule out sarcoidosis, Lyme disease, and tuberculosis which may present with similar manifestations should be considered.

Treatment follows a step-ladder approach similar to JIA. Topical and regional corticosteroid injections are used initially in some cases, although dense pars plana snowbanks and vitreous cells will not typically respond to topical corticosteroids. Besides regional corticosteroids, oral corticosteroids and peripheral retinal cryopexy or laser photocoagulation may be used. For dense pars plana snowbanks, cryopexy may be preferred as laser photocoagulation may not result in adequate uptake. However, cryopexy may be associated with transient inflammation; for this reason, retroseptal corticosteroids (triamcinolone acetonide 40 mg/ml) may be given in patients with pars plana snowbanks and cystoid macular edema. Laser photocoagulation may be applied to pars plana snowbank when uptake is possible and to peripheral areas where retinal ischemia is observed. Immunosuppressive drugs are often required for patients who have recurrent or chronic disease, particularly in patients who have received corticosteroid but either failed a systemic corticosteroid taper or have developed recurrences shortly following regional corticosteroid injections. MTX and mycophenolate mofetil (MMF) are first-line steroid-sparing agents for pars planitis but require laboratory monitoring for serum chemistries, liver enzymes, renal function, and hematologic indices [20]. As in the adult patient, it is incumbent on the prescribing provider to thoroughly assess for and rule out as best possible demyelinating disease prior to initiating anti-TNF therapy prior to utilizing such therapy for refractory cases.

Lyme Disease

Lyme disease is caused by the spirochete *Borrelia burgdorferi* transmitted by infected species of *Ixodes* ticks. It is a multisystem disease involving multiple organ systems. In early stages, the most common ocular finding is a follicular conjunctivitis and episcleritis [53]. The most common intraocular manifestation is intermediate uveitis [54].

Diagnosis of Lyme disease is based on clinical history, presentation, and serologic studies. ELISA is the most commonly used diagnostic serologic test; however, in equivocal cases, Western immunoblotting is recommended [55]. The presence of intraocular inflammation in Lyme disease is regarded as CNS infection requiring systemic therapy. For children, ceftriaxone (50–75 mg/kg per day) in a single daily intravenous dose (maximum, 2 g) is recommended. Alternatively, cefotaxime (150–200 mg/kg per day) may be divided into three or four intravenous doses per day (maximum, 6 g per day), or penicillin G (200,000–400,000 units/kg per day; maximum, 18–24 million units per day) can be divided into doses given intravenously every 4 hours for those with normal renal function [56].

Posterior Uveitis

Toxoplasmosis

Toxoplasmosis is the leading cause of posterior uveitis in all age groups, representing up to 70% of pediatric posterior uveitis in children [57]. The intracellular protozoan *Toxoplasma gondii* may be acquired or congenitally transmitted. Cats are the definitive host and the organisms may exist in three forms: the trophozoite, the bradyzoite (tissue form), and the oocyst (soil form) [58]. Human transmission may occur through ingestion of tissue cysts in raw or undercooked meat, vertical transmission through the placenta, or direct inoculation of oocysts.

Transplacental transmission occurs in cases with primary maternal infection. Approximately 60% of transmission occurs during the third trimester; however, treatment during pregnancy reduces this rate [59]. Transmission in early trimesters often leads to unviable pregnancies or severe congenital disease. Disease severity is inversely related to gestational age the protozoan is transmitted.

Ocular toxoplasmosis may present as an acquired condition or reactivation of congenital disease. Reactivation disease often presents as blurred vision, with clinical findings of local retinochoroiditis adjacent to an old chorioretinal scar. Absence of a scar may suggest acquired disease. Nongranulomatous anterior uveitis with increased intraocular pressure and retinal vasculitis may also be seen in this condition. In immunocompetent hosts, inflammation can be self-limited. Macular lesions were found more often in patients with congenital toxoplasmosis.

Diagnosis is usually clinical, though serologic testing for specific antibodies against *T. gondii* may be helpful. In the first year of life, the presence of IgA and IgM may be indicative of prenatal or postnatal infection. Polymerase chain reaction assays of aqueous and vitreous samples are sensitive and specific for establishing a diagnosis.

Treatment may differ between adults and children. Treatment is typically recommended for newborns, children with active lesions regardless of location, and immunocompromised patients. Pregnant women with acquired disease should also receive treatment. Women infected with *T. gondii* before 25 weeks are given an alternating regimen of pyrimethamine, sulfonamides, and spiramycin. Treatment is continued during the first year of life. Clindamycin or trimethoprim-sulfamethoxazole can be substituted for pyrimethamine. Prenatal treatment should be approached with caution given the potential teratogenic side effects.

Toxocariasis

Toxocariasis is a parasitic infection caused by exposure to the nematode *Toxocara canis* and *T. cati* which complete their life cycle in their primary hosts, dogs and cats, respectively. Ingestion of larvae can occur through undercooked meat, oral-fecal route, or exposure to larvae in sandboxes or litter dishes. After ingestion of the ova, *Toxocara* grows into a larva in the intestinal tract and disseminates via portal circulation [60]. Organisms reach the eye through choroidal, ciliary, or retinal circulation. The disease is most often unilateral and painless, affecting children ages 2–9 years.

Major manifestations of *Toxocara* infection include diffuse vitritis (nematode endophthalmitis), posterior pole granuloma, and peripheral granuloma. Peripheral granuloma is the most common manifestation and is thought to arise as a later manifestation of acute inflammation.

Peripheral granulomas can cause distortion of the fovea secondary to macular dragging or even retinal detachment. Nematode endophthalmitis is the least common form of ocular involvement.

Systemic manifestation of *Toxocara* can result in visceral larva migrans, a condition consisting of fever, hepatosplenomegaly, pulmonary symptoms (mimicking asthma), and eosinophilia [60]. Immunologic diagnosis can be made by an elevated ELISA titer, though the test is not definitive with ocular toxocariasis. One study reported only 45% of patients with ocular toxocariasis titers had levels higher than 1:32 [61]. Cytologic aqueous fluid evaluation for eosinophils or *Toxocara* antibodies can be sampled to provide evidence of ocular involvement [62].

Treatment for ocular toxocariasis includes topical, periocular, and systemic corticosteroids. The use of antihelminthic medications has been described for ocular toxocariasis [63]; however, there is no treatment algorithm that is universally accepted [64]. If identified on examination, laser photocoagulation of motile larvae may be considered [65]. Corticosteroids should be considered concurrently with antihelminthic agents to prevent the exacerbation of intraocular inflammation.

Behcet Disease

The clinical features and course of Behcet disease (BD) in children are similar to those in adults [66]. Though there is no consensus on what age pediatric and adult BD should be defined, some report that disease onset before 16 is indicative of pediatric BD. [67] In children, oral ulcers are typically the initial manifestation of BD. Skin, joint, neurologic, gastrointestinal, vascular, pulmonary, renal, and cardiac involvement have all been reported in children.

In 60% of BD children, ophthalmic manifestations were noted, including conjunctivitis, scleritis, uveitis, disc edema, retinal vasculitis, and optic neuropathy. Cases may present as both severe uveitis or retinal vasculitis [68]. As in adults, inflammatory involvement of the posterior eye segment requires immediate systemic treatment, usually consisting of a combination of systemic corticosteroids and an immunosuppressive drug. Azathioprine, cyclophosphamide and chlorambucil, cyclosporine, MTX, and MMF are immunosuppressive therapies used in conjunction with corticosteroids for BD. If this regimen remains ineffective or a sight-threatening course of the disease occurs, biologic agents such as interferon-α or TNF-α antagonists (infliximab or adalimumab) may be indicated also in children to preserve vision.

Vogt-Koyanagi-Harada Syndrome and Sympathetic Ophthalmia

Vogt-Koyanagi-Harada (VKH) and sympathetic ophthalmia (SO) are rare but reported causes of uveitis in children [69]. The disorder is characterized by bilateral panuveitis, exudative retinal detachment, meningismus, vitiligo, alopecia, and poliosis. Acutely, high-dose systemic steroids, orally and/or intravenously, are efficacious in the acute reduction of inflammation. Corticosteroid-sparing agents such as MTX, MMF, and/or CSA can be added in relapsing cases. Recently, biologics including adalimumab and infliximab have been reported in limited case series and case reports for pediatric VKH [70, 71].

VKH and SO share similar pathogenesis in that patients may have systemic T-cell responses to melanocyte antigen. Adalimumab and infliximab also have been found to be effective in case reports as steroid-sparing agents in patients with SO, the former in a patient refractory to methotrexate and topical corticosteroid [72] and the latter in a patient refractory to methotrexate, mycophenolate mofetil, cyclosporine A, and daclizumab [73].

Biologic Therapy in Pediatric Uveitis: Additional Considerations

Biologic agents differ from the chemically derived drugs described earlier in their source and complexity. Unlike most drugs produced by chemical reactions, biologic agents are derived from human or animal sources (i.e., produced in biologic systems). They have complex structures with amino acids or nucleic acids. The Food and Drug Administration (FDA) has recommended industrial guidelines for manufacturers to assess the safety and effectiveness of biologic products in pediatric uveitis [74].

Over the last decade, biologic agents have gained popularity with uveitis specialists and rheumatologists as an alternative for patients with refractory disease or intolerance to traditional immunosuppressive therapies. For conditions such as JIA and Behcet disease, TNF-alpha inhibitors are increasingly used and have demonstrated efficacy for pediatric and adult uveitis [22, 75–77]. Off-label use of biologics has been extensively reported in pediatric uveitis, though higher doses have been reported, primarily with the tumor necrosis factor-alpha inhibitor infliximab [31].

Biologic agents that are FDA approved in pediatric disease include infliximab (Crohn's disease >6 years old), adalimumab (JIA >4 years old), abatacept (JIA >6 years old), and tocilizumab (systemic juvenile idiopathic arthritis >2 years old). However, daclizumab is no longer manufactured in the United States. To date, the only biologic agent FDA approved for adult uveitis as a clinical indication is adalimumab although other agents including infliximab, rituximab, and newer agents including tocilizumab and abatacept have also been reported and previously discussed [78, 79]. Adalimumab recently received FDA approval for the treatment of adults with noninfectious intermediate, posterior uveitis and panuveitis; all other biologic and nonbiological agents are utilized off-label for the treatment of noninfectious uveitis, with the exception of patients with a systemic associated disease with FDA approval.

Future Directions in Therapy for Pediatric Uveitis

As newer biologic agents and immunologic therapies are developed for rheumatologic and autoimmune conditions, the use of these systemic medications for pediatric indications including uveitis offer promising approaches; however, short- and long-term systemic monitoring are often needed to ensure safety, particularly given the infectious and immunologic side effects that have been observed with biologic and nonbiological agents. As our understanding of the genetic and immunologic background of specific pediatric uveitis improves, it is likely that more targeted therapies will be utilized to directly address the mechanisms at play in individual disease conditions [80].

References

1. Cunningham ET Jr. Uveitis in children. Ocul Immunol Inflamm. 2000;8:251–61.
2. Suhler EB, Lloyd MD, Choi D, et al. Incidence and prevalence of uveitis in Veterans Affairs Medical Centers of the Pacific Northwest. Am J Ophthalmol. 2008;146:890–6.
3. Zierhut M, Michels H, Stubiger N, Besch D, Deuter C, Heiligenhaus A. Uveitis in children. Int Ophthalmol Clin. 2005;45:135–56.
4. Levy-Clarke GA, Nussenblatt RB, Smith JA. Management of chronic pediatric uveitis. Curr Opin Ophthalmol. 2005;16:281–8.
5. Malinowski SM, Pulido JS, Folk JC. Long-term visual outcome and complications associated with pars planitis. Ophthalmology. 1993;100:818–24.
6. Rosenberg KD, Feuer WJ, Davis JL. Ocular complications of pediatric uveitis. Ophthalmology. 2004;111:2299–306.
7. Nagpal A, Leigh JF, Acharya NR. Epidemiology of uveitis in children. Int Ophthalmol Clin. 2008;48:1–7.
8. Deschenes J, Murray PI, Rao NA, Nussenblatt RB. International Uveitis Study G. International Uveitis Study Group (IUSG): clinical classification of uveitis. Ocul Immunol Inflamm. 2008;16:1–2.
9. Wentworth BA, Freitas-Neto CA, Foster CS. Management of pediatric uveitis. F1000Prime Rep. 2014;6:41.
10. Michels H, Schuchmann L, Truckenbrodt H, Renz K. Rheumatic iridocyclitis in childhood – differentiation on the basis of clinical and immunological parameters. Klin Padiatr. 1982;194:104–8.
11. Thorne JE, Woreta FA, Dunn JP. Risk of cataract development among children with juvenile idiopathic arthritis-related uveitis treated with topical corticosteroids. Ophthalmology. 2010;117:1436–41.
12. Slabaugh MA, Herlighy E, Ongchin S, van Gelder RN. Efficacy and potential complications of difluprednate use for pediatric uveitis. Am J Ophthalmol. 2012;153:932–8.
13. Buchman AL. Side effects of corticosteroid therapy. J Clin Gastroenterol. 2001;33:289–94.
14. Sood AB, Angeles-Han ST. An update on the treatment of pediatric chronic non-infectious uveitis. Curr Treatm Opt Rheumatol. 2017;3:1–16.

15. Smith JA, Mackensen F, Sen HN, et al. Epidemiology and course of disease in childhood uveitis. Ophthalmology. 2009;116:1544–51, 51.e1
16. Petty RE, Southwood TR, Baum J, et al. Revision of the proposed classification criteria for juvenile idiopathic arthritis: Durban, 1997. J Rheumatol. 1998;25:1991–4.
17. Chia A, Lee V, Graham EM, Edelsten C. Factors related to severe uveitis at diagnosis in children with juvenile idiopathic arthritis in a screening program. Am J Ophthalmol. 2003;135:757–62.
18. Wolf MD, Lichter PR, Ragsdale CG. Prognostic factors in the uveitis of juvenile rheumatoid arthritis. Ophthalmology. 1987;94:1242–8.
19. Kotaniemi K, Kautiainen H, Karma A, Aho K. Occurrence of uveitis in recently diagnosed juvenile chronic arthritis: a prospective study. Ophthalmology. 2001;108:2071–5.
20. Zierhut M, Doycheva D, Biester S, Stubiger N, Kummerle-Deschner J, Deuter C. Therapy of uveitis in children. Int Ophthalmol Clin. 2008;48:131–52.
21. Armaly MF. Statistical attributes of the steroid hypertensive response in the clinically normal eye. I. The demonstration of three levels of response. Invest Ophthalmol. 1965;4:187–97.
22. Hawkins MJ, Dick AD, Lee RJ, et al. Managing juvenile idiopathic arthritis-associated uveitis. Surv Ophthalmol. 2016;61:197–210.
23. Heiligenhaus A, Michels H, Schumacher C, et al. Evidence-based, interdisciplinary guidelines for anti-inflammatory treatment of uveitis associated with juvenile idiopathic arthritis. Rheumatol Int. 2012;32:1121–33.
24. Simonini G, Paudyal P, Jones GT, Cimaz R, Macfarlane GJ. Current evidence of methotrexate efficacy in childhood chronic uveitis: a systematic review and meta-analysis approach. Rheumatology (Oxford). 2013;52:825–31.
25. Sijssens KM, Rothova A, Van De Vijver DA, Stilma JS, De Boer JH. Risk factors for the development of cataract requiring surgery in uveitis associated with juvenile idiopathic arthritis. Am J Ophthalmol. 2007;144:574–9.
26. Bou R, Adan A, Borras F, et al. Clinical management algorithm of uveitis associated with juvenile idiopathic arthritis: interdisciplinary panel consensus. Rheumatol Int. 2015;35:777–85.
27. Amin RM, Miserocchi E, Thorne JE, Hornbeak D, Jabs DA, Zierhut M. Treatment options for juvenile idiopathic arthritis (JIA) associated uveitis. Ocul Immunol Inflamm. 2016;24:81–90.
28. Bichler J, Benseler SM, Krumrey-Langkammerer M, Haas JP, Hugle B. Leflunomide is associated with a higher flare rate compared to methotrexate in the treatment of chronic uveitis in juvenile idiopathic arthritis. Scand J Rheumatol. 2015;44: 280–3.
29. Ramanan AV, Dick AD, Jones AP, et al. Adalimumab plus methotrexate for uveitis in juvenile idiopathic arthritis. N Engl J Med. 2017;376:1637–46.
30. Correll CK, Bullock DR, Cafferty RM, Vehe RK. Safety of weekly adalimumab in the treatment of juvenile idiopathic arthritis and pediatric chronic uveitis. Clin Rheumatol. 2018;37:549–53.
31. Tambralli A, Beukelman T, Weiser P, Atkinson TP, Cron RQ, Stoll ML. High doses of infliximab in the management of juvenile idiopathic arthritis. J Rheumatol. 2013;40:1749–55.
32. Smith JA, Thompson DJ, Whitcup SM, et al. A randomized, placebo-controlled, double-masked clinical trial of etanercept for the treatment of uveitis associated with juvenile idiopathic arthritis. Arthritis Rheum. 2005;53:18–23.
33. Calvo-Rio V, Santos-Gomez M, Calvo I, et al. Anti-interleukin-6 receptor tocilizumab for severe juvenile idiopathic arthritis-associated uveitis refractory to anti-tumor necrosis factor therapy: a multicenter study of twenty-five patients. Arthritis Rheumatol. 2017;69:668–75.
34. Tappeiner C, Mesquida M, Adan A. Evidence for tocilizumab as a treatment option in refractory uveitis associated with juvenile idiopathic arthritis. J Rheumatol. 2016;43:2183–8.
35. Mesquida M, Molins B, Llorenc V, et al. Twenty-four month month follow-up of tocilizumab therapy for refractory uveitis-related macular edema. Retina. 2018;38:1361–70.
36. Tappeiner C, Miserocchi E, Bodaghi B, et al. Abatacept in the treatment of severe, longstanding, and refractory uveitis associated with juvenile idiopathic arthritis. J Rheumatol. 2015;42:706–11.
37. Adrovic A, Barut K, Sahin S, Kasapcopur O. Juvenile spondyloarthropathies. Curr Rheumatol Rep. 2016;18:55.
38. van der Linden S, Valkenburg HA, Cats A. Evaluation of diagnostic criteria for ankylosing spondylitis. A proposal for modification of the New York criteria. Arthritis Rheum. 1984;27:361–8.
39. Hoover DL, Khan JA, Giangiacomo J. Pediatric ocular sarcoidosis. Surv Ophthalmol. 1986;30:215–28.
40. Jasper PL, Denny FW. Sarcoidosis in children. With special emphasis on the natural history and treatment. J Pediatr. 1968;73:499–512.
41. Weinreb RN. Diagnosing sarcoidosis by transconjunctival biopsy of the lacrimal gland. Am J Ophthalmol. 1984;97:573–6.
42. Rodriguez GE, Shin BC, Abernathy RS, Kendig EL Jr. Serum angiotensin-converting enzyme activity in normal children and in those with sarcoidosis. J Pediatr. 1981;99:68–72.
43. Gedalia A, Molina JF, Ellis GS Jr, Galen W, Moore C, Espinoza LR. Low-dose methotrexate therapy for childhood sarcoidosis. J Pediatr. 1997;130:25–9.
44. Lopalco G, Fabiani C, Sota J, et al. IL-6 blockade in the management of non-infectious uveitis. Clin Rheumatol. 2017;36:1459–69.
45. Lu L, Shen M, Jiang D, et al. Blau syndrome with good responses to tocilizumab: a case report and focused literature review. Semin Arthritis Rheum. 2018;47:727–31.

46. Mackensen F, Smith JR, Rosenbaum JT. Enhanced recognition, treatment, and prognosis of tubulointerstitial nephritis and uveitis syndrome. Ophthalmology. 2007;114:995–9.
47. Mackensen F, Billing H. Tubulointerstitial nephritis and uveitis syndrome. Curr Opin Ophthalmol. 2009;20:525–31.
48. Gion N, Stavrou P, Foster CS. Immunomodulatory therapy for chronic tubulointerstitial nephritis-associated uveitis. Am J Ophthalmol. 2000;129:764–8.
49. Jabs DA, Nussenblatt RB, Rosenbaum JT, Standardization of Uveitis Nomenclature Working G. Standardization of uveitis nomenclature for reporting clinical data. Results of the First International Workshop. Am J Ophthalmol. 2005;140:509–16.
50. Pederson JE, Kenyon KR, Green WR, Maumenee AE. Pathology of pars planitis. Am J Ophthalmol. 1978;86:762–74.
51. Nussenblatt RB, Whitcup SM, Palestine AG. Uveitis: fundamentals and clinical practice. 2nd ed. St. Louis: Mosby; 1996.
52. Tang WM, Pulido JS, Eckels DD, Han DP, Mieler WF, Pierce K. The association of HLA-DR15 and intermediate uveitis. Am J Ophthalmol. 1997;123:70–5.
53. Mikkila HO, Seppala IJ, Viljanen MK, Peltomaa MP, Karma A. The expanding clinical spectrum of ocular lyme borreliosis. Ophthalmology. 2000;107:581–7.
54. Karma A, Seppala I, Mikkila H, Kaakkola S, Viljanen M, Tarkkanen A. Diagnosis and clinical characteristics of ocular Lyme borreliosis. Am J Ophthalmol. 1995;119:127–35.
55. Rosenbaum JT, Rahn DW. Prevalence of Lyme disease among patients with uveitis. Am J Ophthalmol. 1991;112:462–3.
56. Wormser GP, Dattwyler RJ, Shapiro ED, et al. The clinical assessment, treatment, and prevention of Lyme disease, human granulocytic anaplasmosis, and babesiosis: clinical practice guidelines by the Infectious Diseases Society of America. Clin Infect Dis. 2006;43:1089–134.
57. Giles CL. Uveitis in childhood – part III. Posterior. Ann Ophthalmol. 1989;21:23–8.
58. Nussenblatt RB, Belfort R Jr. Ocular toxoplasmosis. An old disease revisited. JAMA. 1994;271:304–7.
59. Wong SY, Remington JS. Toxoplasmosis in pregnancy. Clin Infect Dis. 1994;18:853–61; quiz 62.
60. Schantz PM, Glickman LT. Toxocaral visceral larva migrans. N Engl J Med. 1978;298:436–9.
61. Schantz PM. Toxocara larva migrans now. Am J Trop Med Hyg. 1989;41:21–34.
62. Shields JA, Lerner HA, Felberg NT. Aqueous cytology and enzymes in nematode endophthalmitis. Am J Ophthalmol. 1977;84:319–22.
63. Dinning WJ, Gillespie SH, Cooling RJ, Maizels RM. Toxocariasis: a practical approach to management of ocular disease. Eye (Lond). 1988;2(Pt 5):580–2.
64. Shields JA. Ocular toxocariasis. A review. Surv Ophthalmol. 1984;28:361–81.
65. Fitzgerald CR, Rubin ML. Intraocular parasite destroyed by photocoagulation. Arch Ophthalmol. 1974;91:162–4.
66. Krause I, Uziel Y, Guedj D, et al. Childhood Behcet's disease: clinical features and comparison with adult-onset disease. Rheumatology (Oxford). 1999;38:457–62.
67. Treudler R, Orfanos CE, Zouboulis CC. Twenty-eight cases of juvenile-onset Adamantiades-Behcet disease in Germany. Dermatology. 1999;199:15–9.
68. Kone-Paut I. Behcet's disease in children, an overview. Pediatr Rheumatol Online J. 2016;14:10.
69. Soheilian M, Aletaha M, Yazdani S, Dehghan MH, Peyman GA. Management of pediatric Vogt-Koyanagi-Harada (VKH)-associated panuveitis. Ocul Immunol Inflamm. 2006;14:91–8.
70. Jeroudi A, Angeles-Han ST, Yeh S. Efficacy of adalimumab for pediatric Vogt-Koyanagi-Harada syndrome. Ophthalmic Surg Lasers Imaging Retina. 2014;45(4):332–4.
71. Khalifa YM, Bailony MR, Acharya NR. Treatment of pediatric Vogt-Koyanagi-Harada syndrome with infliximab. Ocul Immunol Inflamm. 2010;18(3):218–22.
72. Kim JB, Jeroudi A, Angeles-Han ST, et al. Adalimumab for pediatric sympathetic ophthalmia. JAMA Ophthalmol. 2014;132(8):1022–4.
73. Gupta SR, Phan IT, Suhler EB. Successful treatment of refractory sympathetic ophthalmic in a child with infliximab. Arch Ophthalmol. 2011;129:250–2.
74. Regulations requiring manufacturers to assess the safety and effectiveness of new drugs and biological products in pediatric patients – FDA. Final rule. Fed Regist 1998;63:66631–66672.
75. Interlandi E, Leccese P, Olivieri I, Latanza L. Adalimumab for treatment of severe Behçet's uveitis: a retrospective long-term follow-up study. Clin Exp Rheumatol. 2014;32(4 Suppl 84):S58–62.
76. Calvo-Río V, Blanco R, Beltrán E, et al. Anti-TNF-α therapy in patients with refractory uveitis due to Behçet's disease: a 1-year follow-up study of 124 patients. Rheumatology (Oxford). 2014;53(12):2223–31.
77. Vallet H, Seve P, Biard L, et al. Infliximab versus adalimumab in the treatment of refractory inflammatory uveitis: a multicenter study from the French Uveitis Network. Arthritis Rheumatol. 2016;68(6):1522–30.
78. Papo M, Bielefeld P, Vallet H, et al. Tocilizumab in severe and refractory non-infectious uveitis. Clin Exp Rheumatol. 2014;32(4 Suppl 84):S75–9.
79. Marrani E, Paganelli V, de Libero C, et al. Long-term efficacy of abatacept in pediatric patients with idiopathic uveitis: a case series. Graefes Arch Clin Exp Ophthalmol. 2015;253(10):1813–6.
80. Lin P, Suhler EB, Rosenbaum JT. The future of uveitis treatment. Ophthalmology. 2014;121(1):365–76.

Index

P. Lin, E. Suhler (eds.), *Treatment of Non-infectious Uveitis*,
https://doi.org/10.1007/978-3-030-22827-9

MIX
Papier aus verantwortungsvollen Quellen
Paper from responsible sources
FSC® C105338

If you have any concerns about our products,
you can contact us on
ProductSafety@springernature.com

In case Publisher is established outside the EU,
the EU authorized representative is:
Springer Nature Customer Service Center GmbH
Europaplatz 3, 69115 Heidelberg, Germany

Printed by Libri Plureos GmbH
in Hamburg, Germany